■ Practical Management of the Balance Disorder Patient

A Singular Audiology Text
Jeffrey L. Danhauer, Ph.D.
Audiology Editor

■ PRACTICAL MANAGEMENT OF THE BALANCE DISORDER PATIENT

Neil T. Shepard, Ph.D.

Steven A. Telian, M.D.

DEPARTMENT OF OTOLARYNGOLOGY
UNIVERSITY OF MICHIGAN MEDICAL SCHOOL

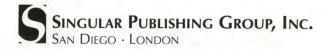
SINGULAR PUBLISHING GROUP, INC.
SAN DIEGO · LONDON

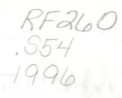

Singular Publishing Group, Inc.
401 West A Street, Suite 325
San Diego, California 92101-7904

19 Compton Terrace
London N1 2UN, U.K.

Typeset in 10/12 Times by So Cal Graphics
Printed in the United States of America by McNaughton & Gunn

Library of Congress Cataloging-in-Publication Data

Shepard, Neil T.
    Practical management of the balance disorder patient / Neil T. Shepard, Steven A. Telian
      p.   cm.
    Includes bibliographical references and index.
    ISBN 1-879105-84-5
    1. Dizziness.   2. Vestibular apparatus—Diseases.   3. Equilibrium (Physiology)   I. Telian, Steven A.
II. Title.
    [DNLM: 1. Vestibular Diseases—diagnosis.   2. Vestibular Diseases—therapy.   3. Vestibular
Diseases—rehabilitation.   WV 255 S547p 1996]
RF260.S54   1996
617.8'82—dc20
DNLM/DLC
for Library of Congress   96-5970
                                                        CIP

■CONTENTS

■ PREFACE

*T*his new textbook provides a practical and systematic approach to the patient with balance disorders. It emphasizes an understanding of how the overall balance system functions to aid in effective evaluation and treatment and provides reliable tools for guiding therapy even when the exact diagnosis may be elusive. Topics covered include a practical presentation of the basics of vestibular system function, the use of clinical information in diagnosis and treatment planning, rehabilitation of the dizzy patient, and surgical patient selection. The authors distill years of clinical experience and research into an intermediate textbook that will serve the needs of any clinician engaged in the treatment of the dizzy patient, including the otolaryngologist, neurologist, physical therapist, and audiologist. In addition, vestibular testing specialists who seek a deeper understanding of these patients to aid in the administration and interpretation of vestibular test results will find the book particularly appropriate to their needs.

The authors intend for this text to provide for a philosophical approach to the complex management of the balance disorder patient. While at an intermediate level, the text will be helpful to the beginning professional in this area when used in combination with other texts. *The Handbook of Balance Function Testing* (1993), edited by Drs. Jacobson, Newman, and Kartush, would be a recommended accompanying resource. For more experienced clinicians, this text is intended to serve as a reference to supplement their current knowledge and experience.

It is the hope of the authors that this text will add to the growing body of literature on the assessment and management of the patient with a balance disorder, in a manner that will improve care for these patients and reduce the frustration felt by clinicians dealing with this complex problem.

■ ACKNOWLEDGMENTS

*T*he authors are thankful for the loving support of our families during this project, particularly our wives, Janis Shepard and Diane Telian. Their patience and devotion have served as a consistent source of strength and encouragement throughout our careers.

We would also like to acknowledge the contributions of our mentor and friend, John L. Kemink, M.D. Dr. Kemink's leadership abilities and vision for a world-class program in vestibular disorders were responsible for bringing both of us to the University of Michigan. He provided us with the academic freedom and the nurturing environment needed to allow the vestibular program to flourish. His untimely death at the hand of a delusional patient cut short a brilliant career, and reminds us to delight in the joy that each day can bring. As we reflect on his compassionate listening skills, as well as his ability to blend clinical wisdom and extraordinary surgical ability to help his patients, we are reminded of the honor that can be brought to the practice of medicine.

■ BASIC ANATOMY AND PHYSIOLOGY REVIEW

EXTENT OF THE PROBLEM

The majority of patients afflicted with an acute balance disorder recover spontaneously with only symptomatic treatment from the medical community (Igarashi, 1984; Pfaltz, 1983). For reasons that are poorly understood some of these patients develop chronic balance system problems requiring significant investments from a variety of medical and surgical specialists to evaluate and manage their disorder.

Vertigo and balance disorders constitute a significant public health problem in the United States. Estimates of the number of persons in this country seeking medical care for disequilibrium or vertigo range as high as 7 million per year. Approximately 30% of the U.S. population have experienced episodes of dizziness by age 65 (Roydhouse, 1974). There are no indications that the problem of balance disorders is diminishing, particularly as the population ages (Herdman, 1994a; Kroenke & Mangelsdorff, 1989). Another compelling issue relates to the increased incidence of falls with aging. Balance disorders and dizziness are important risk factors for falls in this population. Among community-dwelling elderly between ages 65 and 75 who do not report any major health problem or acute balance disorder, at least 25 to 35% report a significant fall annually. For persons over 75 years old, those reporting a significant fall at least once per year rises to 32–42%. The rates become significantly higher for those who have any type of impaired mobility including acute or chronic balance disturbances. While most falls do not result in serious injury, 18.6 of 1000 falls for those 60–65 years of age, and 55 out of 1000 falls for those over 65 years require medical attention. It is estimated that falls are the leading cause of death from injuries in those over 65 years of age. Since it can be inferred from epidemiological studies that balance disorders increase the probability of an injurious fall, the management of balance disorders in the elderly population becomes a critical issue (Blake, Morgan, & Bendall, 1988; Campbell, Reinken, Allan, & Martinez, 1981; Prudham & Evans, 1981; Tinetti, Speechlay, & Ginter, 1988).

The balance system is more complex than the auditory system, primarily because of the motor component. Thus, the evaluation and interpretation of disorders in this system are also complex, leading to difficulty in management of patients with balance disorders. A key element in the management of the balance disorder patient is the distinction between the acute and chronic conditions. While priorities for management will be detailed in later Chapters, promoting a better understanding of this important concept is one of the key purposes served by this text. Chronic balance disorders can result by one of two general mechanisms. One is the patient who suffers from repeated insults from an unstable lesion within the vestibular system, such as from Ménière's disease. The other is the patient who has suffered an acute lesion, and although the lesion is stable (the function of the peripheral vestibular system is not changing as it does with a disorder like Ménière's disease), the anticipated central compensation processes (reviewed in detail in Chapter 2) have failed or are only partially complete, leaving the patient with functional disability months or years after the onset. These chronic patients have a variety of complaints, the most common of which are brief spells of vertigo or unsteadiness provoked by head movement. This is in contrast with the patient who suffers an acute onset of symptoms with various forms of disequilibrium and neurovegetative complaints that began for the first time within the last 72 hours. Most of these acute patients will make a spontaneous recovery without medical intervention. The diagnostic studies and management tools selected should vary significantly depending on the acute or chronic nature of the patient's complaints. Various combinations of medical, surgical, and physical therapy managements will be used, depending on the potential explanations for persistent symptoms in the chronic balance disorder patient.

The emphasis of this text will be directed toward the diagnosis and management of the chronic balance disorder patient. The text is intended for members of any professional discipline providing care for persons with balance disorders. The acutely vertiginous patient will be discussed briefly and management suggestions will be offered to reduce the possibility of chronic dysfunction. The interested reader will be referred to recent information available in other textbooks and medical journals that discuss clinical and laboratory evaluation, surgical and medical treatment, and vestibular rehabilitation programs. It is a combination of the other literature sources and this text together that form a firm resource for the professional working with the balance disorder patient. It is not the intent of this text to serve as a single detailed source for all aspects of the evaluation and treatment of the balance disorder patient. The authors hope that the integration of information from a variety of sources provided herein will result in more accurate diagnosis and effective treatment of balance disorder patients.

An important aspect of laboratory evaluation is the proper interpretation of test results. Our approach will be to integrate the interpretation of presenting clinical signs and symptoms with diagnostic test results to assist the reader to determine the extent, site, and compensation status of a lesion, as well as its functional impact on the patient. This requires proper understanding of individual test results, but allows for alteration in interpretation based upon other findings and the presenting signs, symptoms, and past medical history. This approach avoids rigid interpretation of test results leading to incorrect diagnosis and is required by the complexity and redundancy of the balance system.

ANATOMICAL AND BASIC PHYSIOLOGICAL CONSIDERATIONS

Anatomically and physiologically, what is the "balance system"? No single structure subserves balance function. Rather, the system consists of multiple sensory inputs from the vestibular end organs, the visual system, and the somatosensory/proprioceptive systems. The input information is then integrated at the level of the brain stem and cerebellum with significant influence from the cerebral cortex, including the frontal, parietal, and occipital lobes. The integrated input information results in various motor and perceptual outputs. Only a brief overview of the major elements of the input and output structures and their basic physiological functioning will be provided here, with other literature providing detailed descriptions, to which the interested reader is referred (Arenberg, 1993; Baloh & Honrubia, 1990; Harada, 1988; Leigh & Zee, 1991; Pompeiano & Allum, 1988; Ryu, 1986; Shimazu & Yoshikazu, 1992; Taguchi, Igarashi, & Mori, 1994; Woollacott & Shumway-Cook, 1989).

Ocular Motor Control and Perceptions of Motion

Figure 1–1 shows a schematic illustration of the membranous labyrinth (more detailed figures are found in the references listed above), including the vestibular and auditory structures of the inner ear. This membranous structure is housed within the bony labyrinth in the petrous portion of the temporal bone, where it is secured by connective tissue and is bathed in perilymph. Endolymph is contained within the membranous structure where the specialized sensory neuroepithelium is located. The vestibular apparatus consists of two groups of specialized sensory receptors: (a) the three semicircular canals—lateral (or horizontal), posterior, and superior, each of which originates from the utricle and terminates in a dilated end (ampulla) that also attaches into the utricle; and (b) the two otolithic organs—the utricular macula and the saccular macula. The semicircular canals are oriented in approximately orthogonal planes to the other ipsilateral canals. While the two horizontal canals are in parallel planes, the two superior and the two posterior canals are in planes approximately orthogonal to each other. The canals are organized into functional pairs. The two members of each pair are in parallel planes of orientation. The three functional pairs are: (a) The two horizontal canals; (b) the superior canal and the contralateral posterior canal; and (c) the posterior canal and the contralateral superior canal. The otolithic organs also function in a paired format with the two utricular maculae in approximately the horizontal plane and the two saccular maculae in the vertical plane.

Contained within each semicircular canal ampulla and otolithic organ is an arrangement of hair cells that constitute the neuroepithelial transduction mechanism for the vestibular end-organs. These hair cells are situated on a mound of supporting cells in the ampulla called the crista ampullaris, and within the maculae of the otolithic organ. Covering the hair cell projections (stereocilia and kinocilium) within the ampulla is a gelatinous membrane, the cupula. The cupula, having the same specific gravity as the endolymph, is not responsive to static position changes of the head in the gravitational field. On the contrary, the gelatinous covering over the hair cells of the otolithic maculae has calcium carbonate crystals called otoconia imbedded in its fibrous network. The presence of the otoconia increases the specific gravity significantly above that of the endolymph. Thus the maculae are responsive to linear acceleration including the force of gravity as the head is placed in different positions.

The axons of the vestibular portion of the cochleovestibular nerve each display the property of a spontaneous tonic firing rate that is intrinsically generated. In both the semicircular canals and the otolithic organs, the activated hair cells modulate the firing rate of the corresponding vestibular nerve fibers. If the stereocilia are bent toward the kinocilium, an increase (excitation) in the spontaneous neural firing rate results. A decrease (inhibition) in spontaneous firing rate results from shearing action away from the kinocilium. The hair cells on the crista ampullaris are arranged such that the kinocilium for each cell is oriented in the same direction relative to the utricle. This is referred to as *morphological polarization*. This polarization within the horizontal canals causes an excitation of neural activity when cupular movement creates a deviation of the stereocilia toward the utricle (*utriculopetal* endolymph flow) and inhibition of neural activity for shearing of the stereocilia away from the utricle (*utriculofugal* flow). The situation is reversed for the superior and posterior canals, with utriculopetal flow resulting in inhibition and utriculofugal flow causing excitation of the spontaneous firing rate. Therefore, stimulation of any of the three functional pairs by angular acceleration in their plane of orientation causes an increase in neural firing rate on one side and a decrease on the contralateral side (an example of this is given in Figure 1–2 and will be discussed below). This same paired action scheme occurs in the otolithic organs; however, the morphologic polariza-

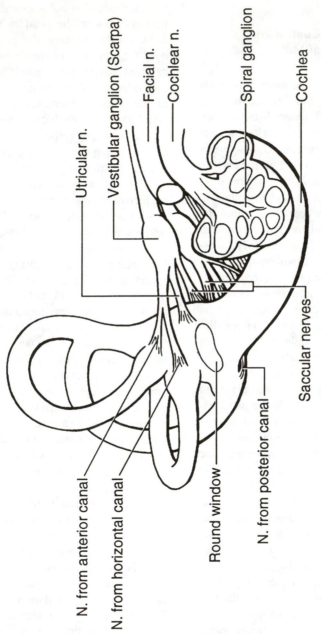

FIGURE 1–1. Illustration of the labyrinth showing the relative orientation of the three semicircular canals to the cochlea and the neural innervation.

Utricular n.

Vestibular ganglion (Scarpa)

Facial n.

Cochlear n.

Spiral ganglion

Cochlea

N. from anterior canal

N. from horizontal canal

Round window

N. from posterior canal

Saccular nerves

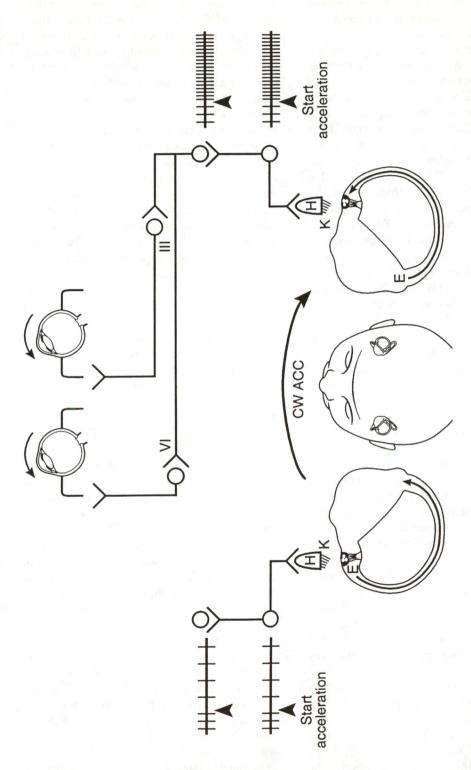

FIGURE 1–2. The orientation of the semicircular canals in the human skull. To each side of the head are enlargements of the horizontal canals illustrating the relative flow of endolymph (E) in each for a clockwise acceleration (CW ACC) of the head. The relative shearing of the sterocilia of the hair cells (H) to the position of the kinocilium (K) is shown. The neural firing rate from each side on the vestibular portion of the VIIIth cranial nerve is shown marked with start acceleration. For the right side the neural connections from the hair cells to the ocular motor nuclei (nuclei of cranial nerve III) and the nuclei of the abducens nerve (cranial nerve VI) are shown. The vestibulo-ocular reflex compensatory movement of the eyes in response to the acceleration is illustrated.

tion of the hair cells is significantly more complicated, allowing for sensitivity to linear acceleration in any direction.

The asymmetrical neural input from the vestibular nerves is interpreted by the central nervous system as either angular or linear acceleration. In addition, the asymmetry resulting from action of the semicircular canals causes a compensatory reflex eye movement in the plane of the canals being stimulated, known as the first of Ewald's three laws (Baloh & Honrubia, 1990; Ewald, 1892). This compensatory reflex movement of the eye is produced by the *vestibulo-ocular reflex* (VOR), and is opposite to the direction of acceleration. To lesser extent this reflex also occurs for linear acceleration, mediated by the otolithic organs. As the primary system utilized for evaluating balance disorder patients is the VOR from the horizontal semicircular canals, we will concentrate on this response. Figure 1–2 schematically illustrates the VOR from stimulation of the horizontal semicircular canals. In this example the subject is seated in a normal upright position and accelerated to the right rotating about the long axis of the body. Since the membranous horizontal canals are connected to the bony labyrinth within the petrous portion of the temporal bone they also accelerate to the right. The endolymph, however, does not move immediately to the right but lags behind the membranous canal because of visco-elastic and inertial forces created by the capillary fluid mechanics of the canal. This effectively produces a relative flow of endolymph in the direction opposite that of the acceleration. Therefore, the cupula in the right canal is deflected toward the utricle while that in the left is deflected away from the utricle. This action results in an excitation of neural firing rate on the right and an inhibition on the left. The individual perceives rotation to the right and, assuming no visual input (darkness or eyes closed), a reflexive eye movement to the left (mediated by the VOR) is produced. This movement is interrupted by fast compensatory movements (saccades) of the eyes back in the direction of the acceleration. This fast saccadic eye movement is not part of the VOR but a resetting reflex stimulated by the position of the

eye within the orbit. If the acceleration continues, the VOR again produces the slow component eye movement opposite the direction of acceleration. An individual viewing the eyes of the subject or recording their movement notes a repeated jerking motion to the right and a slower motion to the left. This eye movement is called jerk nystagmus and named by the direction of the fast component. In this example, the nystagmus would be right-beating. If the acceleration is stopped and the subject simply continues to spin to the right at a constant velocity, the perception of motion and the jerk nystagmus would slowly decrease over a 20–25 second interval with loss of perceived angular motion and nystagmus. Therefore, without visual input the subject is unable to perceive constant velocity and will detect only acceleration or deceleration. If the subject rotating to the right at a constant velocity for 60 seconds is suddenly brought to a stop, a reversal of the endolymphatic flow shown in Figure 1–2 would occur. The subject would now perceive intense rotation to the left and would demonstrate left beating nystagmus, even though perfectly still. It will again take 20–25 seconds for the perception of motion and the left beating nystagmus to dissipate. It is known that the cupula returns to its equilibrium position in 8–10 seconds. The time for the cupula to return to within 37% of its equilibrium position is referred to as the cupula time constant (normal 6–8 sec), and the time required for the magnitude of the slow-component eye velocity of the nystagmus to reduce to 37% of its original value at the start of the deceleration is called the canal-ocular time constant (normal 15–18 sec). This prolongation of motion perception and nystagmus beyond the time frame expected from the dynamics of the cupula is due to neural firing rate asymmetry that persists within the vestibular nuclei, a phenomenon known as the *velocity storage integrator* (Cohen, Henn, Raphan, & Dennett, 1981; Raphan, Matsuo, & Cohen, 1979; Waespe, Cohen, & Raphan, 1985). The nodulus of the cerebellum plays a major role in the control of the velocity storage integrator. Interaction between the primary afferent neural inputs from the otolith organs and the semicircular canals is apparently mediated through the velocity storage integrator. More specific discussion of the canal-ocular time constant and its clinical utility will be given in Chapter 6.

As shown in Figure 1–2, the VOR of the horizontal canals is mediated by a simple three-neuron arc involving the vestibular nuclei and cranial nerves III and VI. Stimulation of the vertical canal pairs also produces a VOR along analogous brain stem pathways. Oblique (or rotatory) nystagmus can be seen with stimulation of the horizontal canals and one of the vertical pairs. The central nervous system pathways from the vestibular nuclei to the extra-ocular muscles involve the cranial nerves III, IV, and VI, the medial longitudinal fasciculus, and collateral neural inputs from the reticular formation in the brain stem. A detailed description of these brain stem and cerebellar pathways and the neurophysiology of the VOR are discussed thoroughly elsewhere (Baloh & Honrubia, 1990; Harada, 1988; Ryu, 1986; Schwarz, 1986).

The principle function of the VOR is the control of eye position during transient head movements to maintain a stable visual image. In addition to this dynamic control system, several other neural pathways that are independent of head movement contribute to eye movement control. Control of smooth pursuit, saccadic, and optokinetic eye movements assists in maintaining clear visual images and contribute to one's perception of speed and direction of body motion. The smooth pursuit system permits tracking of a visual target with a smooth continuous movement of the eye. This mechanism provides for stable image projection to the fovea of the retina, the region providing for maximum sensitivity and therefore greatest clarity of the image. In order to utilize smooth pursuit, the trajectory of the target must typically be predictable, and the frequency of movement less than approximately 1.2 Hz. Constraints on maximum peak velocity and acceleration of the target also apply. The most efficient range of smooth pursuit function is for frequencies less than 1 Hz. This would be the mechanism most likely used when viewing a single bird flying across a person's visual field or when watching a pendulum swing. While the parameters of frequency, peak velocity, and acceleration all impact on performance, acceleration is the limiting factor for a target moving in a sinusoidal manner. The vestibulo-cerebellum (flocculus, nodulus, and posterior vermis) plays a dominant role in smooth pursuit; the remainder of the cerebellum, portions of the brain stem, and cortical areas also participate under certain conditions (Leigh & Zee, 1991).

As indicated above, the saccadic system of eye movement control provides the fast component during the production of jerk nystagmus. The primary functional goal of the saccadic movements is to reposition a visual target of interest onto the fovea with a single rapid eye motion (Leigh & Zee, 1982, 1991). In order to accomplish this task, supratentorial processes must participate to calculate the strength of the neural signal to be delivered to the extra-ocular musculature needed to stimulate a rapid and accurate single movement of the eyes. In addition to the cortical activity, both the pontine reticular formation and the vestibulo-cerebellum participate in modulating the parameters of movement such as the velocity of the saccade, its latency to onset, and the accuracy of the saccade (Cohen & Buttner-Ennever, 1984; Cohen, Matsuo, Fradin, & Raphan, 1985; Zee & Robinson, 1978). When a target of interest is moving outside the operating parameters of the smooth pursuit system, the saccade system facilitates the tracking ability by superimposing jerk movements onto the smooth movements. The difference between the position of the target on the retina and the desired position on the fovea is known as *retinal slip*. It provides one of the cues hypothesized in the calculation of the saccade movement parameters (Zee & Robinson, 1978).

The *optokinetic response* is a combination of smooth pursuit and saccade mechanisms, and may be produced by repeated movements across a stationary subject's visual field, moving the subject in a stationary visual field, or both. Evidence from research does suggest that the optokinetic system is more than a simple superimposition of smooth pursuit and saccade systems (summary in Leigh & Zee, 1991). The optokinetic response is a perception of movement and produces *optokinetic jerk nystagmus* (OKN, nystagmus produced by the movement of objects in the visual field) similar in character to that of the VOR. Right-beating OKN results from objects crossing from right to left in a subject's visual field. While there is some indication of a separate "optokinetic control system," eye movement experts generally agree that the smooth pursuit and saccade control centers in the brain stem and cerebellar pathways mentioned above are the predominant control mechanisms (Honrubia, Baloh, & Khalili, 1989; Rahko, 1984; Ventre, 1985; Zasorin, Baloh, Yee, & Honrubia, 1983). Because of this control interaction it is suggested that a way to study the true optokinetic system is with optokinetic afternystagmus studied in the dark (discussed further in Chapter 6) (Leigh & Zee, 1991). The main purpose of the optokinetic system is to provide for clear visual images during sustained head movements. The perception of motion that can be generated with optokinetic stimulation is so powerful that the vegetative symptoms of motion sickness (nausea, emesis, etc.) can be produced without actual movement of the subject. This response is exploited commercially in amusement park attractions that simulate motion. The production of nystagmus and the perceptions of motion may suggest some direct interaction between the vestibular system and the optokinetic system. It has been demonstrated that this occurs not at the level of the periphery, but through the velocity storage integrator in the vestibular nuclei and vestibulocerebellum (Kubo, Igarashi, & Wright, 1981; Waespe, Cohen, & Raphan, 1983; Zee, Yamazaki, Butler, & Gucer, 1981). Although the range of frequency, velocity, and acceleration over which optokinetic responses are stimulated is broad compared to the VOR and smooth pursuit systems, many errors in perception would occur if this were the only perceptual system of motion available. The integration of optokinetics, smooth pursuit, saccade movements, and the VOR for control of accurate visual perceptions will be discussed later.

One last system of oculomotor control is *visual fixation*. This is the active process of maintaining a fixed line of gaze on a target of interest. While this system shares neurological substrate with the smooth pursuit system, evidence suggests that it is a separate control system (Leigh & Zee, 1991). When a subject is asked to gaze at a specific target in the primary position, the size and frequency of microsaccadic movements of the eyes is reduced compared to primary gaze without a specific target of interest. When gaze is directed laterally or vertically, the initial movement and placement of the target on the fovea is a property of the saccade system; however, the maintenance of gaze for a prolonged period involves the visual fixation system together with mechanisms referred to the saccade system for eccentric gaze.

Postural and Motor System Control

A schematized concept of the major anatomical structures and pathways involved in static and dynamic postural control activities is shown in Figure 1–3. The interested reader is referred to other sources for details of both anatomy and physiology of these pathways (Truex & Carpenter, 1969). The cerebral cortex influences lower motor centers via projections through two pathways. The first are long fibers of the corticospinal tract, the *pyramidal system*, which plays a major role in the control of fine, isolated, versatile movements that set the basis for skill aquisition. The tracts of the pyramidal system orginate in the cells of the cerebral cortex, with all tracts passing through the medullary pyramid and extending the full length of the spinal cord. The cells and axons of the pyramidal system are referred to as the *upper motor neurons*. The signals passed through the pyramidal tracts initiate volitional movements. Approximately 55% of the fibers end in the cervical cord, with the remainder distributed to the thoracic and lumbosacral segments. This implies the pyramidal system control over the upper extremities is much more extensive than that over the lower.

The second pathway for cerebral cortex projections is the *extrapyramidal system*. This system consists of four large brain stem nuclei and the basal ganglia. The four brainstem nuclei functionally related to the basal ganglia are the subthalamic nucleus, the subtantia nigra, red nucleus, and the brain stem reticular formation. These pathways provide the mechanisms for

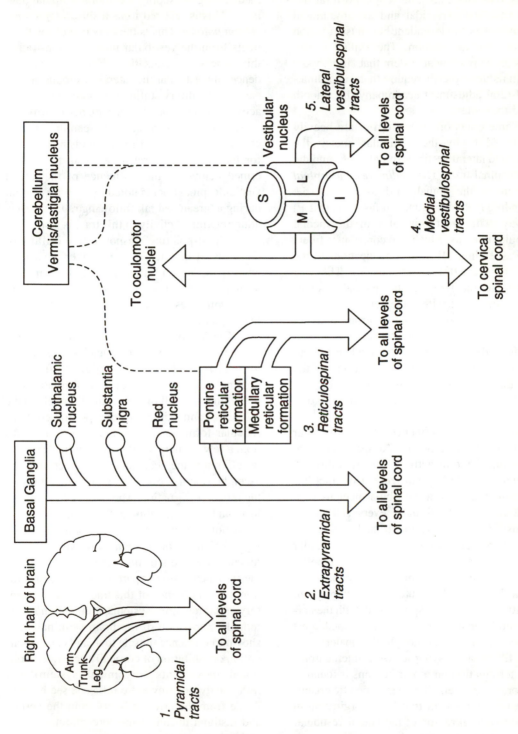

FIGURE 1–3. The five pathways involved in the control of coordinated limb and body movements. S, superior vestibular nucleus; M, medial vestibular nucleus; L, lateral vestibular nucleus; I, inferior vestibular nucleus.

large gross movement patterns that are primarily reflexive and constitute major postural adjustments. The pyramidal and extrapyramidal systems are not independent but must function in a coordinated fashion. The skilled movements of the pyramidal system that are nonpostural in nature typically require that a coordinated postural adjustment accompany the smooth skilled movement.

Three tracts originate from or are heavily contributed to by the vestibular nuclei: the medial and lateral vestibulospinal tracts, and the reticulospinal tract. The *medial vestibulospinal tract* enters the spinal cord as part of the descending medial longitudinal fasiculus (MLF) pathway. This tract originates in the medial vestibular nucleus, which also contributes fibers to the ascending MLF, with connections to the nuclei of the extra-ocular muscles. The vast majority of the fibers in the medial vestibulospinal tract end within the cervical cord via synaptic connections to interneurons and not directly on motor neurons. Given the projections from the medial vestibular nucleus to both the ascending and descending portions of the MLF, this tract may play a major role in the cervical-vestibulo-ocular reflexes, coordinating eye-head movements.

The principal influence of the vestibular system and the specific areas of the cerebellum on the spinal motor activity is carried through the *lateral vestibulospinal tract*. This tract has its origin in the lateral vestibular nucleus with contributions from virtually every cell in the nucleus. The lateral vestibular nucleus receives its inputs not only from the primary vestibular afferents of the VIIIth nerve, but also cerebellar efferents from the vermis and the fastigial nuclei. The tract distributes inputs throughout the entire length of the spinal cord, with the cervical and lumbar segments receiving the largest number of fibers. Although the majority of these fibers also synapse with interneurons, direct termination on motor neurons is found in the thoracic segment. There is a specific organization to this tract, in that fibers orginating in the rostroventral region of the lateral vestibular nucleus supply the cervical region; fibers originating in the dorsocaudal region supply the

lumbosacral segments; and those in the intermediate region supply the thoracic spinal segment. This is referred to as a *somatotopic projection pattern*. This is the only one of the three tracts from the vestibular nuclei demonstrating this type of organization. Experimental evidence suggests that the lateral vestibular nuclei exert a facilitory influence upon the reflex activity of the spinal mechanisms controlling muscle tone. This influence is seen in the muscles of the distal lower limbs and is responsible for the *functional stretch response* to be described below. Further influence of the lateral vestibulospinal tract is noted by activity present during a threatened fall following rapid accelerating rotation. Activity in this tract is also noted in the "past-pointing" response (the drifting of the arms to the side of the weaker peripheral end-organ, in an uncompensated peripheral asymmetry, when up and down movements are made with eyes closed. This will be discussed in Chapter 3).

The last of the tracts with strong indirect input from the vestibular nuclei is the *reticulospinal tract*. These fibers originate from the pontine and medullary reticular formations in the brain stem. All of the vestibular nuclei have efferent connections to the pontomedullary reticular formation of the brain stem. In addition, a few primary vestibular neurons, cerebellar efferents, the accessory optic tract, and the ascending spinal tracts also provide inputs to the reticular formation. The fibers of the reticulospinal tract originating in the pontine reticular formation constitute the majority of the descending MLF in the brain stem. However, the pontomedullary fibers of the reticulospinal tract in the spinal cord are not part of the MLF. In addition to the influence of this tract on the respiratory and circulatory systems, stimulation of the reticular formation of the brain stem has been shown to influence muscle tone and cause facilitation or inhibition of cortically generated volitional movements (pryamidal system) and reflex activities (myototic reflexes, see below). Aside from the efferent fibers from the vermis and fastigial nuclei of the cerebellum, afferent paths to these two areas are from the secondary vestibular neurons arising from the vestibular nuclei, the ascending spinal pathways, and the pontomedullary reticular formation of the brain stem. This significant network of input and output pathways that interconnect the cerebellum, reticular formation, and the vestibular system is hypothesized to play a major role in the maintenance of equilibrium and coordination of locomotor activities (Mori & Takakusaki, 1988; Pompeiano, 1994).

In reviewing static and dynamic postural control, three general movement control systems need be considered (see Table 1–1). The *myototic reflex* is stimulated by an externally generated pull on a muscle, causing stimulation of tendon and muscle stretch receptors. This is mediated through spinal cord pathways, just as a deep tendon reflex. The purpose of this reflex appears to regulate muscle force thereby maintaining stability at a joint. It is a localized, stereotyped response to the external stimulus. The typical latency of this response is in the range of 40 milliseconds. Although it assists in postural movements by maintaining joint stiffness, it is not directly responsible for coordinated movements across a joint (Gurfinkel, Lipshitz, & Popv, 1974).

Second, the *automatic muscle response (functional stretch response)* is stimulated by an external event via the somatosensory input pathways. While mediated through spinal pathways, its amplitude and onset are modulated through brain stem and subcortical pathways including the basal ganglia. This response provides for coordinated limb and trunk movements across the joints (coordinated body segment movements about a joint, such as hip or ankle). While it is usually a stereotyped response, it demonstrates adaptability if the environmental context requires an adjustment of the typical reflex movement. Like the myototic response, the latency to onset is relatively fixed at about 100 msec. This coordinated muscle response provides for the corrective action to recover from a destabilizing perturbation of the center of mass, such as when an individual is lightly bumped from behind while standing (Nashner, 1976, 1977; Nashner, Woollacott, & Tuma, 1979).

The third level is *volitional movement.* These are mediated at all levels including cortical sensory and motor areas. These are responsible for learned, purposeful movements. Consequently, the latency to onset is highly variable yet typically longer than 140 msec (Nashner & Cordo, 1981). By definition, these movements have to be highly adaptable.

Vestibular, Visual and Somatosensory System Contributions to the Functional Stretch Response

Horak and collagues (Horak & Nashner,1986; Horak, Diener, & Nashner,1989; Horak, Nashner, & Diener, 1990) have demonstrated that stereotyped responses to unexpected forward or backward translations of the surface on which a subject stands can be described by strategies based on the principal joint around which the body rotates. The *ankle strategy* involves primary rotation about the ankle, whereas the *hip strategy* has the hip joint as the primary point of rotation. Figure 1–4 A and B

TABLE 1–1. Organization of Movement Control.

Movement Type	Pathways	Purpose	Latency
Reflex (myotatic stretch)	Spinal cord	Regulate joint stiffness	= 40 msec
Automatic	Brain stem, Subcortical	Coordinate movements Across joints	= 100 msec
Voluntary	Brain stem, Cortical	Generate purposeful movements	Variable
			>150 msec

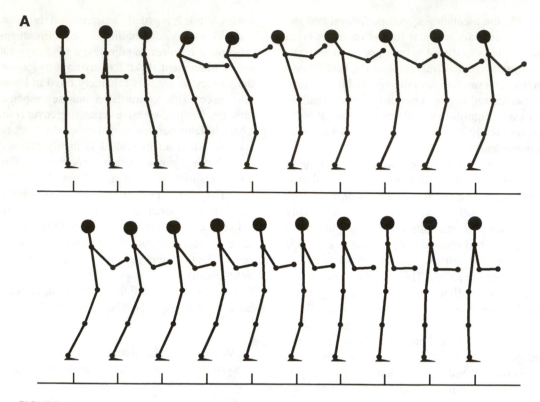

FIGURE 1–4. Computer reconstruction of a subject with eyes closed standing on a movable platform. An unexpected anterior translation of the platform is given, causing a small backward sway. The movements of the body were monitored by an opto-electric system allowing for determination of the movements of multiple body segments. Each tic mark represents 0.1 seconds of time, with the tic mark at the

illustrate both strategies in a series of computer reconstructed body segments of a subject reacting to a sudden unexpected anterior translation of the support surface. Each figure represents 0.1 seconds in time. Part A shows an ankle strategy and part B demonstrates a hip strategy. The strategy used in a given situation is dependent on the magnitude of the perturbation of the center of mass, and the conditions of the support surface (width relative to size of the foot and the amount of friction between the foot and the support surface). In Part B, the subject is standing on a 5-cm wide beam instead of a flat support surface. The functional impact of strategy selection will be discussed in Chapter 2, while the present discussion centers on how these stereotyped responses are stimulated. Horak and Nashner (1986) have suggested that the functional stretch response is stim-

ulated by the dorsiflexion (closure of ankle angle) or plantarflexion (opening of the ankle angle) movement at the ankle, mediated via stretch receptors in the tendons and muscles. Additionally, recent investigations by Allum et al. (Allum, Honegger, & Schicks,1993; Allum, Schicks, & Honegger, 1994), using first normals and then patients with bilateral peripheral labyrinthine paresis, have elucidated how the strategies are stimulated and which components of the input systems contribute to this process. The following conclusions were reached:

1. The timing of the ankle and hip strategies are distinct and the selection of the strategy to be used based on afferent inputs appears to occur within the first 100 msec following the perturbation.

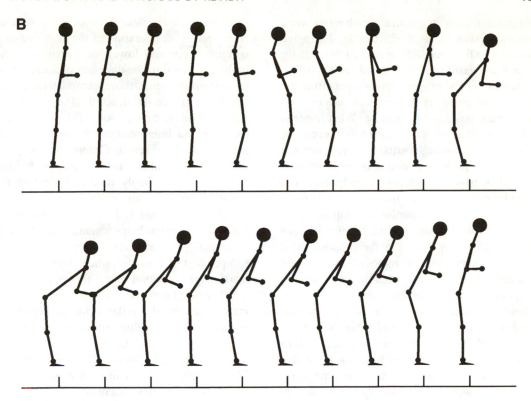

top left representing time zero. **Part A** demonstrates the recovery action with dominant movement about the ankle. The subject in A was standing on a flat firm surface larger than the foot. In **part B**, the recovery action is shown for the subject standing on a 5-cm-wide beam under the center of the foot. Note in B the principal movement is about the hip.

2. Determination of the velocity of the upper leg (thigh including hip) and the knee joint angle are suggested as candidates to provide the information needed to select between the ankle and hip strategies.

3. The trigger to produce a functional stretch response appears to be limited to the ankle angle for rotational stimuli but involves both the ankle and knee for certain types of translational movements.

4. The onset latencies and most of the muscle response timing patterns in the functional stretch response are not influenced by the vestibular end organs.

5. Labyrinthine function appears to heavily influence the muscle amplitudes within either strategy, specifically by enhancing the muscles of the lower limbs (tibialis anteri-or, soleus, and quadriceps) while suppressing the amplitude of the para-spinal muscles.

6. If information from the ankle and knee are unavailable, the default appears to be the hip strategy.

It should be noted that, while some differences in suggested mechanisms appear to exist between this work and similar studies by Horak and Nashner (1986), the magnitudes and velocities of the experimental perturbations were different. This may simply indicate that the responses and trigger mechanisms are task specific, as suggested in other postural control studies (Alexander, Shepard, Gu, & Schultz, 1992).

The work of Allum and colleagues suggests that the vestibular end-organ activity is not used to initiate the functional stretch reflex when proprioceptive inputs are available. Extensive research in this area (Allum et al., 1993, 1994b; Horak & Nashner, 1986; Horak et al., 1990) indicates that the proprioceptive inputs from the lower limb joints are the principal cues to stimulate the repositioning response. What happens when proprioceptive/somatosensory cues are not available? Is the functional stretch response absent? The answer is no, as is easily demonstrated in persons with severe peripheral neuropathies of the lower limbs. These persons respond with a well-coordinated respositioning response with a delayed onset. Similar findings are noted in normals when the proprioceptive input is experimentally removed by transient ischemia. It can be shown that the same muscles responsible for the ankle strategy functional stretch response activate in response to a perturbation, but with a 50–75 msec delay (Nashner & Grimm, 1978). This response is noted with or without visual input. This would suggest that when lower limb joint inputs are not available, the vestibular end-organ activity can be used to stimulate the response, but a delay is introduced.

How much of the response to a perturbation of the center of mass is influenced by prior experience and the knowledge that a perturbation will eventually take place? This question is very important since clinical posturography paradigms do provide the patient with information about the task to be studied. Work by Maki and Whitelaw (1992) indicates that knowledge about the task has a minimal effect other than possibly to optimize the use of the selected strategy, but has no effect on the selection of the strategy or the magnitude of the actual response. Prior experience with the task was suggested to increase arousal of the subject without substantial impact on performance.

Vestibular, Visual, and Somatosensory System Contributions to Volitional Movements

Several specific reflexes are related to *vestibular system function* that are thought to assist in the acquisition and execution of learned purposeful movements. First is the *vestibulo-spinal reflex*. As with the vestibulo-ocular reflex, acceleration of the head causes a specific upper and lower limb response. The limbs ipsilateral to the direction of acceleration are extended, while those contralateral to the acceleration are contracted (Pompeiano & Allum, 1988; Roberts, 1968). This reflex is the basis for the interpretation of certain clinical tests, to be discussed in Chapter 3. The pathways for this reflex use the lateral vestibulospinal tract probably mediated through the vertical semicircular canals and otolithic organs. The second is known as the *righting reflex*. This reflex helps maintain the head in horizontal gaze orientation relative to gravity, independent of trunk movement, within the limits of range of motion of the neck in the sagittal and lateral planes. It is suggested by experimental data that this reflex is mediated primarily through the otolithic organs and the medial vestibulospinal tract (Berthoz & Pozzo, 1988; Pozzo, Berthoz, & Popov, 1994). Figure 1–4B illustrates this reflex with a series of computer reconstructed body segments of a subject reacting to a sudden unexpected anterior translation of the support surface. Each frame is 0.1 sec apart. Note how the head moves in directions opposite the trunk in order to maintain the horizontal gaze orientation. It is important to note that this figure is an example of the perturbation with the subject's eyes closed. This behavior would be the same with the eyes open. Two additional reflex activities, the tonic neck reflex and the labyrinthine reflex, impact upon static but not dynamic situations. The significance of their contribution to active postural control in the adult is debatable; however, the work of Fukuda (1983) presents a line of reasoning worthy of consideration. The tonic neck reflex is seen in the early weeks of infancy and is stimulated by neck torsion. The ipsilateral limbs extend while the contralateral contract. This behavior is evident in situations where an angular acceleration may be absent from the volitional movement (typically a learned skill). Thus it has been suggested that the tonic neck reflex may not disappear after a few weeks of life, but may simply be reduced in its ability to produce these limb movements. The tonic neck reflex is mediated via muscle stretch receptors in the neck through the reticulospinal and probably the medial vestibulospinal tract. These same cervical afferent inputs may be responsible for another reflex of minor influence in the normal adult system, the cervico-ocular reflex, to be discussed in Chapter 2.

The labyrinthine reflex is stimulated by the position of the head relative to the gravity vector. Thus, this reflex is the property of the otolith organs and the lateral vestibulospinal tract. It is easily demonstated in animals, and can be seen in human activities, especially related to athletics and dance. If a cat is held upside down it will extend all limbs, yet contract them when the head is stabilized in the normal upright orientation (see Figure 1–5). This reflex may assist humans in developing certain learned skills in sports that require limb extension or contraction, such as skating, gymnastics, and spring board diving (Fukuda, 1983).

The visual system, while important, is not critical to volitional postural control unless one of the other two systems is unavailable or disrupted by pathology. A significant body of literature illustrates the influence visual stimuli may have over postural control (Berthoz, Lacour, Soechting, & Vidal, 1979; Courjon & Jeannerod, 1979; Diener et al., 1986; Fitzpatrick, Burke, & Gandevia, 1994; Nashner & Berthoz, 1978; Ring, Matthews, Nayak, & Isaacs, 1988) This seems especially true if objects equal to or greater than a subject's height are within five meters. Typically the visual influence occurs in the form of optokinetic visual stimuli. This can be seen by observing individuals standing alongside a train on the adjacent platform. As the train begins to move, the persons tend to lean in the direction of the train movement for a brief period. This movement involved their perception of drifting in a direction opposite the train motion is due to the optokinetic effect in their peripheral vision. The effect is most prominent if the persons are within 5–10 feet of the train as the motion is initiated. As we stand or walk through an area of congestion with other people or vehicles moving about, the optokinetic effect is continuous. For the majority, this effect is selected out and does not have an adverse impact. However, this situ-

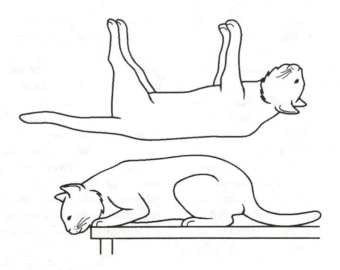

FIGURE 1–5. The demonstrated limb responses of the cat for the head in two different positions relative to the pull of gravity. The extension or contraction of the limbs is attributed to the tonic labyrinthine reflex, a response to changes in otolithic stimulation.

ation produces significant symptoms for certain balance disorder patients. The optokinetic effect when the subject is still is an object-motion influence, such as in the train example. For some individuals, head or eye motion with the objects in the visual field stationary can be equally stimulating. The most common example involves the subject walking through the aisle of a store and scanning the objects on the shelves, the "grocery store effect." For many who are sensitive to visual motion stimuli, the symptoms of dysequilibrium can be stronger than those stimulated by head movement. This result of optokinetic stimulation is probably a consequence of the modulation of peripheral vestibular primary afferent inputs by the visual input (accessory optic tract) at the level of the vestibular nuclei in the velocity storage integrator (Cohen, Uemure, & Takemore, 1973; Lafortune, Ireland, & Jell, 1991; Waespe et al., 1983; Zee, Yee, & Robinson, 1976). In normal individuals, the ability to dissociate peripheral and foveal vision allows you to read and walk through a crowd while adjusting your path and gait speed to avoid other moving or stationary objects. In addition to the optokinetic effect produced primarily through the peripheral visual inputs of the accessory optic tract, direct foveal stimulation by a stationary object can impact on quiet volitional stance. Experimental evidence from normals has shown that if the afferent proprioceptive and somatosensory inputs from the plantar surface of the foot, the ankle region, and the tendon and muscle stretch receptors are interrupted, quiet volitional stance may be maintained in a normal fashion if the eyes are open and the subject fixates on an object. If the eyes are closed, the subject goes into a high-frequency (1 Hz), low-amplitude sway pattern. It is hypothesized that the decreased sensitivity of the vestibular labyrinth at low-acceleration, low-frequency head movements accounts for the "1 Hz sway" pattern. In other words, the peripheral vestibular system is unable to completely act as a substitute for the missing proprioceptive/somatosensory system for a task in this acceleration/frequency range (Mauritz & Dietz, 1980). Yet with the eyes open the stance is quiet, suggesting visual influence facilitating postural control is preferred over labyrinthine input when usual foot support surface cues are not available for quiet stance. The general low-frequency range of the visual system (less than 1.2 Hz for smooth pursuit and fixation) would lend itself more to this task than that of the vestibular end-organ (0.8–5 Hz), which is better suited for initiating the functional stretch response (a response to a perturbation with stronger head acceleration, and higher frequency activity) in the absence of proprioceptive input, discussed in the previous section.

When walking or attempting quiet stance, cutaneous proprioceptive and somatosensory inputs assist in our postural control and volitional movements. This appears to be more highly utilized than vestibular and visual inputs for stance and posture, with the others increasing their influence as the skill level or complexity of the task increases and/or desired speed of execution increases. This is clearly illustrated by observing the contrast in normal stance and disrupted (mildly ataxic) gait of an individual without peripheral vestibular inputs in a dark environment. An increase in the size of the base of support is typically noted, with individuals widening the separation of their feet as they walk to prevent a fall, yet giving the ataxic appearance to their gait. However, if the subject is asked to stand quietly, a much simpler task, with the feet together and the eyes closed, this can many times be done within a range considered normal. Therefore, when evaluating patients with chronic complaints that involve balance disturbance, it is imperative to account for the influence of each of the input systems.

2

■ FUNCTIONAL PHYSIOLOGY AND COMPENSATORY MECHANISMS

*T*his Chapter will describe how the balance system functions to facilitate the activities of daily life. A solid grasp of this information, along with the basic physiology, sets the stage for understanding the methods of evaluating the dysfunctional balance system in patients. First, we will concentrate on the function of individual systems and then discuss the all important issue of *systems integration*, or how these systems are combined to help us function in routine daily activity. The effects of aging on these functional components will be addressed, followed by a discussion of the compensation process in response to a balance system insult.

From a functional point of view the balance system has three primary goals:

1. To rapidly correct any inadvertent displacement of the center of mass from its equilibrium position over the base of support (the feet when standing) to prevent a fall, either from (a) a volitional movement or (b) from an unexpected perturbation in the center of mass
2. to provide accurate perceptions of body position in the environment along with perceptions of direction and speed of movement
3. to control eye movements in order to maintain a clear visual image of the external world while the individual, the environment, or both are in motion.

Clearly the vestibular labyrinth has a critical role in accomplishing the three goals of the system. It is erroneous, however, to conceive of the system as limited to the vestibular end-organ. A more accurate representation of the balance system involves multiple sensory inputs (vision, proprioception, and vestibular) with coordinated, automatic outputs involving the muscles of postural control. This input/output system utilizes a mechanism known as *stimulus-coded response pairing*, such that any combination of stimuli produces a predictable stereotyped muscle response. This is true for the maintenance of upright posture, as well as the control of eye movements. Understanding the complexity and integrated nature of the balance system suggests that while the evaluation of vestibular end-organ function is necessary, it is often not sufficient to fully characterize a patient's status.

PERCEPTIONS AND INTEGRATED EYE MOVEMENT CONTROL

To this point we have considered the function of the major components of the ocular motor system: the vestibular end organs, the vestibulo-ocular reflex, and the oculomotor system. We have stressed that these systems do not function as independent entities but as an integrated unit. Take for example, the vestibular system's ability to provide perceptions of motion and control of eye movement during head motion. The semicircular canals function as integrating accelerometers that are relatively independent of frequency from 0.8 to 5 Hz. The vast majority of head movements produced by routine activities fall within this range. The system continues to be responsive to head accelerations above and below this frequency range, but is decreasingly efficient for frequencies below 0.8 or above 5.0 Hz (Baloh & Honrubia, 1990; Schwarz, 1986; Wall, 1990). Passive head movements in man-made vehicles can produce both zero acceleration conditions with constant velocities (such as a smooth airplane flight) and nonzero accelerations at frequencies far outside the typical operating range (jet fighter aircraft or liftoff of a space craft escaping earth gravitational pull). We usually have no difficulty describing the direction, speed, or orientation of our movement as long as visual input is available from the stationary world. Such judgments depend upon the optokinetic system, effectively expanding the range of frequencies and magnitude of movements we can accurately perceive. While proprioceptive inputs such as pressure sensations, vibrations, or even wind against our skin assist in orientation, it is the combination of our vestibular and optokinetic systems that provides perceptions of motion relative to gravity and the stationary world.

Changes in environmental context should produce appropriate changes in the harmonious output responses to the three input cues. However, they also may place the inputs into direct conflict with each other. It is theorized that congruent information is maintained under these circumstances, while conflicting information is selectively suppressed, as the visual and somatosensory inputs are compared to the input arising from the vestibular end-organ (Barin, 1987). Obviously, some time is required for this process to take place. During this interval, the sensory conflicts are analyzed and the automatic reaction from the stereotyped muscle response can be modified. This phenomenon is illustrated when you are stopped at a traffic signal and the vehicle in your peripheral visual field begins to creep forward. The reflex is to rapidly apply the brakes in response to a false sensation of backward motion. This linear vexion (perception of linear motion when none is taking place) illustrates a sensory conflict between the visual input and actual head movement. The optokinetic visual input produced an inaccurate perception of motion, triggering a learned but incorrect automatic response. It is quickly apparent that you are not moving backwards and the brake is released. If the same event is repeated immediately, the incorrect response will not be produced. Such sensory conflicts are common during daily activities. While most conflicts are produced by visual input, others occur through the somatosensory pathways. This may occur when standing or walking on an irregular or easily compressible surface (such as gravel, mud, or a soft rug). The normal balance system handles these conflicts with only minor disruptions in activity. The ability to modify the automatic muscle output responses produced by a particular stimulus in changing environmental contexts reflects the adaptive properties of the balance system. This capacity allows an alteration in the stimulus-coded response to correct a destabilizing automatic reaction after the initial stimulus presentation.

Functional activities of the vestibulo-ocular and oculomotor portions of the balance system are similar to those of the postural control system, except that activity in the extraocular muscles are now the outputs of interest. Stimulus-coded response pairs also govern the vestibulo-ocular reflex (VOR) and the oculomotor control systems, and show similar properties of context dependency and adaptive plasticity (Bronstein, 1992; Furst, Goldberg, & Jenkins, 1987; Melvill, Berthoz, & Segal, 1984; Melvill, Guitton, & Berthoz, 1988; Melvill & Mandl,

1981; Möller, Ödkvist, White, & David, 1990; Möller, White, & Ödkvist, 1990; Zee, 1994). The primary functional task of the VOR and oculomotor control systems is to stabilize a visual image when the head is in motion. When visual inputs are available, the smooth pursuit function of the oculomotor system stabilizes the visual surroundings during movements up to just under 0.5 Hz, providing a gain (ratio of eye velocity to target velocity) of 1.0. The smooth pursuit system breaks down at higher frequencies, with poorer gains above 1 Hz. The reflex eye movements mediated by the VOR demonstrate a gain (ratio of eye velocity to head velocity) near 1.0 for head motions within the frequency range from 1 to 5 Hz. Below 1 Hz, and especially below 0.1 Hz, the gain is substantially lower (0.3 to 0.6) when measured in the dark. Thus, whereas either mechanism could not maintain stable gaze position independently, the combination of both mechanisms can maintain a clear visual image from stationary head position through movements up to 5 Hz. The need for both systems to work cohesively is illustrated when a pathologic process destroys both vestibular end organs. This creates a symptom known as *oscillopsia*, wherein the visual surroundings seem to oscillate or bounce whenever the head is moving with a frequency above 0.5 Hz. Since most normal head motions are between 0.5 and 4 Hz, this condition can be most disruptive in daily activities. The smooth pursuit system can accommodate the visual needs of the patient with increasing effectiveness as the frequency of motion decreases below 0.5 Hz.

The functional goal of the system of saccadic eye movements is to rapidly replace a visual target onto the fovea of the eye. When the head is stationary and target motion exceeds the limits of the smooth pursuit system, saccadic movements begin to appear. These rapid eye movements are stimulated by a phenomenon known as *retinal slip*, wherein the image of interest moves off the fovea toward the periphery of the retina. Whenever the target motion is less predictable or the limits of the smooth pursuit system are dramatically exceeded, more saccadic activity is required. Whenever the head is in motion (with or without concomitant target motion), some saccadic activity appears to be essential to maintain visual fixation (Cohen & Buttner-Ennever, 1984; Cohen et al., 1985).

All of the oculomotor control systems are used in harmony as we attempt to visualize targets of interest during daily activities. This is illustrated in Figure 2–1. Part A shows a target of interest moving from primary gaze to the far right lateral position. To continue to observe the target, the subject first produces a rightward saccade replacing the target on the fovea. Next the head is brought into alignment with the angle of vision while the target is stabilized on the fovea for continuous viewing. To accomplish this, a combination of smooth pursuit and the vestibulo-ocular reflex are used. Once the head and eyes are again stationary, the task of maintaining gaze falls to the visual fixation system. During the head movement for alignment with the target, a corrective saccade of less than 5 degrees is noted. This suggests that the combination of smooth pursuit and VOR were insufficient to maintain perfectly stable gaze, resulting in some retinal slip of the image and a small saccadic correction (Tomlinson,1988). Such combined eye movements with examples of the minor corrective saccades are shown in Figure 2–1B, where a subject repeatedly looks back and forth between a target on the right and one on the left. This is the process used as we survey the visual world throughout the day. The ability to perform these visual capturing tasks quickly and accurately depends on the proper function of both the vestibular and oculomotor systems. Abnormalities in any of these systems can produce functional disability for any task requiring coordinated movements of the head and eyes, such as driving a rapidly moving car. This activity demands that the driver constantly evaluate the visual surroundings and occasionally glance for information from the dashboard. Knowing the complexity of these seemingly simple tasks helps the clinician to understand why patients with chronic vestibular dysfunction may feel hopelessly insecure about driving, even when they are not experiencing active bouts of vertigo.

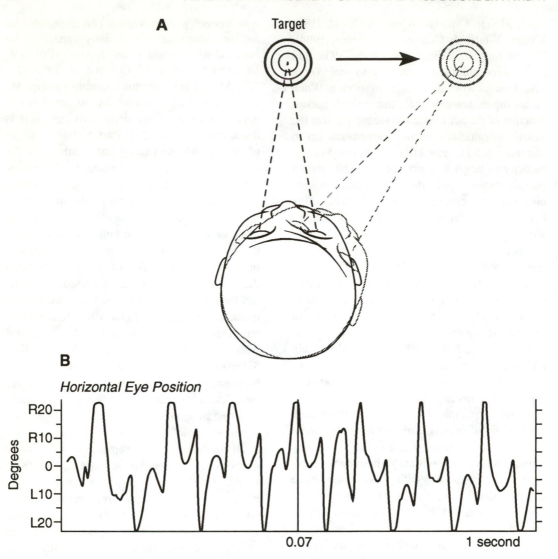

FIGURE 2–1. A. Illustrates the movement of the subject in order to maintain visualization of a target that moves first to the right and then back to the left. **B.** Graph of the horizontal eye postion in degrees as a function of time associated with the task given in part A. The movements were recorded with standard electro-oculargraphic techniques, with electrodes placed at the lateral canthi and a ground (common) on the center forehead. The plot shows that the eyes move first with a saccade and then return smoothly to the center of the orbit position as the head moves to align with new target position.

MAINTENANCE OF POSTURAL CONTROL

Volitional Control of Static and Dynamic Posture

As indicated in the introduction to this Chapter, two important purposes of the postural control system are volitional maintenance of the center of mass over the support surface, and the ability to reposition the center of mass over the support surface after an unexpected perturbation. Functionally, postural control is maintained during volitional activities by the mechanisms discussed in Chapter 1. These activities range from quiet stance to very complex and highly skilled athletic movements. In the clinical setting, we typically focus our diagnostic interest in the evaluation of static stance and gait. In daily activities, we must be able to reweight the influence of the three sensory inputs contributing to balance depending on the environmental context. This is evident as we manipulate our way through a crowd of people; arise in a dark room and begin walking on a thick carpet; step unexpectedly onto a slanted surface; go from a well-lit environment into one of darkness; or walk on an irregular surface. The strategy of input weighting used by adults has been conceptualized in various models (Nashner, 1979; Nashner & McCoullum, 1985). From a modeling point of view, these activities may be seen as varying the gain of a set of input amplifiers. The manner of setting the gain is the analogy used for weighting of the inputs, forming the strategies used for the task. Of interest functionally is the evidence that children under the age of 7.5 years cannot automatically suppress conflicting input cues from the visual system or the proprioceptive/somatosensory system by adjusting the weighting of the various inputs as adults do. Those below age 5 perform in a manner that reflects a completely different scheme for weighting the inputs. The years between age 5 and 7.5 appear to be a transition period, where the child gradually adopts a more adult strategy (Forssberg & Nashner, 1982). Responses to unexpected perturbations in the center of mass showed automatic postural adjustments in this age group that were similar to the adult except for increased variability. These findings imply that automatic postural adjustments and the context-dependent weighting of the three sensory inputs are processes that we organize separately. The implication is that the automatic postural adjustments mediated by functional stretch receptors is a hierarchically lower process that matures before the adaptive process. At the other end of the age spectrum, anecdotal experience suggests an increased reliance on foot support surface cues among individuals over 70 years of age, implying a change in the weighting strategy. In formulating methods for clinical evaluation of volitional stance and gait, issues such as the use of multiple inputs, system redundancy, and age-related postural strategy selection must be considered.

Reaction to Unexpected Perturbations in Center of Mass

The second major functional goal of the postural control system is to evaluate the magnitude of an unexpected deviation of the center of mass from its equilibrium position and to produce an appropriate corrective reaction. There is no specific sensory system for detecting center of mass position. Therefore, we rely on the same three sensory input mechanisms to provide this information. The primary somato-sensory/proprioceptive inputs used for this task are changes in ankle, knee, and hip angles when standing and walking. This sensory information is integrated with visual and vestibular inputs, and stimulates automatic coordinated muscle contractions that produce the desired postural response. This stimulus-coded response pairing appears to produce stereotyped muscle responses to a given input in most individuals (Allum & Pfaltz, 1985; Horak & Nashner, 1986; Nashner, 1979, 1983; Nashner & Berthoz, 1978). Although a large number of muscle response combinations could theoretically be used for any given stimulus, the goal of rapid reaction time is best served by a limited set of automatic responses, eliminating the need to consciously consider and select the optimal choice (Nashner & McCoullum, 1985). As discussed in Chapter 1, even though all three sensory inputs are available to provide orientation, the somatosensory input from changes in the ankle angle seems to be the dominant cue that triggers the automatic muscle responses while standing. The ankle stretch receptors seem to exclusively determine responses for plantarflexion (opening the ankle angle), and a combination of ankle, knee, and possibly hip receptors contribute to responses from dorsiflexion (closing of the ankle angle). Visual and vestibular end organ inputs participate more by modulating the response than by stimulating it, unless the somatosensory input is disrupted or the automatic response is inherently destabilizing

(Allum, 1983; Allum & Pfaltz, 1985;). The response to changes in joint angle is mediated through afferent pathways involving the spinal cord, brain stem, and cerebellum. These inputs extend to motor cortex projections and are followed by the efferent responses returned through the spinal tracts to the appropriate musculature (Keshner, Woollacott, & Debu, 1988; Woollacottl, von Hosten, & Rosblad, 1988). This was described in Chapter 1 as the myototic reflex and the automatic functional stretch response. Collectively, these are called the *automatic long loop pathways.*

In addition to the stimulus-coded responses of this system, the response generated is contingent on the environmental context. Thus, the system can be characterized as context dependent, or *feed-forward.* This term implies that the stereotyped response pattern is selected prior to a perturbation, based on the current environmental context. This is illustrated in Figure 2–2 where a subject standing on a flat surface larger than the foot is subjected to a sudden posterior perturbation of the support surface. This induces a forward sway to which an automatic

response is generated. The processed electromyographic response from the major lower limb musculature is plotted as a function of time. In Figure 2–2A, a distal to proximal progression of muscle response occurs, starting with the gastrocnemius, putting the subject back into position by pivoting around the ankle joint (ankle strategy). This response uses force exerted by the toe and ball of the foot against the floor as part of the mechanics to reposition the center of mass. In Figure 2–2B, the same posterior surface perturbation is provided, resulting in the same degree of dorsiflexion at the ankle angle and similar inputs to the visual and vestibular organs. However, this time the subject is standing on a beam that does not allow for toe or heel contact with the support surface. As pictured, the muscle response is entirely altered, with simultaneous contraction of the quadracepts and abdominal muscles resulting in a rotational motion at the hip joint (hip strategy). This represents a different stimulus-response pair when the same provocative stimulus is presented in a different environmental context (Horak & Nashner, 1986). Use of either

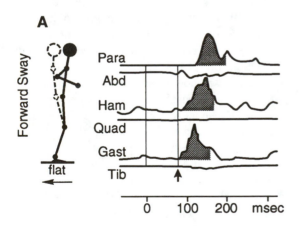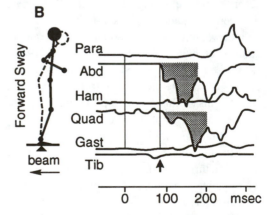

FIGURE 2–2. Illustrated is the initial (solid Figure) and the reaction position (dotted Figure) of a subject standing on a platform that gives a small posterior perturbation. **A.** The subject is on a flat firm surface larger than the foot. **B.** The subject is standing on a 5-cm-wide beam. In both A and B, the activity from lower limb muscles recorded by surface electrodes (EMG response has been filtered and rectified) as a function of time is shown. Para, paraspinal muscles; Abd, abdominal muscles; Ham, hamstring muscles; Quad, quadracept muscles; Gast, gastrocnmious muscle; Tib, tibialis anterior muscle. (Horak & Nashner, 1986).

the hip or ankle strategy can replace the center of mass following a perturbation. In the ankle format, vertical pressure is applied against the support surface under the toes or the heel of the foot to cause the repositioning. In the hip strategy, a horizontal shear force at the foot results from the movement of the upper body. The force is oriented toward the direction of the body sway, thus pushing the body back into a stable position. When standing on a beam or a compressible surface it is difficult to apply enough vertical pressure under the heel or toe to accomplish the recovery. In these settings, use of the hip strategy is more appropriate. The hip strategy is also more effective when the magnitude of the perturbation is large. It generates a greater restoring force than the ankle strategy, but requires significantly greater energy expenditure. When the support surface is slippery, there is insufficient friction between the surface and the foot, and use of the hip strategy is likely to produce a fall. Therefore, using an ankle strategy or taking a corrective step would better facilitate recovery of stance. An extensive discussion of the practical aspects of postural control is given by Nashner (1993a).

Feedback information is certainly used by the postural control system, yet the system does not respond as an immediate feedback network. In point of fact, the context dependency and automatic, stereotyped stimulus-response pairing of the system can prove to be destabilizing in some situations. Say for example the subject from Figure 2–2A has experienced five of the posterior perturbations without falling. If the portions of the surface supporting the toes and heels are rapidly removed during the next perturbation, the subject will be left standing on a beam as in Figure 2–2B. Initially, he will respond inappropriately. If the system was one of immediate feedback, the muscle response shown in Figure 2–2B would be expected. Instead, an initially destabilizing response like that in Figure 2–2A is demonstrated on the first trial, followed by the appropriate corrective response to prevent a fall. Repeated trials of this event produce a progressive change in muscle response from that seen in Figure 2–2A to that of 2–2B by the fifth trial (Nashner & Grimm,

1978). This example nicely demonstrates that the postural control system is also able to modify its responses as an adaptive learning system.

SYSTEMS INTEGRATION

As previously discussed, changes in joint (ankle, knee, hip) angle are the dominant input cues for triggering correction of the center of mass after an unexpected perturbation. However, if somatosensory input is compromised, utilization of the visual and vestibular end organ inputs must increase. When visual information is available, it provides the information needed to compensate for the lack of accurate somatosensory information from the distal lower limbs. For example, even a patient with severe, bilateral vestibular paresis may be able to step from a firm surface onto a soft, uneven area during daylight hours without difficulty. Yet at night, the patient may fall because all three systems are disrupted to some degree. If the individual has functioning vestibular endorgans, then the darkness and the disruption of the somatosensory cues is less threatening. This phenomenon can also be illustrated from balance function testing using posturography. The subject stands on a platform that suddenly tilts the toes up. The initial automatic muscle response is stimulated by dorsiflexion of the joint angle, and is the same as if forward sway was induced by a backward translation of the support surface (see Figure 2–3). This response of contracting the gastrocnemius, followed by hamstring and paraspinal muscles, is destabilizing in this setting, throwing the subject backwards. After a delay of approximately 40–70 msec, a stabilizing muscle response from the antagonist muscles (the tibialis anterior and the quadraceps) helps to reposition the center of mass and prevent a fall. This stabilizing response is hypothesized to be a vestibulospinal response correcting the initial automatic somatosensory response. A last example of this continuous evaluation of the various inputs to the postural control system is the individual with severe peripheral neuropathy involving the lower limbs. Quiet, upright stance can be main-

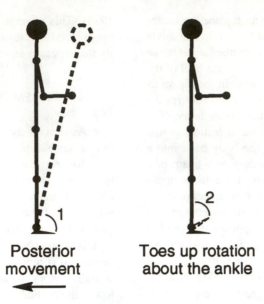

Posterior movement   **Toes up rotation about the ankle**

FIGURE 2–3. Two means of causing a dorsi-flexion manuever (closing of the ankle angle) at the ankle. The first is with a posterior movement of the surface, inducing forward sway (left Figure); and the second is by simply tilting the toes upward. Angle 1 is equal to angle 2.

tained until vision is disrupted. Then a high-frequency (about 1 Hz), low-amplitude sway pattern in the saggital plane appears until accurate visual cues are restored. In this case, vision is acting as a substitute for the somatosensory and proprioceptive inputs that typically would be used to maintain stable stance. In a normal subject, the vestibular apparatus probably serves as an internal reference against which the inputs from vision and somatosensory are compared to guide future decisions in the same stimulus-context situation.

EFFECTS OF AGING

This section will briefly review the changes in balance system function that result from aging. The discussion will be organized to discuss changes in the individual functional elements such as vision, reflex timing, somatosensation, and proprioception. Then consideration will be given to global changes in ocular motor,

VOR, and postural control performance. The reader must bear in mind that the literature on aging may be confounded by the inclusion of individuals with subtle pathology in a supposedly normal elderly population (Manchester et al., 1989). In a similar manner, the definition of normal aging used by different investigators will impact on their conclusions. In spite of these qualifiers, conclusions can be derived that are generally reliable, with differences noted in the detailed results and magnitude of effects observed. The reader desiring more details on this subject is referred to several works reviewing this important area (Alexander, 1994; Lalwani, 1994; Woollacott & Shumway-Cook, 1989). This discussion of changes in the aging balance system has two specific foci in this text: First, to impress on the clinician that a multi-system evaluation is warranted when dealing with balance disorders in the elderly; and second, to suggest the need for age-specific normative data for the performance tests used to characterize balance disorder patients.

Functional Elements

Aging impacts virtually all aspects of the individual sensory and motor components of the balance system. In the visual system, declining visual acuity, depth perception, contrast sensitivity, sensitivity to glare, and dark adaptation are all reported to occur. Degenerative changes due to generalized atrophy in the vestibular system are seen in the otolithic organs, vestibular neuroepithelium, vestibular nerve, vestibular nuclei, and areas of the vestibulo-cerebellum. In a summary of this work, Lalwani (1994) points out that the changes include demineralization and fragmentation of the otoconia along with a slow decline in the number of hair cells and ganglion cells in the peripheral system. Since the specialized neural hair cells of the mamalian peripheral vestibular system are nonmitotic, the loss of sensory elements throughout the life span cannot be replaced. Therefore, the effects of aging together with exogenous factors can be responsible for dramatic changes in the vestibular system over time.

As with the other input sources of the balance system, the somatosensory system has also been shown to undergo degenerative changes with aging. Positioning sense, general sensation, and threshold for motion detection at a joint all show changes with age. Muscle strength in the lower limbs as measured by isometric and isokinetic torque is noted to decline with age. Loss in the power and work output of the muscles is also apparent. These declines, together with a reduction in the rate of development of maximum muscle force, could certainly impact on many aspects of postural control. Additional complicating musculoskeletal system factors include decreases in the range of motion and increases in the stiffness at various joints (Alexander, 1994).

Although studies of normal elderly are able to demonstrate statistically significant changes in the above individual components compared to younger subjects, these changes in isolation may not be clinically significant. However, a combination of subclinical problems may result in mild functional 'disability. Beyond this, experimental and clinical evidence suggests a decline in the ability to integrate the three sensory inputs for maintenance of posture (Alexander, 1994). Work by Baloh, Jacobson, and Socotch, (1993) implies a decrease in the ability to utilize visual input to influence the vestibular system in a normal older population. Another important aspect is that of cognitive function. As age advances, performance on tasks requiring cognitive processing slows. This is especially true for information integration and the preparation of responses. As decision points in a task requiring motor output are approached, slowing is again noted with increasing age (Stelmach & Worringham, 1985).

Ocular-Motor Control

For years, investigators have shown age effects on the various systems for oculomotor control (Baloh et al., 1993; Peterka, Black, & Schoenhoff, 1990a; Mulch & Petermann, 1979; Zackon & Sharpe, 1987). The effect that is most clinically significant is seen in the smooth pursuit system, both for horizontal and vertical movements (Dener, 1994). This is especially important given the advent of computerized electronystagmography (ENG) evaluations, where paradigms stress the pursuit system by testing across a reasonable physiological range (see Chapter 5). This type of evaluation will accentuate degradations in performance with age as shown for optokinetics (Baloh et al., 1993). The principle effect is a decrease in the ability to use smooth pursuit eye movements to track a target with a predictable trajectory. A progressive increase in the number of saccadic corrections needed to follow the target is noted. Figure 2–4A and B demonstrate this effect by showing the rightward and leftward velocity gain values, a measure of the "smoothness" of the conjugately recorded eye movement tracings (standard electro-oculography, see Chapter 4), as functions of increasing target frequency and increasing age. Figure 2–4C also shows the effect of increasing target frequency and age on the phase (how much the eye lags behind the target) of the eye movement. These data come from recent work

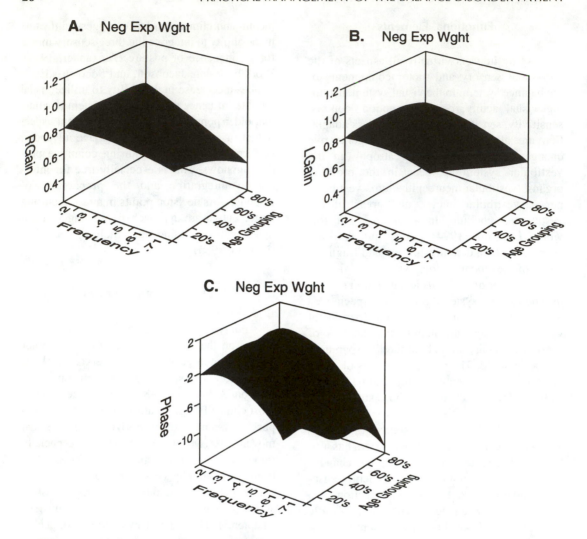

FIGURE 2–4 The effects of age of the subject and frequency of target movement (sinusoidal tracking task in the horizontal plane) for three output parameters of conjugate movements of the eyes. The eye movements were recorded via electro-oculographic techniques (see Chapter 4). **A.** Velocity gain (velocity of the eye divided by the velocity of the target) of the conjugate, horizontal eye tracking for eyes moving rightward. **B.** Velocity gain of the conjugate, horizontal eye tracking for eyes moving leftward. **C.** Phase (in degrees) of eye movements (relative timing of the eye movement compared to target movement; negative numbers mean the eyes are lagging behind the target) not specific for direction left or right. (See Chapter 5 for further explanations of velocity gain.)

in our laboratory (Smith-Wheelock, Shepard, & Lawson, submitted) recording the pursuit and saccadic eye movements in healthy subjects from ages 20 through 90 years. Our data, as well as others (Pitt & Rawles, 1988; Sharpe & Zackon, 1987; Sonderegger, Meienberg, & Ehrengruber, 1986), demonstrate statistically significant declines in velocity, latency, and accuracy for reactionary and volitional saccadic movements with advancing age. Statistically significant correlation coefficients between saccade performance parameters and age were noted for eye movements recorded both individually and conjugately. However, strength of association measures suggested that no more than 7% of the variance in these parameters can be accounted for by age. Similar results also were obtained when statistical tests of differences between age group were performed. These data imply that while the maximum velocity, accuracy, and latency parameters of saccade performance worsen with age, age itself does not appear to be a clinically significant variable. Whether the recordings of saccade movements are binocular (conjugate) or individual eye recordings appears to be more important. The implications of this finding will be discussed in Chapter 5.

As optokinetic function and smooth pursuit are strongly related, an age effect would be expected for optokinetics given the highly significant effect of age on pursuit tracking. This is indeed what the literature reflects (Baloh et al., 1993; Mulch & Petermann, 1979; Perterka et al., 1990a). This effect is statistically significant and probably clinically important as well. As with pursuit tracking, the nature of the testing paradigm for optokinetic nystagmus may accentuate the age effect. Baloh et al. (1993) report a velocity saturation effect that accounted for the decline in eye velocity with increasing target velocity in older age groups. In light of these findings, age-specific normative data for the clinical assessment of oculomotor function is imperative for smooth pursuit, desirable for optokinetics, but may not be required for saccade testing.

Vestibulo-Ocular Reflex and Its Interaction with Visual System Input

The vestibulo-ocular reflex has been shown to decrease in gain as a function of age (Goebel, Hanson, & Fishel, 1994; Mulch & Petermann, 1979; Paige, 1992; Peterka et al., 1990a, 1990b). This decrease has been demonstrated for both thermal caloric stimuli, as well as rotational stimuli across a broad frequency range (0.01-6 Hz). The changes observed in the VOR are probably accounted for by the pathologic changes in the vestibular end-organ itself (Peterka et al., 1990a). Yet, the magnitude of the effect, at least in the high frequencies, may be explained by the natural adaptive plasticity (changes in function to improve performance

resulting from exposure to a given stimulus) of the central nervous system components of the VOR. This plasticity allows for adjustments in gain determined by the visual input mismatch during head movement, like that experienced each time new corrective lenses are obtained (Zee, 1994). Similar adjustments may also occur with gradual minor changes in peripheral system performance. However, adaptive plasticity and other visual-vestibular interaction activities, such as visual enhancement or suppression of the VOR, are noted to deteriorate in the elderly (Baloh et al., 1993; Paige, 1992). Therefore, while the central adaptive properties work to preserve the relationships between head movement and coordinated eye movement, age effects may limit if not eliminate this function. For example, caloric responsiveness diminishes with age, and while statistically demonstrated in a population study, clinical significance in the individual case is doubtful. Thus, age-specific normative data are probably not required (Peterka et al., 1990b). However, for rotational stimulation, at least at the lower frequencies (less than 1 Hz) clinically evaluated, evidence suggests that normative data should be normalized for age. The effects of age seem to influence the parameter of phase lead (timing relationship between head movement and eye movement, see Chapter 6) more significantly, while the central adaptive processes may adjust for deterioration in gain (the velocity of the eye movement divided by the velocity of the head movement, see Chapter 6) produced by the slow degenerative changes in peripheral vestibular function (Paige, 1992). For low frequency rotational stimuli, phase lead is found to increase with age while gain decreases (Paige, 1992; Peterka et al., 1990b). The implication is that age-related normative data for phase would improve the accuracy of clinical evaluation of VOR function in older age groups. It is less likely that age-specific normative data for gain would be as important.

Static and Dynamic Postural Control

Significant attention has been paid to the effect of aging on postural control. The interested reader is referred to Alexander (1994) for an extensive review of the work in this area. A major driving force behind this research is the increased rate of falls with aging (Tinetti et al., 1988). As yet, in spite of the general changes noted with postural control in the "normal" elderly, an actual cause-and-effect relationship between the postural control changes and rate of falls has not been established. In summary, most investigators have been able to show statistically significant changes compared to younger controls under two conditions: when the support surface was altered to require standing either on a beam or a compressible surface, or when significant unexpected perturbations in the center of mass were introduced (Alexander, 1994). During quiet stance with the eyes open or closed, healthy elderly subjects show trends for population differences compared to younger subjects, but the differences are minimal. With more challenging support surfaces and perturbations, the reported differences ascribed to age are an increase in myoelectric activity in response to anterior translations of the support surface; increased variability in performance with increased number of fall reactions; and a greater use of upper body movement similar to the *hip strategy* discussed above.

In recent work by Alexander et al. (1992), these same questions of changes in postural contol response to an unexpected backward perturbation of the center of mass was studied in "super-healthy" elderly subjects, a select group of very healthy and active older persons. The population was highly screened to eliminate subclinical disease that might have confounded the effects of age. Extensive kinematic data were used to characterize the body movements. The major findings were: significant differences in postural control were noted only for the challenging situation of beam standing and significant anterior translations of the support surface; greater use of upper body segments with increased rotational magnitudes and variability were noted in the elderly, primarily for beam standing tasks; and, decreased control of head stabilization in space (the righting reflex discussed earlier) was suggested for the elderly. Although the findings were similar to those in the prior literature, the magnitude of the differ-

ences were small and appeared to be specific to particular tasks. The nature of the differences were also noted to not be destabilizing for these elderly subjects. In contrast, the differences on the most difficult tasks seemed to invoke changes in performance that made the elderly subjects less likely to loose balance, at the expense of greater energy expenditure. It is interesting to speculate whether changes observed in this select group were due to the anatomical and physiological changes noted for functional deficits discussed above, or at least in part due to a behavioral change produced by fear of falling. This behavioral influence would probably be subconscious, yet may reflect the prevailing perceptions regarding falls and their consequences in the elderly.

COMPENSATION FOR VESTIBULAR LESIONS

The vestibular system is the only special sensory system in which unilateral loss of function can seriously threaten the long-term survival or well-being of an organism. In humans, injury to the central or peripheral system may result in considerable disability. Fortunately, most disease processes involving the vestibular labyrinth are self-limited, and spontaneous functional recovery can be expected. This is due to the remarkable ability of the central nervous system to recover after a labyrinthine injury, a process known as *vestibular compensation*. Failure to recover from a peripheral labyrinthine insult may be due to continued dysfunction in the vestibular end-organ itself or to failure of central vestibular compensation. Being alert to this critical distinction and its clinical implications is crucial for successful management of the dizzy patient. Excellent detailed discussions regarding vestibular compensation after unilateral peripheral lesions are available in the literature (Curthoys & Halmagyi 1995; Smith & Curthoys 1989).

Recovery From Acute Vestibular Lesions

The vestibular labyrinth transduces linear and angular acceleration of the head into afferent neural impulses that provide the brain with information necessary to maintain gaze stability and postural control during active movement of the head. The information from each peripheral system must be concordant with that from the other side in order for the system to function properly. In the setting of an acute disruption of labyrinthine or vestibular nerve activity, the vestibular nuclei will receive discordant information from the two peripheral organs, resulting in vertigo, nystagmus, and a host of undesirable vegetative symptoms such as nausea and vomiting. Some vestibular diseases, such as Ménière's disease, produce a transient electro-chemical or biomechanical disturbance of labyrinthine function resulting in a spell of vertigo that resolves once the disturbance has been rectified. In such cases, the resolution of symptoms results from a return to baseline peripheral vestibular function rather than from an adjustment in the central nervous system. Other types of vestibular injury such as vestibular neuritis, acute labyrinthitis, and labyrinthine injuries from otologic surgical complications or temporal bone fractures produce a significant disruption in the functional capacity of the vestibular periphery.

The response to a permanent vestibular lesion occurs through one or more of several potential recovery mechanisms. The goal is to achieve stability of gaze and postural control both under static and dynamic conditions by whatever means are available. One such mechanism is restitution of normal peripheral function, as might be seen after successful anti-inflammatory treatment of vestibular neuritis if there is no evidence for ongoing pathology. If this does not occur, the patient is dependent on the process of vestibular compensation. This process can be generally defined as changes which occur in the central nervous system following a vestibular lesion by which an optimal functional state is reestablished.

There are several important neurophysiologic dimensions contained within the overall concept of vestibular compensation. These include adaptation of input-output responses in both the vestibulo-ocular and vestibulo-spinal pathways, sensory substitution, or substitution of alternative motor responses. Using the vestibulo-ocular reflex as an example, there is

spontaneous nystagmus after acute unilateral loss of vestibular function because of the imbalance in inputs coming to the two vestibular nuclei. After a period of adaptation, the spontaneous nystagmus disappears. The individual is then free of vertigo when the head is still and is said to be "compensated" under static conditions. However, when the head is in motion, the alteration of the vestibular inputs in response to changes in head acceleration produce outputs in terms of eye movements that are inappropriate and destabilizing with reference to the visual environment. Thus we say that the patient is "uncompensated" with respect to the dynamic condition. The ability of patients to spontaneously compensate under dynamic conditions is quite variable. Adaptation may be excellent in some individuals, yet it is unusual to find those who have recovered from a significant vestibular injury with no vestiges of instability or disorientation under the most challenging head motion or balance tasks.

Habituation is another key feature in the process of compensation for peripheral injury. This neurophysiologic concept is best defined as a reduction in the pathologic response to a specific movement, brought about by repeated exposure to the provocative stimulus. It can be thought of as a subset of adaptation for responses to dynamic conditions. Habituation should be distinguished from fatigability, a transient phenomenon characterized by a slow decline of afferent neuronal impulses to a constant or repetitive stimulus. This distinction is best illustrated by the patient with benign paroxysmal positional vertigo in whom the response intensity declines when the Hallpike maneuver is repeated. This latter process is not felt to contribute to long-term habituation or compensation.

If there is complete bilateral loss of peripheral vestibular function, adaptation of the VOR is not possible and sensorimotor substitution is required. Animals seem to have a strong cervico-ocular reflex that manifests itself clearly in this setting, although this reflex seems to be less prominent in humans. Those with bilateral loss become highly dependent upon visual and proprioceptive inputs to maintain postural control. Gaze stability is compromised in this setting, leading to the symptom of oscillopsia during head movements that are at frequencies and speeds greater than the operational limits of the smooth pursuit system. These individuals may substitute alternative motor strategies for the VOR, such as the use of saccadic eye movements instead of slow phases or cognitive strategies in which gaze overshoot is prevented by preplanned volitional eye movements to accompany anticipated head movement.

Incomplete Compensation and Decompensation

It appears that the initial central compensation process is enhanced by head movement but delayed by inactivity. Thus, if the patient adopts an inactive life-style and avoids rapid head movements because of the unpleasant symptoms produced, the process of compensation may never be optimized. This phenomenon often accounts for those patients who have persistent motion provoked vertigo years after an otherwise uneventful recovery from a vestibular injury or ablative vestibular surgery. The effectiveness of vestibular compensation also appears to be hindered by preexisting or concurrent central vestibular dysfunction.

Although remarkably reliable overall, central vestibular compensation appears to be a somewhat fragile, energy-dependent process. Even after it is apparently complete, it is not uncommon to observe periods of symptomatic relapse due to decompensation. This may be triggered by a period of inactivity, extreme fatigue, change in medications, general anesthesia, or an intercurrent illness. A relapse of vestibular symptoms in this setting does not necessarily imply ongoing or progressive labyrinthine dysfunction, but often just a temporary lapse of vestibular compensation.

Adaptive Plasticity and Vestibular Compensation

The unique capacity of the central nervous system for adaptation to changes in the sensory environment is known as *adaptive plasticity*. Adaptive plasticity is a critical factor in the process of recovery from a permanent vestibular injury in that it permits the individual to adapt to the sensorimotor deficits produced by asymmetric peripheral vestibular afferent activity. The acute phase of vestibular compensation constitutes the initial response to a labyrinthine injury and occurs within the first 24 to 72 hours. This portion of the process results in correction of the static symptoms of unilateral vestibular injury, including intense vertigo, vomiting, and spontaneous nystagmus. The chronic phase of compensation accounts for correction of the dynamic symptoms of a vestibular injury, such as disequilibrium when walking and vertigo/disorientation during activities that require active head movement. In an otherwise healthy individual, this would be expected to take place over a 1–6 week interval.

Mechanisms of Vestibular Compensation

It is not known what specific factors trigger the process of vestibular compensation. The concept of error signals has been advanced to explain this phenomenon. These may include the simple loss of synaptic input from the VIIIth nerve to the vestibular nucleus, factors related to the degeneration of the nerve, and abnormal sensory inputs that result from the loss of peripheral function. For example, the physiologic stimulus for dynamic adaptation of the VOR appears to be *retinal slip*, the instability of the visual image on the retina during head motion. However, it seems that recovery from static asymmetry in the VOR (as measured by spontaneous nystagmus) does not depend on visual experience. This finding illustrates the important distinction between the properties of static and dynamic compensation. Beyond this, one must remember that after compensation occurs, the error signals are largely resolved. Therefore the mechanisms to maintain compensation are most likely different from those initially employed to achieve it. In fact, the compensated vestibular system appears to be somewhat fragile and susceptible to decompensation by fatigue, medication, and associated illness. The status of compensation also seems to be influenced by the level of arousal and input from the visual and somatosensory environment (Mathog & Peppard, 1982). There are several sensory inputs that seem to play a role in successful compensation for vestibular lesions. Visual input does expedite but is not essential for the elimination of spontaneous nystagmus. On the other hand, as mentioned above, compensation of dynamic gain deficits in the VOR is significantly impaired under circumstances of visual deprivation. Cervical inputs resulting from the static head tilt after labyrinthectomy in animal models seem to facilitate the recovery of static postural symptoms, since recovery can be delayed by restraint in the neutral head position. However, in humans with bilateral loss of labyrinthine function, the cervical-ocular reflex gain and latency are highly variable and the reflex probably contributes minimally to gaze stability.

Input from the remaining labyrinth probably has no influence on the maintenance of static compensation. A secondary contralateral labyrinthectomy performed after compensation from the first procedure produces static symptoms as profound as those that would be expected if there had been no prior deficit. This observation is known as *Bechterew's phenomenon* and suggests that resolution of spontaneous nystagmus and the other static symptoms after the initial labyrinthectomy is due to a restoration of tonic activity in the ipsilateral vestibular nucleus that is independent of input from the contralateral intact labyrinth or vestibular nucleus. In fact, the resting activity in the nucleus on the side of the original labyrinthectomy remains constant even if the vestibular commissure is transected. In addition, resting activity typically is restored in both vestibular nuclei after bilateral labyrinthectomy. On the other hand, commissural input from the intact labyrinth appears to be essential for dynamic compensation of gaze stability.

Neurochemical Changes

Despite the fact that the deafferented vestibular nucleus shows only a limited recovery of response to active head motion, lesions in this structure may prevent compensation or cause decompensation to occur. Thus, the regeneration of the resting activity in the ipsilateral nucleus seems to be essential to the establishment and maintenance of compensation. Little is known about how this resting activity so critical to the acute phase of compensation is restored. As there are no clear neurophysiologic influences from outside the nucleus or anatomic changes within the nucleus within the brief time course of behavioral recovery, neurochemical factors probably play a key role. Research in animal models has demonstrated that multiple pharmacologic preparations may influence vestibular compensation, including excitatory and inhibitory amino acids, cholinergic substances and their antagonists, adrenergic substances and other monoamines, polyamines, and neuropeptides. Denervation supersensitivity to neurotransmitters or changes in pre- or postsynaptic neuronal activity are most likely to provide the explanation for the restoration of an appropriate spontaneous firing rate in the ipsilateral vestibular nucleus. There may in fact be an automatic mechanism ubiquitous within the central nervous system that corrects for a prolonged reduction in tonic activity of a neuron, such that no mechanism unique to the vestibular system would be required. Thus, identification of general mechanisms underlying denervation supersensitivity may help to unlock our understanding of vestibular compensation (Smith & Darlington, 1991).

One substance with particular clinical relevance is the inhibitory amino acid gamma-amino-butyric acid (GABA). This compound mediates commissural input between the vestibular nuclei and inhibitory input to the vestibular nuclei from the cerebellar Purkinje cells. The administration of benzodiazepines such as diazepam (Valium®) acts to potentiate the action of GABA. Diazepam administration has been shown to decrease tonic activity in vestibular neurons and to decrease the response of these neurons to rotational stimuli in the cat (Sekitani, Ryu, & McCabe, 1971). Thus some authors have suggested that administration of diazepam should retard compensation (Schaefer

& Meyer, 1981). Animal data has not always supported this concept. An early study in cats showed no delay in return of medial vestibular nucleus activity with diazepam use after labyrinthectomy (Bernstein, McCabe, & Ryu, 1974). The authors (Berstein et al., 1974) also noted some behavioral benefits in the treated group and suggested that this may have resulted from elimination of the devastating symptoms of acute vestibular loss, leading to earlier locomotion and head motion, promoting compensation. Peppard (1986) also noted in cat experiments that while the antihistamine dimenhydrinate (Dramamine®) delayed VOR compensation, diazepam had little effect. A study utilizing squirrel monkeys documented an increase in early disequilibrium along with the expected reduction of nystagmus intensity in response to diazepam (Ishikawa & Igarashi, 1984). However, the study found no apparent differences in physiologic parameters at three weeks post-labyrinthectomy and documented a fairly dramatic benefit in the diazepam treated group as measured by time required for return to baseline performance on a locomotor balance task.

SUMMARY

The acute phase of vestibular compensation results in the elimination of static symptoms such as intense persistent vertigo, spontaneous nystagmus, and ataxia due to disruption of postural control. This process occurs rapidly in mammals, usually within three days. It seems to depend primarily upon a resetting of tonic activity in the ipsilateral vestibular nucleus. Although the cerebellum was previously thought to be essential in this process, more recent research has called this idea into question. The process

seems also to be independent of transcommissural input from the contralateral vestibular nucleus. The time course of the recovery from static symptoms is too fast to invoke mechanisms involving reactive synaptogenesis. Most likely there are critical neurochemical changes, including but perhaps not limited to denervation supersensitivity, that mediate a return of neural activity on the injured side.

The chronic phase of vestibular compensation after a unilateral vestibular lesion accounts for the elimination or reduction of symptoms caused by disturbances in the dynamic aspects of gaze stability and postural control. These include bursts of vertigo associated with rapid motion of the head, positional vertigo persisting after initial recovery from a vestibular lesion, and disequilibrium during ambulation or more challenging locomotor tasks. This process is less reliable than static compensation, and the time course is considerably more variable. Multiple sensory inputs contribute to this process, and there is a critical need for intact input from the remaining contralateral labyrinth and vestibular nucleus. Adaptive plasticity in the central nervous system plays a large role in dynamic compensation, and the trigger for the plasticity seems to be error messages generated by the sensory asymmetries produced by conflicting inputs generated by head movement. There is evidence for modification of neural activity in several areas of the brain stem and cerebellum that appears to assist the development of dynamic compensation, as well as to support its maintenance. Administration of pharmacological agents or endogenously occurring neurotransmitters may retard or enhance compensation, and some have also been demonstrated to produce decompensation in previously recovered animals.

3

▪ THE NEUROTOLOGIC HISTORY AND PHYSICAL EXAMINATION

THE NEUROTOLOGIC HISTORY

A complete clinical history is probably the single most important portion of the diagnostic evaluation of the balance disorder patient. The differentiation between the various peripheral vestibular disorders is particularly dependent on historical information and the conclusions that the physician draws from the interview. Most vestibular disorders cannot be distinguished from one another simply by vestibular testing or other diagnostic interventions. Failure to properly discriminate these disorders on historical grounds may be the source of considerable ongoing distress for the patient, and may lead to improper management by the physician. Because subsequent treatment decisions will be based on the clinical diagnosis, it is particularly appropriate to spend additional time during the history to clarify important features. In addition, balance function study results are best interpreted in light of a proper clinical history.

Importance of the Chief Complaint

The main reason that the patient is seeking medical attention for his or her balance distur-

bance should be identified. Although little specific diagnostic information may be gained, it is often helpful to hear an account of the patient's perception of his or her illness prior to pursuing more specific questions. One can often gain a sense for how much functional disability the vestibular symptoms have produced. The psychosocial impact of the illness may also become clear in the patient's initial comments. Sometimes patients will volunteer that their symptoms are trivial or have resolved completely, but they simply want to make sure that they have not suffered a stroke or developed a brain tumor. If the patient is not permitted to share this information freely, important aspects of the individual's care may be overlooked.

Using the History to Establish the Diagnosis

Once the patient has shared the main concerns raised by his or her condition, the first specific questions should be phrased to gain information regarding the initial onset of symptoms. The characteristics and intensity of the balance disturbance at that time provide useful insight for the differential diagnosis. If the patient can recount specifics surrounding the symptom onset such as date and time of day, along with the activity interrupted by intense vertigo, the physician can be reasonably certain that the patient has suffered a significant peripheral labyrinthine insult. Surprisingly, if the physician does not specifically inquire, patients who are preoccupied with recent symptoms and disability may neglect to report a very profound vestibular crisis that occurred initially. If the onset was more insidious, and the patient is unable to provide any account of an initial event, an acute peripheral disorder is less likely. Other important issues to discuss at this stage of the interview include the association of physical trauma, barotrauma, or an intercurrent illness prior to the onset of vertigo. Patients should also be asked about previous remote episodes of vertigo.

It is very important to question the patient regarding the association of a hearing loss or other auditory symptoms with the onset of vertigo. A complete audiometric assessment should be performed early in the evaluation. The presence of an associated sensorineural hearing loss, whether stable, progressive, or fluctuating, is the single strongest incriminating factor in identifying a pathologic labyrinth (Shone, Kemink, & Telian, 1991). The presence of other otologic symptoms such as aural fullness and tinnitus may also be helpful in lateralization. Head trauma associated with disequilibrium and fluctuating sensorineural hearing loss may suggest an oval or round window fistula. A history of previous otologic surgery or familial hearing loss is also important.

Differential Diagnosis of Vertigo: Historical Features

The clinical history is also central in determining the best specific clinical diagnosis in the dizzy patient. This section reviews features of each important vertigo syndrome that are critical in differential diagnosis. Detailed descriptions of the specific clinical entities discussed here, along with discussions of less common disorders that may cause vertigo, are available in standard reference materials (Baloh & Harker, 1993; Kveton, 1994; Schessel & Nedzelski, 1993).

Vestibular Neuritis

This diagnosis is characterized by an acute vestibular crisis followed by gradual improvement. The acute crisis involves severe vertigo that may last several hours up to 3 days. At times the initial vertigo may not be quite as intense or protracted. The key features that distinguish this diagnosis are the characteristic time course, absence of associated auditory symptoms, persistence of the vertigo even when motionless, and failure to return rapidly to normal. Gradual improvement and complete recovery is anticipated. Sometimes central nervous system compensation for this lesion may be incomplete, and mild positional or motion-provoked vertigo may persist for many years.

Viral Endolymphatic Labyrinthitis

This condition produces an acute vestibular crisis with a history similar to vestibular neuritis. However, the vertigo is accompanied by a sudden loss of hearing usually within a few hours before or after the onset of vertigo. The recovery period should be similar to that seen in vestibular neuritis. The hearing loss may recover or persist.

Benign Paroxysmal Positional Vertigo

This diagnosis is suggested when the patient describes vertigo that is primarily provoked by head motion or particular body positions, and further history does not reveal an extended vestibular crisis at onset. Even if the symptoms were very intense and frightening, they do not persist more than 30 seconds, and they resolve if the patient remains motionless. Often patients will report that they were able to press forward with their usual activities even on the first day of symptoms. Such behavior would be unexpected in a patient suffering from vestibular neuritis or labyrinthitis.

Ménière's Disease

If the patient experiences recurrent, spontaneous spells of intense vertigo lasting several hours and accompanied by hearing loss, tinnitus, and aural fullness, Ménière's disease is suspected. This condition causes intermittent periods of labyrinthine dysfunction, with most patients reporting normal balance between spells. The cause of this disease is unknown, although hereditary factors may play a role. In most cases studied histopathologically, this disease has been associated with the presence of endolymphatic hydrops, suggesting that inner ear fluid dynamics are altered. This finding has led to the introduction of several medical and surgical interventions that are unique to Ménière's disease.

Delayed Onset Vertigo Syndrome

This diagnosis is made when episodic vestibular symptoms, similar to those in Ménière's disease, develop months or years after a sensorineural hearing loss of any cause. For example, this condition may develop after a congenital hearing loss, an idiopathic sudden or progressive loss, or following a "dead ear" complicating a stapedectomy, even if vertigo was absent or negligible at the onset of the hearing loss. Some authors feel that this syndrome is a variant of Ménière's disease, with endolymphatic hydrops developing as a sequela of prior otologic pathology. Thus, this syndrome is sometimes called *delayed endolymphatic hydrops*. The diagnosis is confirmed by documenting the hearing loss and making certain that there is no evidence for dysfunction in the normal ear. Rarely, the vertigo develops from changes in the previously normal ear. In such cases the diagnosis is "delayed contralateral endolymphatic hydrops."

Labyrinthine Complications of Otitis Media

This diagnosis is established by an association with documented acute or chronic suppurative otitis media. Toxic labyrinthitis (sometimes called *serous* labyrinthitis) is diagnosed when acute or chronic otitis media is complicated by vestibular dysfunction without a significant associated sensorineural hearing loss. Suppurative labyrinthitis, a rare but more serious bacterial infection of the labyrinth that may result from otitis media, is diagnosed when there is an acute vestibular crisis accompanied by a profound sensorineural hearing loss and fever. Patients with cholesteatoma may develop a labyrinthine fistula from erosion of the otic capsule, usually the dome of the horizontal semicircular canal. This typically results in intermittent vertigo, and should be suspected whenever a patient with cholesteatoma reports dizziness of any kind. Some patients with a labyrinthine fistula from cholesteatoma can elicit vertigo by pressing their finger into the ear canal.

Perilymph Fistula

If an abnormal communication exists between the inner and middle ear, allowing the loss of perilymph, dizziness and/or hearing loss may result. This diagnosis must be suspected when inner ear symptoms follow trauma, barotrauma, stapes surgery, or an event requiring significant straining, such as weight lifting or childbirth. Most otologists do not entertain this diagnosis unless such a history precedes the onset of symptoms. The possibility that perilymph fistula can develop spontaneously without a significant injury is controversial (Shea 1992). This condition will remain a diagnostic puzzle until a reliable standard for the intraoperative confirmation of a fistula is available, allowing the development and validation of preoperative diagnostic predictors.

Acoustic Neuroma

These benign tumors arise from the Schwann cells lining the axons of the cochleovestibular nerve. In light of their cell of origin, as well as the fact that they almost always arise from the vestibular portion of the nerve, it has been suggested that a more appropriate name is *vestibular schwannoma*. Generally, these tumors cause hearing loss or tinnitus without vestibular symptoms. If balance symptoms occur, they tend to be mild and intermittent. Acoustic neuromas rarely cause acute vestibular crises, but they may produce syndromes that mimic many other vestibular diagnoses. Thus, acoustic neuroma and other tumors of the cerebellopontine angle should always be suspected when evaluating patients with vestibular complaints.

Vertebrobasilar Vascular Insufficiency

The vertebrobasilar system provides arterial blood flow to the essential structures of the vestibular system, including the inner ear, VIIIth nerve, brain stem, and cerebellum. This system originates from the right and left vertebral arteries that arise in the neck, travel through the transverse processes of the cervical vertebrae, and enter the skull at the foramen magnum. They give off branches to the brain stem and cerebellum before merging into the single basilar artery, located ventral to the brain stem. The anterior inferior cerebellar artery arises from the basilar artery and provides blood flow to the labyrinth, along with a portion of the brain stem and cerebellum. Given the structures supplied by these vessels, it is not surprising that reduced blood flow in the vertebrobasilar system may cause vertigo. Transient symptoms may accompany generalized arterial hypotension from any cause, including cardiac arrhythmias and orthostatic hypotension. Although most significant hemorrhagic or thrombotic vascular accidents involving the posterior fossa circulation are fatal or neurologically devastating, milder events may produce more subtle findings. They are usually accompanied by abnormalities on the neurologic exam other than vertigo and nystagmus, such as diplopia, ataxia, dysarthria, and dysphagia. In such cases, urgent radiographic imaging is appropriate. Some patients with diabetes mellitus or atherosclerosis have balance complaints and may be discovered to have multiple small ischemic areas in the brain stem. Others may have intermittent vertebrobasilar insufficiency associated with postural changes, certain head positions, or exercise. Rarely, the subclavian steal syndrome results in insufficient posterior fossa perfusion when the arm is exercised. This condition arises when there is an obstruction in the circulation to the left arm proximal to the site where the vertebral artery arises. The increased demand for blood flow in the arm during exercise results in retrograde (backward) flow through the left vertebral artery, literally stealing blood that was intended for the brain and inner ear.

Demyelinating Disease

Vertigo or dizziness is an initial symptom in 5 to 15 % of patients with multiple sclerosis. Nearly 50% of patients with this disease become vertiginous at some time during the course of the illness. Vertigo may be transient or permanent and is usually accompanied by nystagmus. If a patient with dizziness reports additional focal neurological signs that are separated in time and anatomic location, a demyelinating disease must be considered. Although the diagnosis is primarily clinical, vestibular testing, cerebrospinal fluid studies, magnetic resonance imaging, and various evoked potential studies are helpful in confirmation.

Epilepsy

Temporal lobe seizures may be heralded by a vertiginous aura. Loss of consciousness usually follows, although motor or sensory phenomena sometimes develop without altered consciousness. Electroencephalography and various brain imaging studies establish the diagnosis.

Migraine

Patients with migraine sometimes develop vertigo as an aura prior to a classic migraine headache (Harker, 1994; Harker & Rassekh, 1988;). The diagnosis in these cases is generally straightforward. However, other patients present with spells of episodic vertigo without subsequent headache, obscuring this diagnosis. In these cases, the spells are similar in duration and intensity to those in Ménière's disease, yet without associated hearing loss, tinnitus, or aural fullness. A personal or family history of classic migraine may help suggest this etiology. Typically, all diagnostic tests of inner ear function are normal, as are radiographic findings. An early stage of endolymphatic hydrops selectively affecting the vestibular portion of the inner ear could be an alternative explanation in such cases.

Using the Clinical History to Guide Treatment Decisions

Most patients with acute vertigo will improve with supportive, expectant management. When this is not the case, they may present for evaluation after several months or years of dizziness. The patient should be asked to describe the progression of symptoms over time, along with the nature and duration of typical spells. Specifically, one wishes to know if the spells are continuous or occur in discrete episodes. If the symptoms are episodic, it is extremely important to distinguish whether they are spontaneous or motion-provoked. If the symptoms are brief and predictably produced by head movements or body position changes, the patient most likely has a stable vestibular lesion, but has not yet completed central nervous system compensation. Those who describe these symptoms sometimes also note a chronic underlying sense of disequilibrium or light-headedness. The chronic symptoms may be quite troublesome, but any intense vertigo should be primarily motion-provoked. These patients are suitable candidates for vestibular rehabilitation, to be described in a later chapter. For now, it is simply important to point out that historical information is essential in deciding who might benefit from rehabilitation therapy.

If the episodic spells described by the patient are longer periods of intense vertigo that occur spontaneously and without warning, this is probably progressive or unstable peripheral dysfunction. One must also suspect a progressive labyrinthine lesion if the vertigo is accompanied by fluctuating or progressive sensorineural hearing loss. Such patients are managed with medical therapy, and if this fails, they constitute the best candidates for surgical intervention. Such patients are not candidates for vestibular rehabilitation, except as an adjunctive postoperative modality.

Additional history regarding current or prior use of medications should be elicited. Many patients are under the mistaken impression that vestibular suppressants will prevent spells of vertigo and take them habitually. When additional spells intervene, the physician sometimes prescribes additional medication. Because oversedation from these centrally acting drugs may retard central nervous system compensation for vestibular lesions, one should consider tapering or discontinuing these medications whenever possible. Medications that must be continued should be directed toward particular symptoms that specifically interfere with the patient's recovery process. A rational plan of use should be outlined with the patient in order to avoid psychological or physiologic dependency.

Other psychosocial aspects can be important in understanding the patient's situation. Some offices ask new patients with dizziness to complete a self-administered questionnaire to elicit historical information of a delicate nature that may be difficult to obtain in a face-to-face interview. Complicating features of anxiety, depression, or excessive dependence on psychotropic medications should be identified. It is desirable to understand the degree of functional disability produced by the patients' vestibular complaints, especially with respect to their professional and favorite social activities. The stability and commitment of their psychological support system should also be evaluated. Some individuals are more distressed by the lack of empathy and understanding from family or co-workers than by the symptoms themselves. Patients who are actively pursuing litigation or disability compensation payments may be disinclined to pursue potentially curative treatment, such as vestibular surgery or a vestibular rehabilitation program.

Classification of Chronic Vestibular Symptoms

The importance of distinguishing the nature of a chronic vestibular complaint can be illustrated by considering the following example: A patient with unilateral deafness seeks medical attention complaining of disabling vertigo. A careful clinical history regarding the onset of his symptoms suggests a severe viral labyrinthitis 2 years ago, involving a previously normal ear. He reports experiencing a sudden profound sensorineural hearing loss during a viral illness, with the simultaneous onset of incapacitating vertigo lasting 2 days. Imaging studies were negative. Now the patient is seeking medical attention because of severe vertigo and associated inability to perform his occupational duties. Two very different situations, distinguishable only by the clinical history, may result in such a complaint. The patient may note that although the intense vertigo resolved within 2 days, any rapid head motion since that time has been associated with a brief but intense burst of vertigo lasting up to 10 seconds, preventing his work with heavy manufacturing equipment. This suggests an uncompensated labyrinthitis, best treated with vestibular rehabilitation and weaning from long-term vestibular suppressants. On the other hand, the patient might report a satisfactory recovery from the initial vertigo, resulting in a symptom-free interval for several months. Then he began to experience intense spells of spontaneous vertigo that last for 30 minutes to 2 hours, requiring him to be removed from the workplace twice a week. This suggests a delayed endolymphatic hydrops resulting from the prior labyrinthitis, a syndrome that should be treated quite differently. If medical therapy with salt restriction and diuretics was ineffective, a labyrinthectomy would almost certainly relieve his symptoms. In the first scenario, a labyrinthectomy is not only unnecessary, but is unlikely to be successful.

Even when an exact diagnosis cannot be established, it is helpful to attempt to classify the nature of the dizziness in such a way that a rational therapeutic approach can be selected. The authors find the following nondiagnostic categories helpful in guiding therapeutic decisions:

Uncompensated Peripheral Lesions

Any of the peripheral vestibular conditions listed earlier may lead to chronic complaints if the central nervous system does not make appropriate adjustments during the compensation stage. If the history suggests uncompensated vestibular function following resolution of a recognized acute clinical syndrome, this is the preferred diagnosis. These patients are best treated with vestibular rehabilitation.

Decompensated Peripheral Lesions

Central vestibular system decompensation may occur even after satisfactory initial compensation during periods of immobility, illness or fatigue. Sometimes decompensation may occur for no apparent reason. Such episodes of decompensation may produce a significant relapse in symptoms and must be distinguished

from progressive or episodic peripheral dysfunction. Vestibular rehabilitation should be reinstituted for these patients. Surgical intervention will generally not benefit those who suffer from occasional decompensation.

Intermittent Peripheral Dysfunction

Patients with Ménière's disease or delayed onset vertigo syndrome will describe periods of intense vertigo. These debilitating spells are followed by a return to perfectly or nearly normal balance function. This is strong evidence for intermittent dysfunction, and these syndromes are treated with symptomatic medical management or surgery. Some patients with migraine equivalents may report symptoms that mimic this category of inner ear disorders. The diagnosis of migraine should be considered when no historical features or test results emerge to document inner ear dysfunction.

Progressive Labyrinthine Dysfunction

Many patients with Ménière's disease will go on to develop a permanent hearing loss and chronic vestibular complaints due to progressive damage to labyrinthine structures. Certain other progressive conditions, such as syphilitic labyrinthitis or Cogan's syndrome, may produce similar patterns. If available, specific medical therapy directed toward the cause of the labyrinthine problem is indicated initially. Once the lesion has stabilized, vestibular rehabilitation may play a role. If the condition is unilateral and the ear cannot be stabilized, surgery may be appropriate.

Mixed Central and Peripheral Dysfunction

Patients who suffer from nonspecific vestibular complaints, especially after head injury, are sometimes found to have evidence for both central and peripheral dysfunction. This group is very difficult to treat due to diagnostic confusion involving issues such as perilymph fistula, poor central nervous system compensation, associated cognitive problems, and the frequent association of crippling chronic headaches and reactive depression. Furthermore, it is not unusual to find that litigation or a disability compensation claim is pending in head injury cases. Such unresolved issues may prevent the elucidation of an accurate history, and may interfere with the patient's incentive for recovery.

Multifactorial Disequilibrium of Aging

The combination of an aging vestibular system, failing vision, and musculoskeletal degeneration can lead to significant disturbances of balance function, as discussed in Chapter 2. Although it may be unsatisfying to inform such patients that there is no specific cure for their symptoms, the clinician must recognize that their functional capacity often can be meaningfully improved with a properly designed program of vestibular rehabilitation.

Pure Central Disorders

Even when serious intracranial pathology has been ruled out by radiographic imaging studies, the history and test results may suggest a central cause for vestibular symptoms. In such cases, referral for a complete neurological evaluation is appropriate. Once this has been completed, vestibular rehabilitation may be appropriate provided that the condition is not progressive in nature.

Psychiatric Disorders

There is a strong tendency toward vestibular complaints among those who suffer from panic disorder and related anxiety disorders such as agoraphobia (Jacob 1988). The exact explanation for this relationship is uncertain. Presumably there is a neurobiologic basis for these symptoms, perhaps at the level of the pontine reticular formation. Sometimes the patient has difficulty distinguishing the dizziness from the anxiety attacks since they occur together. In fact, they probably comprise a positive feedback cycle, resulting in escalating symptoms. In addition, dizziness may be a nonspecific complaint that complicates clinical depression. Fail-

ure to recognize and treat these psychiatric problems can lead to considerable wastefulness in the health care system, along with unnecessary delay in proper treatment and frustration for the patient.

THE NEUROTOLOGIC PHYSICAL EXAMINATION

Otologic Examination

The physical examination of the vestibular disorder patient should begin with a careful otoscopic examination. This may reveal acute otitis media, chronic suppurative otitis media with or without cholesteatoma, or evidence of previous otologic surgery. Mass lesions of the temporal bone are rare, but may cause vestibular complaints. Vertigo or nystagmus with pneumatic otoscopy is suggestive of fistulization of the inner ear, syphilis, or Ménière's disease. In the vast majority of dizzy patients, the otoscopic examination is normal.

Cranial Nerve Examination

A complete head and neck examination including assessment of cranial nerve function should be performed. Hypesthesia (reduced sensation) of the external auditory canal skin (Hitselberger's sign) or an absent corneal reflex may be signs of an acoustic neuroma. Facial nerve paralysis in association with acute vestibular complaints suggests an infection, such as herpes zoster oticus, or an intrinsic lesion of the temporal bone. Facial paralysis is very unusual in cases of acoustic neuroma prior to surgical removal. Skull base lesions may disrupt inner ear function along with any of the cranial nerves of the jugular foramen.

Neurotologic Examination for Vestibular Disorders

A fairly comprehensive neurologic exam is appropriate when evaluating patients with vestibular complaints. The clinician will naturally focus on specific neurotologic findings such as nystagmus, but other neurologic properties essential to balance such as cerebellar function and distal lower extremity strength and proprioception also should be assessed.

When describing observed spontaneous or positional nystagmus, its characteristics including type, direction of the fast component, and presence or absence of fixation suppression should be noted. Nystagmus produced by peripheral vestibular lesions is generally horizontal or rotary jerk nystagmus, with a slow component mediated by the vestibulo-ocular reflex and a fast compensatory component. The direction of the nystagmus may assist in the identification of the abnormal ear. As most vestibular lesions are paretic in nature, they produce a nystagmus with the fast phase beating away from the involved ear. Pure vertical or pure rotary nystagmus is almost certainly produced by pathology within the central nervous system.

Office Tests of Balance System Function

A variety of test procedures may be used in the office setting to assess the balance disorder patient. These, like the laboratory studies to be discussed in Chapters 4–7, assist in the identification of the extent and site of the lesion. These straightforward clinical tests are essentially variations of the related laboratory studies but have less ability to quantify the outcomes. The theoretical basis behind many of these tests are well founded in the physiological considerations discussed in Chapters 1 and 2. Due to the subjective nature of these tools, the validity and

reliability of these tests are reduced compared to the formal laboratory studies. Unfortunately, little clinical research exists to define the sensitivity/specificity and test reliability for these procedures. The interested reader is referred to work by Baloh and Honrubia (1990), Leigh and Zee (1991), Shumway-Cook and Horak (1986), and Halmagyi and Curthoys (1988).

The remainder of this chapter will be devoted to the office studies that have been found to be most reliable and valid for evaluating extent and site-of-lesion when compared to formal laboratory studies of balance function. It is important to stress that this comparison is not from controlled clinical research, but only based upon anectodal experience. Where data on performance characteristics of the tests is available, it will be discussed. When selecting clinical tests to be performed in the office evaluation of the balance disorder patient, it is useful to organize them according to the components of the balance system that they evaluate. Tables 3–1, 3–2, and 3–3 provide this type of organization. Certain oculomotor, vestibulo-spinal and postural control tests, together with other routine tests of neurological function (finger to nose, finger to finger, pronator drift, and rapid alternating movements of hands and/or feet), provide evidence for motor system abnormalities identified in Table 3–4. As information emerges from the neurotologic history and routine office test results, other studies that are not routinely performed may be used to further evaluate a specific potential abnormality.

Ocular Range-of-Motion/Gaze Stability

Simple oculomotor function is examined by having the patients gaze at an object about

---

TABLE 3–1. Office Tests of Ocular Motor Function/Gaze and Spontaneous Nystagmus

- ◼ Ocular Range-of-Motion/Gaze Stability
- ◼ Monocular Eye Cover (Latent Nystagmus)
- ◼ Spontaneous Nystagmus
  - ◾ Frenzel Lenses
  - ◾ Ophthalmoscope
- ◼ Horizontal and Vertical Pursuit Tracking
- ◼ Reactionary & Volitional Horizontal and Vertical Saccades
- ◼ Optokinetic Nystagmus

TABLE 3–2. Office Tests for Vestibulo-Ocular Reflex Function

- Oscillopsia Test
  - Passive Head Rotation
  - Ophthalmoscope
  - Snellen Chart
- Halmagyi Head Thrust
- Head-Shaking Nystagmus
- Nystagmus Provoked During Pneumatic Otoscopy
- Rapid Positioning: Hallpike Maneuver
- Positional Nystagmus—Frenzel Lenses
- Post-Rotary Nystagmus Decay Time Constant—Frenzel Lenses
- Minimal Ice-Water Calorics—Frenzel Lenses

TABLE 3–3. Office Tests of Vestibulo-Spinal Reflex and Postural Control Function

- Musculoskeletal Assessment
  - Ankle, Knee, and Hip Joint Range-of-Motion
  - Ankle, Knee, and Hip Joint Stength
  - Sensation in the Distal Lower Limbs
  - Deep-Tendon Reflexes
- Past-Pointing
- Romberg
- Tandem (Sharpened) Romberg
- Modified Clinical Test for Sensory Interaction of Balance
- Fukuda Stepping Test
- Casual Gait—With and Without Reciprocal Horizontal Head Movements

TABLE 3–4. Motor Control System Abnormalities

Pyramidal	Extrapyramidal	Cerebellar
Spasticity	Rigidity	Hyptonia
Clasp Knife	Cogwheel/Leadpipe	Intention Tremor
Poor Fine Motor	Dysrhythmia	Dysmetria
+ Clonus	Dysdiadochokinesis	Ataxic Gait
+ Babinski	Bradykinesia	
Hyperreflexia	Shuffle Gait	
Spastic Gait		
Pronator Drift		

18 inches from their nose and follow the object with eye movements only. It is best to slowly direct the movement laterally by 35–40 degrees, vertically by 30–35 degrees, and to each of the upper and lower right and left quadrants by 25–30 degrees off the sagittal plane. If conjugate eye movement is not observed, or if monocular or binocular motion is restricted, this finding needs to be investigated for a possible historical explanation. If an explanation is not available, this finding should be followed with appropriate diagnostic testing. The restricted and/or disconjugate eye movement must be accounted for when interpreting other office and laboratory studies that rely upon eye movements. A pause in the motion of the object in the primary and each eccentric end point for a minimum of 15–20 seconds allows for visualization of any gaze-evoked nystagmus (formerly known as "gaze paretic nystagmus," Leigh & Zee, 1991). Physiologic end-point nystagmus is often present and can be differentiated from

gaze-evoked nystagmus since it does not persist beyond a few seconds. If persistent gaze-evoked nystagmus is noted in any position, all of the gaze positions should be repeated with a longer pause to assure the examiner that episodic nystagmus in other positions of gaze has not been missed. An example of this would be in Periodic Alternating Nystagmus (PAN) where nystagmus may be present for several minutes and then absent for an equal period of time (Leigh and Zee, 1991). In addition, primary position, right and left lateral, up center, up right, and up left positions should be evaluated with Frenzel lenses. These are 20-diopter lenses with lighting on the patient's side (Figure 3–1) that help to remove the ability of the patients to fixate on an object and suppress their nystagmus. When using the Frenzel lenses, the patient is simply asked to move his or her eyes in the desired directions without a visual target. When the patient is viewing in the primary position with the lenses in place, this constitutes investigation for *spontaneous nystagmus*. For a discussion of the use of the ophthalmoscope to investigate

spontaneous nystagmus and gaze-evoked nystagmus, the interested reader is referred to Leigh & Zee (1991). The characteristics of the nystagmus with and without visual fixation are used to differentiate gaze-evoked nystagmus of peripheral vestibular origin from centrally generated gaze-evoked nystagmus. There are situations, such as a mass lesion in the cerebellar pontine angle that can present with characteristics of both peripheral and central gaze evoked nystagmus. The criteria for making the distinction between central and peripheral gaze evoked nystagmus are the same as for the laboratory version of this test, and are as follows (Barber & Stockwell, 1980; Daroff, Troost, & Dell-Osso, 1978; Leigh & Zee, 1991; Stockwell, 1983):

1. If of central origin, nystagmus does not typically appear in the primary position and the nystagmus beat may change direction with different eye positions with fixation.
2. If of central origin, the magnitude of the nystagmus remains the same or decreases when visual fixation is removed.

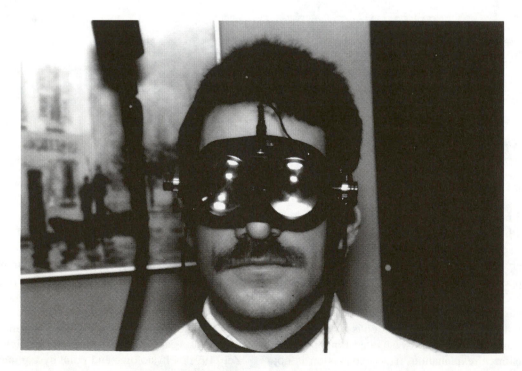

FIGURE 3–1. Frenzel lenses.

3. If of central origin, the slow component velocity of the nystagmus (the compensatory eye movement component to the nystagmus, see Chapter 1) shows a slowing behavior for each beat as the eye moves back toward the primary position; see Figure 3–2A.

4. If of peripheral origin, the nystagmus may increase in magnitude and/or become evident in additional positions of gaze when visual fixation is removed.

5. If of peripheral origin, nystagmus can appear in any of the positions, but is typically direc-

tion-fixed (i.e., always beating in the same direction).

6. If of peripheral origin, the slow-component velocity is typically linear in nature, maintaining a constant velocity as the eye moves back toward the primary position (see Figure 3–2B).

Horizontal and Vertical Pursuit Tracking

During the process of evaluating gaze stability and ocular range-of-motion, pursuit tracking ability should be evaluated. The viewing object

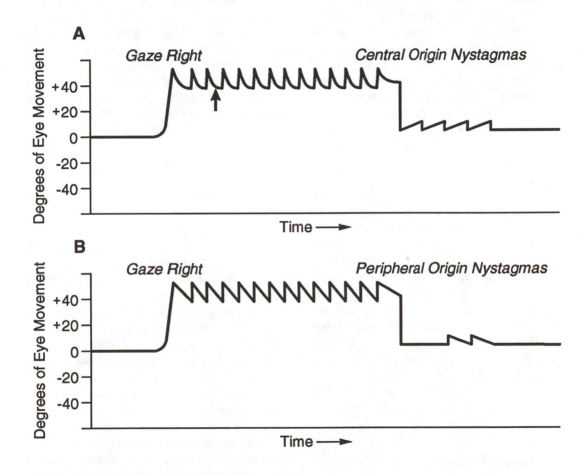

FIGURE 3–2. Plots of horizontal eye position in degrees (positive eyes moving rightward, negative eyes moving leftward) as a function of time. The drawings represent conjugate eye movements. **A.** Right beating gaze-evoked nystagmus of central origin stimulated by gazing 40° to the right. The arrow shows the reduction in speed of the slow-component portion of the nystagmus. As the eyes return to the center position, left beating rebound nystagmus is noted. **B.** Right beating gaze-evoked nystagmus of peripheral origin stimulated by gazing to the right by 40°. As the eyes return to the center position, reduced amplitude of ongoing right beating nystagmus is noted. This is not rebound nystagmus.

used (usually a light or the examiner's finger) is oscillated at a slow pace (less than 0.5 Hz) over a horizontal or vertical excursion of 25–30 degrees to either side of primary position. For the horizontal movements, anything other than a smooth eye movement pursuing the target suggests a central oculomotor control system abnormality, most likely pathology involving the vestibulo-cerebellum. Typically, vertical movements will not be as smooth as horizontal, even in the normal individual. An important pathologic finding that may become evident when evaluating vertical pursuit is the appearance of uncontrolled, repeated horizontal movements of the eyes superimposed upon a disturbance in the smooth tracking of the target. This finding is known as *saccadic intrusions*, and reinforces the suggestion of central oculomotor control involvement. Smooth pursuit, as discussed earlier, is highly sensitive to patient age. The movement of the target must be kept quite slow if elderly patients are expected to display smooth eye movements.

Monocular Eye Cover

With the subject viewing an object at least 18 inches away, cover one eye while observing the other for a vertical adjustment. Then perform the same test covering the other eye. Subtle skew deviation is detected if the uncovered eye adjusts vertically when the other eye is covered. Skew deviation indicates dysfunction in the otolithic input from the peripheral end-organ or in the brain stem's interpretation of the otolith input. This is a part of the ocular tilt reaction that may result from either peripheral or central dysfunction (Dieterich & Brandt, 1994; Halmagyi et al., 1990; Halmagyi, Curthoys, Brandt, & Dieterich, 1991; Halmagyi, Gresty, & Gibson, 1978).

Volitional Horizontal and Vertical Saccades

The patient is instructed to stare at the examiner's nose while the examiner holds up a finger to the right or left of the nose at a point that would require a 30–35 degree eye movement to view the finger. The subject is instructed to look back and forth between the finger and nose on command, constituting a volitional saccade task. The eyes should deviate in a conjugate manner with crisp movements, and stop on the target without repeatedly falling short or passing beyond the target. Apparent slowing and/or dysmetria of the saccade can suggest a lesion in the brain stem or cerebellar region (see Chapter 5). Dysconjugate slowing of the eye that is adducting (moving toward the nose) is suggestive of internuclear ophthalmoplegia. When this finding is confirmed for adduction of both eyes, a diagnosis of multiple sclerosis is strongly suggested. Subtle slowing of vertical or horizontal saccades can be recognized by using a diagonal target pattern. One finger is held approximately 20 degrees to the right and up with the other 20 degrees to the left and down. The patient looks repeatedly between the two fingers. If the saccade speeds are relatively similar (as expected), the eyes will move in a diagonal pattern. However, slowing of the horizontal component leads to alternating vertical then horizontal saccades as the eyes proceed from one target to the next. If the vertical saccade is slowed the movements would be horizontal first then vertical.

Oscillopsia Test

PASSIVE HEAD ROTATION. The patient is instructed to stare at a distant target while the examiner rotates the head in a smooth manner, horizontally through a 20–30 degree arc. The frequency of rotation is initially low (< 0.5 Hz) and gradually increased to 1–2 Hz. If the vestibulo-ocular reflex gain of at least one labyrinth is normal, the eyes will remain stationary in space with the head moving around them. If there is a bilateral peripheral vestibular weakness, the eyes will show repeated saccadic corrections as the subject seeks to maintain visual fixation on the target. When repeated saccadic behavior is noted the patients will typically report that their target is no longer stationary.

SNELLEN CHART. An alternative way to quantify oscillopsia is called the *Dynamic Visual Acuity Test*. The patient is instructed to identify the lowest line on the Snellen eye chart that is possible to read without errors. Then they attempt to repeat reading the chart while their head is being passively rotated in the horizontal plane at 1–2 Hz. Results in our laboratory for 150 consecutive balance disorder patients demonstrate that a mean change of 1 line is expected when there is normal bilateral VOR gain. The variance in this study shows that a change of 3 lines is slightly greater than 2 standard deviations from the mean. Thus, oscillopsia is clinically documented if visual acuity deteriorates with head motion to the degree that the patient can only resolve letters that are 3 or more lines higher on the Snellen chart.

Halmagyi Head Thrust

This test of unilateral vestibulo-ocular reflex gain was introduced by Halmagyi and Curthoys (1988). Their paper provides an excellent description of test administration and the data indicating test validity. Briefly, the patient views a distant object and the examiner suddenly rotates the head to the right or the left through a small arc at a rapid rate. Then the head is rotated in the opposite direction. If the VOR gain is relatively normal on the side the movement is directed toward, the eyes typically remain fixed in space. However, if repeated saccadic corrections of the eye (directed opposite to the head movement) are needed to return to the target, reduced VOR gain on that side is suggested. This test differs from the oscillopsia test in that it is using discrete, sudden head movements in a single direction. This stresses one end-organ at a time, provided the head movement is rapid.

Head Shake Nystagmus

The patients are asked to actively shake their head, as if to say "no!" in a vigorous manner for 15–20 seconds. After they stop, the examiner immediately views their eyes with Frenzel lenses. If nystagmus is observed, and there was no spontaneous nystagmus prior to head shaking, an otherwise statically compensated peripheral lesion has become evident. The nystagmus generated in this fashion is typically brief and will usually beat nystagmus away from the injured side, assuming a paretic lesion. Many times, a brief reversal of the initial nystagmus with beats in the opposite direction may be noted. This test illustrates the utility of Ewald's second law (Ewald, 1892). This law describes the asymmetry in excitational versus inhibitory activity in the semicircular canal system. The reversal of the nystagmus is thought to be an example of short-term central nervous system adaptation (Leigh & Zee, 1991). Sensitivity and specificity of this test has been reported by Jacobson, Newman, and Safadi, (1990). They found performance to be poor for mild to moderate losses of peripheral vestibular system function as measured by bithermal caloric irrigations (senstivity = 27% and specificity = 85%). A thorough discussion of the technique and alternative hypotheses for interpretation are found in other literature (Hain, Fetter, & Zee, 1987; Stockwell & Bojrab, 1993a, 1993b).

Nystagmus Provoked During Pneumatic Otoscopy

While performing pneumatic otoscopic examination, with a good hermetic seal, the examiner asks the patient to visualize a stationary, distant target. As movement of the tympanic membrane is produced by varying pressure in the external auditory canal, the patient is asked to report if movement of the visual target is perceived. If this is a repeatable observation, it suggests the possibility of abnormal coupling between the external canal and the labyrinth (Hennebert's sign, Schuknecht, 1974). While the etiology of such abnormal coupling may vary, a positive test may help to lateralize the pathology to the right or left peripheral system.

Post-Rotary Nystagmus Decay Time Constant

Using a smoothly rotating swivel chair, the patient is gently spun at a constant velocity of 180–200°/sec (approximately 2 sec per revolution) for 8–10 full revolutions, while wearing Frenzel lenses or with the eyes closed. The head must be maintained in the horizontal plane. After the completion of the turns, the chair is brought to a sudden stop. The patients need to be warned that they may experience the strongest sensation of circular movement after the stop. The post-rotary nystagmus is then monitored (using Frenzel glasses) for the length of time required for the nystagmus to cease. This time period approximates the post-rotary time constant (see Chapter 6), typically expected to be greater than 12 seconds. If a shorter value is documented, peripheral vestibular system pathology on the side opposite the direction of rotation is suggested. This would be the labyrinth stimulated by the sudden deceleration from a constant velocity rotation. The test is then repeated in the opposite direction.

Rapid Positioning: The Hallpike Maneuver

This test is a well-known office procedure used primarily to elicit evidence for Benign Paroxysmal Positional Vertigo (BPPV). While the nystagmus produced by BPPV is the most common positive result induced by this maneuver, it is not the only one. Discussions of the various responses, and the therories behind BPPV are provided in several sources (Baloh and Honrubia, 1990; Baloh, Honrubia, & Jacobson, 1987; Brandt & Steddin, 1993; Jacobson, Newman, & Kartush, 1993). The major characteristics of a classic Hallpike response for BPPV are given in Table 3–5. The method of performing the evaluation is given in Figure 3–3. Two important aspects of the technique are: (a) the head should be turned to the 45 degrees off the sagittal plane and the eyes observed for nystagmus prior to any downward movement, to rule out any confounding results from neck torsion; and (b) the head should be held securely with both hands, with the patient using the examiner's arm for support during the movement. Moving the patient by the shoulders may cause a neck injury. Since humans have poor fixation suppresion ability for torsional nystagmus (Leigh & Zee, 1991), this test can be done in a lighted environment without fear of suppressing the response. Frenzel lenses may be used to assist the examiner in viewing the patient's eye movements, but are not mandatory.

This maneuver is also typically part of the standard electronystagmography (ENG) protocol. However, since the test is administered identically in both settings, it will be discussed here. The only alteration used in the ENG is the documentation of evoked eye movements with various recording techniques. If, however, the technique is not one of direct, binocular eye movement recording (such as infrared video or scleral coil techniques), the results of the recording should not be used to interpret the response. Classically, positive Hallpike responses produce a torsional nystagmus with the fast phase directed toward the dependent (underneath) ear. When conventional electrooculography (EOG) techniques are used to record this type of eye movement, the torsional component cannot be detected and only the linear components will be evident. The linear component of the fast phase eye movements associated with a classical Hallpike response are paradoxically directed opposite from that of the torsional movements reported by an examiner visualizing the patient's eyes. For example, a right classical Hallpike response would show counterclockwise torsional nystagmus, the fast component of the nystagmus beating toward the

---

TABLE 3–5. Major Characterstics of Benign Paroxysmal Positional Vertigo

■ Latency to onset of symptoms (nystagmus)—1 to10 seconds after the movement

■ Duration of symptoms (nystagmus)—Less than 1 minute

■ Type of nystagmus—Linear/rotary beating toward the underneath ear by direct observation

■ Following up movement, may see a reversal of nystagmus direction and repeat of symptoms

■ Symptoms and nystagmus are fatigable with a single or multiple repeats

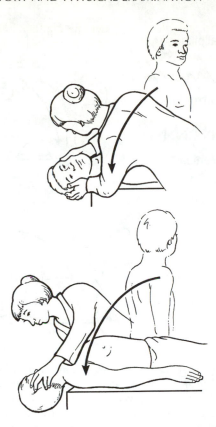

FIGURE 3–3. Illustrations of the technique for the Hallpike manuever, for right side (top) and left side (bottom). Note the patient's eyes are open and fixating on the examiner.

right ear. Yet the recordings for the classical right Hallpike response, as shown in Figure 3–4, show left beating horizontal and up-beating vertical nystagmus. The explanation for this apparent dichotomy comes from understanding the actions of the agonist/antagonist muscle pairs that generate the eye movements (superior and inferior obliques ipsilaterally, and inferior and superior rectus for the contralateral eye). This concept is thoroughly described in the work by Baloh et al. (1987). Thus, it is essential that the Hallpike maneuver be performed as part of the clinical examination, with direct visual observation of the evoked eye movements, rather than deferring this examination to only the recordings made during the ENG battery. The test should also be performed during the ENG battery, since the fatigability (over repeated manuevers) can cause it to be present sometimes and not others, but it should be done with di-

rect visualization by the examiner. Recognition of this feature of EOG recording in a patient with a positive Hallpike response can also be important in the interpretation of other aspects of positional nystagmus, discussed in the next chapter.

As indicated in Table 3–5, the classic Hallpike response includes both symptoms of vertigo and the nystagmus response. It may be useful to recognize that some patients experience vertigo without nystagmus, with the classic latency period, crescendo-decrescendo pattern, and fatigability of response with repeat of movement. When symptoms with these appropriate characteristics are observed without nystagmus, it may be labelled as a *subjectively positive* Hallpike maneuver. If both nystagmus and symptoms are noted, the term *objectively positive* Hallpike maneuver is used. Although primarily descriptive, these terms both imply a

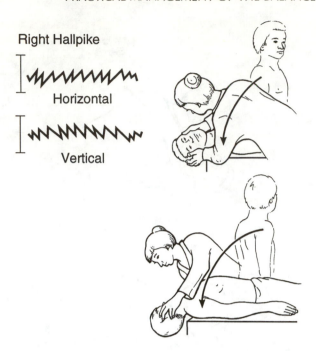

FIGURE 3–4. Repeat of Figure 3–3, illustrating the nystagmus that would be recorded by standard electro-oculographic techniques using electrodes at the lateral canthi of each eye and electrodes above and below the right eye. The horizontal trace shows position of the eye as a function of time (upward movement of the trace implies rightward eye movement). Left beating nystagmus is shown. The vertical trace shows position of the eye as a function of time (upward movement of the trace implies upward movement of the eye). Up beating nystagmus is shown.

diagnosis of Benign Paroxysmal Positional Vertigo and help to describe the relative intensity of the disorder. The distinction is also important from the standpoint of treatment, since the particle repositioning maneuvers depend on the presence of nystagmus to monitor the progression of the treatment procedure. The particle repositioning maneuvers will be discussed in Chapter 10.

Positional Nystagmus

The patient is placed slowly into the supine, head right and head left positions and eye movements are observed with Frenzel lenses. The corresponding right and/or left lateral decubitis positions need to be evaluated to investigate the influence of neck torsion on nystagmus production if nystagmus is noted only in the head right or left positions. The finding of

spontaneous or positional nystagmus in the absence of any central vestibulo-ocular or oculomotor abnormalities suggests peripheral vestibular system disease. Interpretations of ageotropic direction-changing positional nystagmus, especially if transient, must be made with caution if positive unilateral or bilateral Hallpike responses were noted (see Positional Nystagmus in Chapter 4).

Minimal Ice-Water Calorics

The patient is placed with the head and shoulders elevated approximately 30 degrees from the supine position. Each ear is alternately irrigated with 2 cc of cold tap water (approximately 10–20°C). The water is infused over 1–2 seconds and left in the canal for approximately 8 seconds. The eyes are then opened and eye movements observed with Frenzel lenses for qualitative assessment of nystagmus velocity and the direction of the fast phase of the nystagmus beat. The responses from each ear are compared for evidence of possible unilateral weakness.

Past-Pointing

The patient uses outstretched arms with index fingers extended. The examiner has the patients bring their index fingers into contact with the hands of the examiner. The patient then raises their arms above their head and back down to touch the examiner's hands. This maneuver is repeated 2–3 times with the eyes open and then several additional times with the eyes closed. A drift of *both* arms together to the right or the left is taken as an indication of peripheral system involvement. Theoretically, if an uncompensated peripheral lesion is present, the patients' perception of movement as the eyes are closed leads to a compensatory adjustment of their arm motion in the opposite direction, so they will not miss the examiner's hands. In most cases, the bilateral arm drift would be toward the weaker of the two labyrinths, although the pathology may be in the opposite ear if a lesion with an irritative status is present. Classic examples of irritative peripheral lesions are seen with Ménière's disease, where the nystagmus may be beating toward the ear with the disease. In that situation, the diseased ear may present as the one most active (the "stronger"), and the arm drift would most likely be to the opposite, nondiseased ear.

Fukuda Stepping Test

This test proposed by Fukuda (1959) is a variation on the Tretversuch Test (stepping test) of Unterberger (1938) and the Waltzing Test of Hirsch (1940). It is based on the same theoretical considerations as the past-pointing test and was designed to help identify the weaker labyrinth. The patient is asked to march in place with his or her eyes closed. The examiner remains behind the subject, both for protection of the unstable patient and to prevent localization to the examiner's voice. Fifty steps are typically used and the amount of rotation to the

right or the left during the stepping maneuver is estimated. The original work by Fukuda suggested that a rotation greater than 30 degrees implied asymmetrical labyrinthine function, with the patient rotating toward the weaker labyrinth. As with the past-pointing test, this may not be the lesion side if an irritative lesion is present. A large clinical review in a population of subjects with chronic balance disorders was conducted to evaluate the performance of this test when administered after head-shaking. A sensitivity of 50% and specificity of 60% were obtained with a criterion for a positive test being a rotation of 60 degrees or more. A positive result is used to document asymmetrical labyrinthine function, independent of the direction of the turn, but will not always properly identify the weaker side (Shepard, Shepard, & Boismier, 1994).

Modified Clinical Test for Sensory Interaction of Balance (CTSIB)

This test was originally described by Horak and Shumway-Cook (1986). In the form suggested here, the patients' ability to maintain quiet volitional stance is evaluated as they sequentially stand on:

1. A flat firm surface with eyes open
2. A flat firm surface with eyes closed
3. A compressible surface with eyes open and
4. A compressible surface with eyes closed.

The test progressively reduces the sensory input systems available to the patient for maintaining quiet stance. By the fourth condition, only the vestibular system is available to provide accurate cues as to the body's position and movement. This evaluation does not provide for specific site-of-lesion information, but can document which sensory input cues are most important for the patient's postural control, thereby suggesting the sensory system that is most likely to be dysfunctional. Information regarding functional compensation with respect to stance also is obtained. This information can help to decide whether balance retraining should be part of the treatment plan. This test is very similar to the sensory organization protocol of dynamic posturography (EquiTest). A double-blind controlled study investigating customized versus generic vestibular rehabilitation programs also compared this office test to dynamic posturography (El-Kashlan, Shepard, Asher, Smith-Wheelock, & Telian, 1996). The overall result indicated that major patterns of abnormality (see Chapter 7), implying the patient's difficulty using vestibular system information (vestibular dysfunction pattern), and normals were well identified by either test. Statistically significant differences were noted and attributed to the inability of the CTSIB to recognize more subtle abnormalities, or to mislabel as vestibular dysfunction, patterns of abnormality that involved difficulties on conditions using accurate visual or somatosensory system cues. A similar comparison of a modified CTSIB and the sensory organization test from EquiTest is reported by Weber and Cass (1993). They also report very high correlation and high sensitivity and specificity (95 and 90%, respectively) for the modified CTSIB with EquiTest as the gold stan-

dard. These results are consistent with that reported above. They did not look at performance in the detail of the patterns developed from EquiTest.

Although these and other office tests are not designed to replace the quantitative results from balance laboratory studies, they can provide a reasonable first impression of the site and extent of pathology within the balance system, as well as an estimate of the compensation status. This information can then be integrated with the clinical history to decide what further diagnostic evaluations or therapeutic measures may be appropriate. For example, clinicians often are asked to evaluate patients with vertigo who have already had a negative magnetic resonance imaging study of the head. If the history suggests a prior viral vestibular neuritis with residual motion-provoked symptoms, and the clinical examination strongly suggests a left peripheral weakness that is partially compensated, formal balance testing may not be needed to secure the diagnosis or choose the proper treatment.

4

■ ELECTRONYSTAGMOGRAPHY EVALUATION

LABORATORY EVALUATION

The purpose of balance function studies encompasses three major goals. The most traditional goal is site-of-lesion localization, seeking to determine which sensory input elements, motor output elements, or neural pathways may be responsible for the reported symptoms. Such testing also may help estimate the extent of the lesion. Localizing the lesion site (peripheral versus central vestibular pathology, dysfunction in motor output systems, etc.) assists in shaping recommendations for further medical or surgical referrals to assist with the evaluation and management of the patient. Extent and site-of-lesion studies also may help confirm the suspected diagnosis, and in cases of bilateral peripheral vestibular system paresis, it will directly influence the rehabilitative management program for the patient. It is critical to realize that the extent of a peripheral, central, or mixed lesion does not correlate directly to the extent of functional disability experienced by the patient (Beynon & Shepard, 1996; Gavie, Shepard, Goldner, & Niham, 1994). The major reason for this confusing paradox relates to the issue of compensation, already discussed in Chapter 2. When patients are counseled regarding results of laboratory studies examining the extent and site-of-lesion, it is important that this be made clear. Informing

patients who are unable to accomplish routine daily activties that their peripheral system lesion is minimal could lead to significant confusion and inappropriate assumptions concerning the functional and psychological status by the patient, the family, and sometimes by the professional. Recent work on the relation between extent and site-of-lesion tests and the patient's perceived difficulties using the Dizziness Handicap Inventory (DHI) indicates a very poor association (Beynon & Shepard, 1996; Gavie et al., 1994; Jacobson & Newman, 1990; Jacobson, Newman, Hunter, & Balzer, 1991). Further, it appears that the DHI is strongly associated with functional performance and has some predictive power regarding performance of tasks that measure functional capacity, such as walking with and without head movement; rising from a chair or bed; and ascending and descending stairs (Gavie et al., 1994).

The second purpose of laboratory studies of balance system function is the assessment of the patient's functional ability to use the system inputs in an integrated fashion with appropriate coordinated outputs. This is best achieved through testing of postural control, static and dynamic (discussed in Chapter 7). This aspect of testing is quite important since it provides the strongest correlation with functional disability. The patients' perception of their own disability as measured through the DHI also was found to be significantly associated with laboratory studies of postural control (Beynon & Shepard, 1996; Gavie et al., 1994; Jacobson et al., 1991).

The third assessment goal is to determine whether the patient may be an appropriate candidate for a vestibular rehabilitation program. As will be discussed in Chapter 10, the principle features that lead to a recommendation for a vestibular rehabilitation program are the subjective characteristics of the patient's symptoms. The typical symptom complex along with laboratory evidence for a stable, uncompensated vestibular lesion constitute the most common indication for a therapy referral. A wide variety of studies are used to assess the balance system in the broadest sense. Although the use of newer, more expensive technology has led to a better understanding and assessment of the balance system, the principles of these studies can be accomplished, if only qualitatively, even if these units are unavailable (Chapter 3, Office Tests). With a sufficient understanding of the basic physiology of the normal balance system, the assessment of balance function can be accomplished even by laboratories of limited size and financial capability.

A complete neuro-otologic history remains the single most important component in the diagnostic evaluation of the balance disorder patient. Any balance function study results must be interpreted in light of the presenting symptoms and prior medical history. This chapter and the following three will discuss the major components of what is called Basic Balance Function Testing. This evaluation includes electronystagmography, comprehensive ocular-motor evaluation, rotational chair testing, and postural control assessment. For each of these areas the reader is referred to the text by Jacobson, Newman, and Kartush (1993) for details of performing these various tests and basic interpretations. This text will focus on correlating the interpretation of results with the historical information available from the patient to help the clinician make proper clinical judgments. Special situations that are more complex will be discussed to help the reader avoid certain pitfalls in routine activities related to the interpretation of balance testing results.

ELECTRONYSTAGMOGRAPHY

Traditional electronystagmography (ENG), using electro-oculography for eye movement recordings, is a process that provides a means of indirectly estimating eye movements (for discussion of the placement of the electrodes the reader is referred to Barber & Stockwell, 1980). The estimates are reliable whether recorded with eyes open or closed, and in a darkened or well-lighted environment. Changes in eye position are indicated by the polarity of the corneal-retinal potential relative to each electrode placed near the eye (Barber & Stockwell, 1980). Since the vestibular apparatus contributes significantly to the control of eye movements, these movements may be exploited to examine the activity of the peripheral vestibular end organs and their central vestibulo-ocular pathways. Historically, ENG became synonymous with vestibular function evaluation, and now is viewed only as a subset of a more complete test battery. The ENG typically consists of a series of subtests performed with eye movement recordings to assess the function of the vestibular end-organs, the central vestibulo-ocular pathways, and ocular-motor processes, independent of vestibular input. These specific tests of central pathway function will be taken up separately in Chapter 5. In addition to the Jacobson et al. text (1993) and the original ENG text by Barber and Stockwell (1980), the interested reader is referred to other references discussing specific issues related to ENG testing and interpretation (Baloh & Honrubia, 1990; Barber & Sharpe, 1988; Stockwell, 1983).

ENG is useful for all patients with balance disorders. Spontaneous, unprovoked eye movements with eyes closed (spontaneous nystagmus) and eye movements provoked by changes in the orientation of the vestibular end-organs relative to gravity (positional nystagmus) are recorded. The slow-component velocity of the nystagmus is the measurement of interest, as it reflects the portion of the nystagmus that is generated by the vestibulo-ocular reflex. The archaic term *slow-phase* has been abandoned because the novice may confuse this measurement with phase measurements on rotational chair testing. Rapid positioning of the subject into specific head positions (Hallpike maneuvers) are performed to provide evidence for one specific condition—Benign Paroxysmal Positional Vertigo. A measure of the relative responsiveness of one horizontal semicircular canal to the other is typically accomplished through thermal caloric irrigations. The irrigations can be performed by open or closed-loop water irrigation in the external auditory canal or through airflow. The purpose of the irrigations is to produce sequential changes in the temperature of the endolymph within each horizontal canal. This causes asymmetric central vestibular activity resulting in nystagmus mediated by the vestibulo-ocular reflex (explanations for temperature effects are provided in the text referenced above and will not be repeated in this discussion). Quantification of the eye movement recordings resulting from each irrigation are compared to evaluate the relative sensitivity of the peripheral end organ, recognizing that one is predominantly measuring responses generated in the horizontal semicircular canal and superior vestibular nerve. One must note that because of potentially differential effects of pathological processes, the horizontal canal may not be fully representative of the status of the vertical canals. In addition, an apparent weakness on one side could be from labyrinthine, VIIIth cranial nerve, or vestibular nuclei origin. In spite of these limitations and the potential of evoking severe vertigo and emesis, this test remains the only currently available method to selectively determine unilateral vestibular responsiveness. Major variations in the traditional methods for caloric stimulation (not to be discussed in this text) have been proposed that provide for simultaneous stimulation of both external canals (Brookler, 1976, 1990; Furman, Wall, & Kamerer, 1988) or the use of fixed temperatures with increasing length of irrigation time (Kumar 1981; Kumar, Mafee, & Torak, 1982; Torak, 1973).

Let us now consider each of the subtests that comprise the ENG, other than those related to ocular-motor function to be discussed in Chapter 5. The various subtests should always be interpreted in light of the ocular-motor results, as these will often influence the diagnostic impression. Therefore, since we have elected to defer the ocular-motor discussion to Chapter 5, general results (normal vs. abnormal and suspected site-of-lesion) from ocular-motor findings will be used here to assist in the interpretation of the other ENG subtests.

The order in which the ENG subtests are performed has several important constraints that facilitate an accurate and valid study. A typical order is given in Table 4–1. It is suggested that ocular-motor testing be performed first, while the patient is fresh and vertigo has not been provoked by positional changes or caloric irrigations. A salient feature of a positive Hallpike maneuver is its fatigability. Therefore, the Hallpike maneuvers are performed prior to positional testing to avoid fatiguing the response. Because calorics are the most provocative with possible vertigo and nausea, they are best placed at the end of the testing. Another important consideration is the arrangement of the ENG testing facility. Continuous visualization of the patient and the recording device together is important for test accuracy, as well as for patient safety and comfort. An example of the suggested arrangement is shown in Figure 4–1. The room should be set so that the examiner can simultaneously visualize the recording screen or strip chart recorder, the patient, and any visual stimulus in use. This allows the examiner to assess compliance with instructions, while attending to the recording, watching for abnormalities or artifacts that occur.

Spontaneous Nystagmus

This test is performed with the patient sitting, head straight and eyes closed. The purpose is to record eye movements when visual fixation is removed, without any provocative head movements or positions. Jerk nystagmus is the princi-

TABLE 4–1. Order of Electronystagmography Subtests

1. Ocular-Motor Evaluation

2. Rapid Positioning Tests (Hallpike Maneuver)

3. Positional Tests

4. Calorics

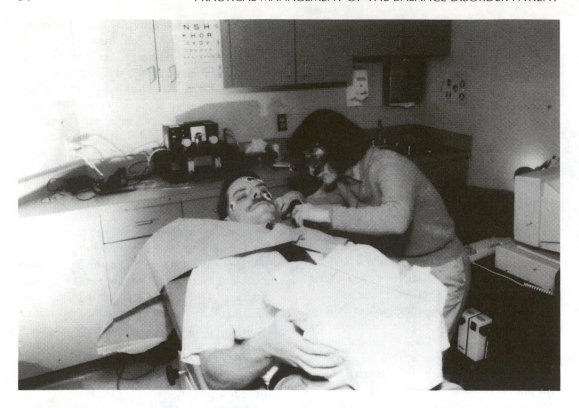

FIGURE 4–1. Electronystamography room arrangement. Caloric irrigation is being illustrated.

ple abnormality of interest in most situations. Other forms of abnormal eye movements, such as pendular nystagmus, may be seen. The interested reader is referred to Leigh and Zee (1991) for a complete review of eye movement abnormalities. In our facility, spontaneous jerk nystagmus is considered abnormal if (a) The slow-component eye velocity is equal to or greater than 6°/sec; (b) if the slow-component eye velocity is 5°/sec or less and clinically significant positional nystagmus is present (Table 4–2); or, (c) the nystagmus changes direction during recording, independent of the magnitude of the slow-component eye velocity (discussions of calculations of slow-component velocity are given in Barber & Stockwell, 1980, and Jacobson et al., 1993).

Clinically significant, direction-fixed nystagmus is interpreted to indicate pathology within the peripheral vestibular system if the extended ocular motor evaluation (see Chapter 5) is normal. In this setting, the presence of clinically significant spontaneous nystagmus, whether direction-fixed or direction-changing, implies

incomplete static compensation (Table 4–3) for a presumed peripheral lesion. This is due to incomplete tonic rebalancing (see discussion in Chapter 2) at the level of the vestibular nuclei in response to asymmetrical peripheral input. When calorics responses prove to be normal, the direction of the nystagmus can be used to suggest either a paretic lesion in the ear opposite to the direction of the fast component or an irritative lesion in the ear on the side of the direction of the fast component. When calorics are abnormal, suggesting a unilateral vestibular weakness, the direction of the nystagmus will imply either a purely paretic lesion or, on rare occasion, the paradoxical paretic labyrinthine lesion with an irritative status. This phenomenon will be discussed with caloric test interpretation.

Hallpike Maneuver

This test was covered completely in Chapter 3, with eye movement examples. No further

TABLE 4–2. Criteria for Clinical Significance: Spontaneous and Positional Nystagmus

■ Slow-component eye velocity (SCv) > 5°/sec
■ SCv < 6°/sec—persistent nystagmus in 4 or more of the 8–11 positions
■ SCv < 6°/sec—sporadic in all positions tested
■ Direction-changing within a given head position

TABLE 4–3. Classification of Peripheral Vestibular System Compensation by Test Results

■ Physiologic Compensation (relative to eye movements)
  ■ Statically Compensated—No clinically significant spontaneous or positional nystagmus
  ■ Dynamically Compensated—No clinically significant directional preponderance from calorics or clinically significant asymmetry by rotary chair
■ Functional Compensation (relative maintenance of quiet volitional stance)
  No clinically significant abnormalities on the sensory organization protocol of dynamic posturography

discussion is needed here, except to remind the reader that a significantly positive Hallpike result, unilaterally or bilaterally, can have an impact on the interpretation of positional nystagmus but should not alter the interpretation of spontaneous nystagmus.

Positional Nystagmus

A complete description of how this test is performed is given elsewhere (Barber & Stockwell, 1980; Jacobson et al., 1993). Briefly, the patient is moved slowly into stationary positions. The eye movements are monitored as in spontaneous nystagmus testing, and should be done with eyes closed. Given the testing done with ocular-motor evaluation (see Chapter 5), the positions do not need to be tested with eyes opened. The more common positions include sitting, head turned right; sitting, head turned left; supine; supine, head turned left; supine, head turned right; right decubitus (right side); left decubitus (left side); and pre-irrigation position (head and shoulders elevated by 30 degrees up from the horizontal plane). In cases where no cervical region injuries or active pathologies are reported, use of head hanging (neck hyperextended) straight, right, and left add three additional positions for testing prior to pre-irrigation position. The purpose of this subtest is to investigate the effect of different head positions within the gravitational field. This is done with eyes

closed, and typically there is no need to repeat this with the eyes open. Positional nystagmus is typically classified by the direction of the fast component of the nystagmus (see Table 4–4). It may be either direction-fixed (always right-beating or always left-beating when present) or direction-changing (both right- and left-beating nystagmus observed during the exam). Direction-changing nystagmus may be subclassified, when appropriate, into geotropic (toward the pull of gravity, toward the underneath ear) or ageotropic (away from the pull of gravity, away from the underneath ear). While ageotropic direction-changing positional nystagmus has been suggested to increase the possibility of a central vestibular system lesion site (i.e., central to the VIIIth cranial nerve), no definitive studies indicate that this association is reliable. A classic example of ageotropic positional nystagmus is that seen secondary to alcohol ingestion. This can cause geotropic positional nystagmus during the first 3–5 hours post ingestion and change to ageotropic for time after 5 hours. This is referred to as Positional Alcohol Nystagmus (PAN I and PAN II). Thus, the clinical interpretation of direction-changing nystagmus may proceed in the same manner as that for direction-fixed. The exception to this situation is when the direction-changing nystagmus is observed while the patient remains in one head position, that is, without a change in gravitational orientation. This is typically interpreted as strongly indicative of central pathway involvement, independent of the ocular motor results, unless an alternative explanation is apparent (discussed below).

Sometimes patients will show perpetuation of their spontaneous nystagmus throughout the positional testing. This is suspected when nystagmus seen with the spontaneous nystagmus test is also present without change, in all positions tested. This should not be interpreted as pathological positional nystagmus. When one observes positional nystagmus that is not simply a continuation of spontaneous activity, one possible explanation involves the interaction between the otolithic organs and the semicircular canals. As the canals are not sensitive to changes in gravitational orientation, nystagmus may result from stimulation of the otolithic organs that in turn influence the neural activity of the semicircular canal inputs (predominantly from the horizontal canal) in the velocity storage integrator within the brain stem (see Chapters 1 and 2). Alternatively, pathological changes in the semicircular canals may cause one or more of them to be sensitive to changes in gravitational orientation by a change in the specific gravity of either endolymph or the cupula. Although these explanations for positional nystagmus primarily involve the labyrinth, an insult to the vestibular portion of the VIIIth nerve also may participate in the generation of such findings. The interpreter must always be alert to the possibility that the interaction of neural activity from the otolithic organs and the semicircular canals may be abnormal secondary to lesions in the brain stem. These may produce positional nystagmus identical to that seen with pure labyrinthine lesions. This concept is not new, given the general understanding that positional nystagmus is a nonlocalizing result. Our approach, as for the interpretation of spontaneous nystagmus, is to place the burden of identification of a central vestibulo-ocular or ocular-motor lesion site on thorough ocular-motor evaluation. If no other concomitant indicators for inner ear pathology, such as tinnitus, aural fullness, fluctuant or rapid loss of auditory sensitivity, are evident, one may safely assume that positional nystagmus is an indicator of peripheral vestibular sys-

tem involvement whenever ocular-motor testing is normal or explained by the patient's age. As with spontaneous nystagmus, the direction of the positional nystagmus may help identify the side of inner ear pathology. The following is an example of such a patient.

CASE 20

A 71-year-old male notes sudden onset of vertigo during 30 years following a motor vehicle accident. There were infrequent spells of vertigo with nausea, lasting several hours at a time, occurring every 1–2 years since the accident. He recently experienced a significant increase in the intensity and frequency 2 months prior to evaluation. He now reports monthly spontaneous spells lasting several hours, along with daily spells of motion-provoked vertigo lasting up to 1 minute caused by head movements. He had constant bilateral tinnitus and aural fullness and complained of fluctuant hearing on the left. Formal audiometrics indicated bilateral, symmetric, high-frequency sensorineural hearing loss with excellent speech discrimination. Test results for the ENG and ocular-motor evaluation were as follows:

ENG: Spontaneous and positional right-beating nystagmus (Figure 4–2) was seen in 6 of 11 positions, ranging from 2–6°/sec. All other findings were normal.

Ocular motor: Normal or explainable by effects of age.

Based on these results, together with the patient's presenting history and symptoms, this ENG would be interpreted to indicate peripheral vestibular system pathology, most likely of labyrinthine origin. Because of the direction-fixed nature of the right-beating nystagmus, the findings would suggest either a left paretic or right irritative lesion. These results should not be interpreted as nonlocalizing, given the normal information from ocular-motor testing. A summary of the approach toward interpretation of positional nystagmus, taking into account history, symptoms, and ocular-motor results, is seen in Table 4–4.

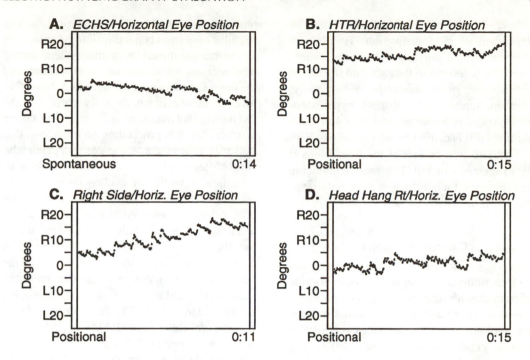

FIGURE 4–2. **A–D** plot horizontal eye position in degrees as a function of time, each showing right beating nystagmus. The time in the lower right corner of each panel is the total elapse time in seconds for that recording, not the total time shown. Each panel represents 7 seconds of tracing. **A.** ECHS—eyes closed head straight. **B.** HTR—eyes closed head turned right, sitting position. **C.** Eyes closed, laying on the right side (right dicubitus position). **D.** Eyes closed, hyperextension of the neck (by approximately 30°) with the head turned to the right.

TABLE 4–4. Positional Nystagmus

■ Direction Fixed—Associated with normal ocular motor findings and history implying peripheral lesion, interpreted as indicating labyrinthine or VIIIth nerve involvement.
■ Direction-Changing
   ■ Geotropic or Ageotropic—Associated with normal ocular motor findings and history implying peripheral lesion, interpreted as indicating labyrinthine or VIIIth nerve involvement. (Anecdotally, ageotropic is the more likely of the two to be associated with a central system lesion site.)
   ■ Direction-Changing Within a Given Head Position—Unless an alternative explanation can be supported (such as effects of benign paroxysmal positional vertigo), this is interpreted to indicate possible central system involvement, most probably brain stem/cerebellar lesion site. Rule out of periodic alternating nystagmus is needed when nystagmus changes direction unrelated in a regular manner to gravitational orientation.

Neck Torsion

Cervical vertigo or nystagmus can be caused by neck torsion. Although infrequently positive in our experience, testing for positional nystagmus can be modified to support or contradict the suspicion of this diagnosis. This is best done by demonstrating consistent positional nystagmus that is direction-fixed for a specific neck torsion condition, regardless of the orientation of the head relative to gravity, with elimination of nystagmus whenever the head is straight relative to the torso. If the problem is due to mechanical compression causing vascular compromise, or from soft tissue injury, it should be independent of head orientation. To evaluate this phenomenon, our protocol has the patient perform neck torsion to the right and the left in three different orientations relative to gravity: sitting up, supine, and with neck hyperextension. Nystagmus has to be present in 4 of the 6 conditions if it is caused by neck torsion to both the right and left, or in 3 of the 3 positions if only to the right or left. It is most convincing when the neck torsion trials are the only positions that provoke nystagmus.

Caloric Irrigations

Descriptions of proper technique for the traditional caloric test paradigms and guidance for routine interpretation are reviewed in standard textbooks (Barber & Stockwell, 1980; Jacobson et al., 1993; Stockwell, 1983). For other less well-known paradigms including bithermal, simultaneous calorics and monothermal calorics with changing irrigation times, the reader is referred elsewhere (Brookler, 1976, 1990; Furman, Wall, & Kamerer, 1988; Kumar 1981; Kumar et al., 1982; Torok, 1973). Our discussion will concentrate on the bithermal, alternating irrigation paradigm and special issues of test administration and interpretation.

The caloric test is the study that is most likely to lateralize a peripheral lesion with objective, repeatable eye movement data. The stimulus employed is nonphysiologic compared to the normal function of the system during head motion, where one side is stimulated and the other is simultaneously inhibited. Nevertheless, the caloric test is the only portion of the test battery that measures unilateral labyrinthine function. Work is proceeding on other tests that also may help evaluate one ear independently. One of these uses acceleration stimuli with recording of vestibular evoked potentials, and another uses a nonphysiologic galvanic stimulation. Additional work continues on assessment of otolith function in balance disorder patients for site and side-of-lesion investigations. A complete discussion of these areas is beyond the intended scope of this text and the interested reader is referred to other sources (Elidan et al., 1991; Elidan, Langhofer, & Honrubia, 1987; Furman & Baloh, 1992; Moore, Hoffman, Beykirch, Honrubia, & Baloh, 1991).

The three primary delivery methods for caloric irrigations are illustrated in Figure 4–3. All are reasonably reliable when the tympanic membrane is intact. When a tympanic perforation or short ventilation tubes are present, the closed loop water irrigation method is preferable. Air calorics in the setting of a tympanic membrane defect may produce paradoxical nystagmus, confusing the interpretation. This is discussed and illustrated by Stockwell (1983). Briefly, blowing air across a moist surface such

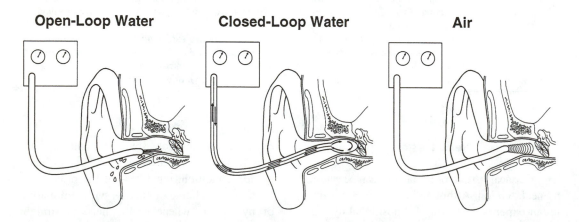

Open-Loop Water   **Closed-Loop Water**   **Air**

FIGURE 4–3. Three techniques for caloric irrigations.

as the middle ear mucosa creates a cooling effect. This may occur even if the air is warm. In general, the most effective medium for reliable temperature transfer is a liquid rather than a gas, although water calorics may be more cumbersome to administer. The examiner needs to be aware that suggested temperatures and length of irrigation time vary depending on the method selected in order to provide for an adequate stimulation. Our routine settings are given in Table 4–5. Suggestions for air calorics also are provided, although they are not performed in our facility. To accommodate patients that are particularly sensitive to the stimulation, decreasing the irrigation time is the best parameter to vary. On the other hand, when patients show significantly reduced responses to caloric stimuli, decreasing temperature by using "ice water" is the better test modification.

In our facility, open-loop water caloric irrigations are routinely used, and closed loop water calorics are performed in those patients with tympanic membrane defects. Therefore, for all examples given in this text, open-loop water irrigations were used for the calorics unless otherwise indicated. Each laboratory should set normative ranges for absolute slow-component eye velocity or any other outcome parameters used for their routine caloric testing. Using the settings given for open-loop water in Table 4–5, our normative data is similar to that reported in several studies attempting to provide normative guidelines (Baloh & Honrubia, 1990; Jacobson et al., 1993; Proctor et al., 1986). For open and closed-loop irrigations, our 95% confidence interval for normal slow-component velocity is between 10–50°/sec, and we expect greater than 20°/sec responses when ice water is used.

The theory behind the mechanism of caloric responses is discussed in detail elsewhere (Baloh & Honrubia, 1990; Barany, 1906; Barany & Witmaack, 1911; Jacobson et al., 1993). Summarizing studies in both terrestrial and weightless environments, there appears to be at least two mechanisms operating. The one that seems to predominate in routine testing involves gravity and the density changes that occur in the endolymph when it is heated or cooled (density decreased or increased, respectively). The head is positioned so that the horizontal canal is oriented parallel to the gravitational vector, with the nose of the patient upward and the head tilted 30° upward from the horizontal plane. During a warm irrigation, the less dense fluid attempts to rise upward. This produces a deviation of the cupula toward the utricle due to the pressure differential across the cupula, causing stimulation of the VIIIth nerve. The reverse action occurs for the more dense area of cooled fluid, causing inhibition. This results in the well-known mnemonic COWS, which refers to the direction of nystagmus: Cold Opposite, Warm Same (relative to the side of the irrigation). When the patient's nose is placed down, so that the plane of the horizontal canal is 180° out of phase with the usual position, the responses are reversed, Cold Same, Warm Opposite. This dependence on gravity can be used to the examiner's advantage in

---

TABLE 4–5. Suggested Parameters for Caloric Irrigation Methods

■ Open-Loop Water
  Temperatures: 30 and 44°C
  Length of Irrigation: 40 seconds
  Flow rate: 300 ml/min
■ Closed-Loop Water
  Temperatures: 25 and 46°C
  Length of Irrigation: 60 seconds
  Pressure of flow: 60–80 mm Hg (flow rate = 150 ml/min)
■ Air
  Temperatures: 28 and 46°C
  Length of Irrigation: 40 seconds, with no perforation
  90 seconds, with a perforation

evaluating a unilateral peripheral lesion with significantly reduced sensitivity. For example, say that a patient had persistent spontaneous right-beating nystagmus at 3–7°/sec throughout the study. Standard bithermal caloric irrigations in the left ear produce no change in the ongoing right-beating nystagmus, yet ice water irrigation on the left seems to increase the right-beating response to between 6–9°/sec, suggesting a possible effect from the left ear. All responses on the right were strong and symmetrical. The question now becomes, is the ice water response due to the influence of the left periphery or simply an untimely variation in the persistent right-beating nystagmus observed throughout the study? It would present a convincing argument for residual left ear responsiveness if the spontaneous right-beating nystagmus could be suppressed or even reversed. As it is impractical to increase the stimulus intensity with warm water, the patient can be turned nose down and the ice water irrigation repeated. If the spontaneous right-beating nystagmus is noted at the beginning of the irrigation but reverses during or after completion of the irrigation, the left periphery is responding. This can be an important finding in the patient with continuing spells of vertigo after an ablative surgical procedure such as vestibular nerve section or transcanal labyrinthectomy. Such evidence may help to verify residual function when it is suspected that the procedure may have been incomplete. On the other hand, if no change was seen with the patient in the nose down position, the question about residual function remaining in the left peripheral vestibular system can *not* be definitively answered. One must remember that only the responses mediated by the horizontal canal and superior vestibular nerve are being measured. In addition, the caloric response represents only one point on the intensity and frequency spectrum within which the semicircular canals respond. Caloric stimulation is equivalent to a very low-frequency rotation between 0.002 and 0.004 Hz. Therefore, lack of a caloric response only indicates that low frequency responses are absent. Rotational chair (discussed in Chapter 6) provides stimulation from 0.01 through over 1 Hz, yet it uses natural angular acceleration of the head, preventing assessment of unilateral function.

The traditional interpretation of caloric stimulation uses a relative comparison of responses on the right versus the left. This is more reliable than use of absolute slow-component eye velocities or other parameters (frequency of beats, amplitude of eye movement) because of significant variability among normals. The formulas (Fitzgerald & Hallpike, 1942) used to provide the percentage comparison of response magnitude (unilateral weakness) and direction bias of eye movement (directional preponderance) are given in Table 4–6. These are typically used by determining the maximum, average slow-component velocity over a 10-second interval of the nystagmus response to each of the four caloric irrigations: right warm (RW), right cool (RC), left warm (LW), and left cool (LC). The use of percentage differences may present a problem when caloric responses produce small slow-component velocities (less than 12°/sec). In this setting, small differences in absolute slow-component eye velocity will produce significant percentage differences. The converse is true with large slow-component eye velocities (greater than 40°/sec). Because most facilities use a fixed percentage difference as a criteria for unilateral weakness and directional preponderance, when eye velocities approach the limits of the normal range, interpretation of unilateral weakness measurements should be made with care. These should always be interpreted in light of the presenting history, signs, and symptoms so as not to give inappropriate weight to the percentage difference at the extremes.

In order to validly compare caloric responses, two assumptions must not be violated. These are:

1. The stimulus delivered to each ear is equivalent.
2. The anatomy of the left and right ear is the same, within normal variations.

If these assumptions are not met, the caloric irrigations may be used only to indicate whether or not the peripheral system is responsive to thermal stimulation. The two sides may *not* be compared meaningfully. The first assumption depends most critically on calibration of the irrigation device and technical care to provide equivalent irrigations. The second assumption is less under the control of the examiner, unless cerumen or other debris that may partially occlude the external auditory canal can be removed prior to the study. Otoscopic inspection of the external canal is mandatory to investigate the possibility of differences that may exist between ears and to evaluate tympanic membrane integrity. In the setting of past otologic surgical procedures, especially mastoidectomy or repair of congenital anomalies, one should be highly suspicious of asymmetrical anatomy. Minor procedures such as ventilation tubes, successful tympanoplasty with minimal thickening of the tympanic membrane, and transmastoid procedures that do not disrupt external or middle ear anatomy generally do not violate the second assumption. Congenital abnormalities such as an atresia plate, a stenotic external canal, or acquired disorders such as a severely atelectatic or absent tympanic membrane may produce falsely asymmetric caloric responses when the labyrinth is actually normal. When it is clear prior to beginning the irrigations that the caloric irrigations cannot be compared, there is no need to use equivalent stimulation times. This is important in ears where the stimulation will be directly in contact with the medial wall of the middle ear secondary to anatomical changes. In such cases, the irrigation should be rather brief, lasting only until the patient reports a sensation of dizziness. If that periphery is normal, a very strong response can be generated with a 3–5 second irrigation time. In addition, the normative data for absolute range of response should not be applied in these cases, as the figures were obtained in subjects with normal anatomy.

A limit for normal values of unilateral weakness and directional preponderance must be established in each laboratory. A number of published works describes these values. It would be sufficient for a facility to test a small number of normal subjects using a described test protocol, and if the observed variability was in agreement with the published figures, the authors' normal values could be used with some confidence. The range of reported normal values varies from 20 to 35%. Our facility considers a difference greater than 24% as significant for both unilateral weakness and directional preponderance.

Due to the variability in absolute responses for reproducible caloric irrigations and the profound influence of the patient's level of alertness (as the patient becomes sleepy the response is lessened, with alertness usually accomplished with simple conversation) (Kileny, McCabe, & Ryu, 1989; Torok, 1970), it is not unusual to obtain three caloric results with very similar values while the fourth may be considerably higher or lower than the others. The outlier is often from the first irrigation performed, due either to an anxious or under- or overalerted status. If this situation results in a significant unilateral weakness or directional preponderance, then the irrigation that produced the outlier value should be repeated. There are times when two of the four irrigations may need to be repeated to substantiate the findings and produce a reliable test result. Figures 4–4 and 4–5 illustrate this situation. In figure 4–4, the results from four irrigations are shown in the four caloric pods. These record the slow-component eye velocity produced over the time course of the response. Each point represents the eye velocity calculated from the raw nystagmus trace for identified nystagmus movements of the eye. The maximum, average slow-component eye velocity over a 10-second interval of maximum response for each irrigation is shown in each pod (refer to Jacobson et al., 1993 for a detailed description of how to calculate these responses from the raw trace). The values given for average maximum values were then combined in the formulas given in Table 4–6 to produce the estimates of unilateral weakness and directional preponderance, given in the figure. These suggest a right unilateral weakness, yet the left warm irrigation is not in line with the others and may account for the observed outcome. Figure 4–5 shows the results after repeat of the left warm caloric irrigation. This result is within normal limits and the right unilateral weakness is no longer suspected. Generally, if a normal response is confirmed by repeating one or more caloric irrigation within a 30-minute

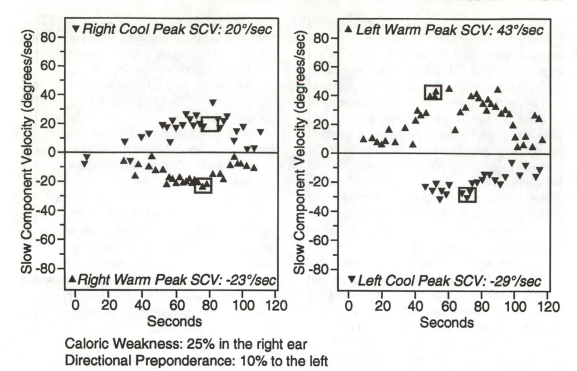

Caloric Weakness: 25% in the right ear
Directional Preponderance: 10% to the left

FIGURE 4–4. Plots of slow-component eye velocity (SCV) from nystagmus provoked by open-loop water irrigations as a function of time. Each triangle represents one slow-component velocity movement of the eye from the nystagmus trace. Responses for the right ear are shown on the left, those for the left ear on the right. The orientation of the triangles represent either cool (30°C), ▼, or warm (44°C), ▲, irrigations. The plots are arranged so that right-beating nystagmus slow-component velocities are on the bottom (right warm, left cool) and left-beating nystagmus slow-component velocities are on the top (right cool, left warm). The velocity values given in top or bottom of each plot represents the average maximum slow-component velocity calculated for the nystagmus beats within the rectangle shown on each plot. These maximum, average slow-component velocity values were used to calculate the caloric weakness and directional preponderance values shown at the bottom of the Figure. Twenty-five percent in the right ear means a 25% weaker reponse on the right compared to the left. Ten percenet to the left, means a 10% greater response for left-beating nystagmus compared to right-beating nystagmus. For purposes of calculations, rightward slow-component velocities are assigned a negative number, leftward are assigned a positive number.

session, the initial abnormal result may be ignored. Repeating caloric irrigations when clinically appropriate will lead to a more valid test result.

Although there are situations where more than four caloric irrigations are needed, there are other times when it is valid to use only two irrigations. It is never desirable to use only two to define a pathologic condition, except where the other two irrigations cannot be performed. Given the following conditions, two warm or cool caloric irrigations are adequate to define a normal result:

1. No clinically significant spontaneous or positional nystagmus was noted in the study
2. The maximum, average, slow-component eye velocity for each ear is greater than 20°/sec when a 40-second caloric irrigation is performed at 300 ml/min flow rate
3. The percentage difference between the responses observed for the two ears is less than 10%.

If all of these conditions are met, the likelihood of having the final result of four irrigations

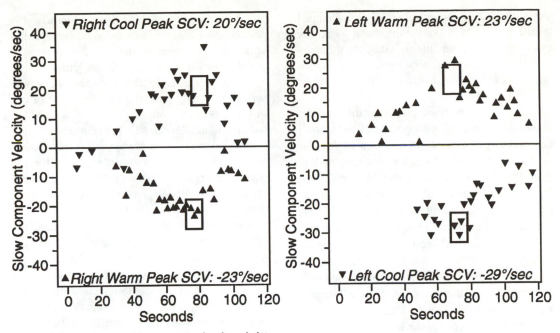

Caloric Weakness: 9% in the right ear
Directional Preponderance: 9% to the right

FIGURE 4–5. See Figure 4–4 legend.

TABLE 4–6. Formulas for Unilateral Weakness and Directional Preponderance

Unilateral Weakness (UW) = (values –100% to +100%)	$\dfrac{(RW + RC) - (LW + LC)}{RW + RC + LW + LC} \times 100\%$
Directional Preponderance (DP) = (values $-\infty$ to $+\infty$)	$\dfrac{(RW + LC) - (LW + RC)}{RW + RC + LW + LC} \times 100\%$

RW, right warm; RC, right cool; LW, left warm; LC, left cool.

documenting a unilateral weakness of 25% or greater, without one irrigation being out of the range of the other three is extremely small. Whenever these conditions are not strictly met, it is suggested that all four irrigations be performed. A more formal review of this same issue with somewhat less conservative criteria for stopping at only two irrigations is reported by Jacobson, Calder, Shepherd, Rupp, and Newman, (1995).

Due to the influence of low eye velocity values on the percentage figures for unilateral weakness and directional preponderance, there are times when use of ice water irrigations are an appropriate alternative to standard cool irri-

gations. If both of the initial warm irrigations result in peak eye velocity values of less than 10°/sec, often we will use ice water for the two remaining irrigations, unless the patient was highly symptomatic with the warm irrigations. As warm and ice irrigations are not equivalent stimuli, care must be taken in interpreting directional preponderance in this setting, especially when a significant unilateral weakness is present, as illustrated by an example later in this chapter. Nonetheless, the values calculated for unilateral weakness will be accurate as they are not influenced by the combination of caloric temperatures, provided the identical procedure is followed for both ears. The benefit of this technique is that larger values of slow-component eye velocity make the unilateral weakness calculation more reliable. In addition, the individual with a mild bilateral paresis will require only four irrigations, instead of six, if ice water is used initially.

The criterion used in our facility for the diagnosis of bilateral peripheral paresis is slow-component eye velocity of less than 10°/sec for all four standard bithermal irrigations, or less than 10°/sec for the warm and 15°/sec for ice water. Using the sum of the four routine irrigations can be misleading, as the sum may be less than 20 if three of the responses are low while one is in the 10–15°/sec range. If an irrigation produces a response above 10°/sec that is repeatable, without persistent spontaneous nystagmus biasing the response, then a bilateral weakness is unlikely. An alternative explanation must be sought for the low response of the other three irrigations, or at least for the weak response in the same ear that generated the normal caloric response. Ice water irrigations can be very helpful to document the absence of a bilateral weakness in this setting, as well as rotational chair or head rotation tests.

When a bilateral weakness is suspected, the clinician must remember that absence of caloric responses, even including the use of ice water, does not necessarily imply complete loss of peripheral vestibular function. Low-frequency rotational chair (discussed in Chapter 6) should be used to further define the extent of the bilateral reduction in peripheral sensitivity. At a minimum, simple head on body rotation with routine ENG recording should be used to verify that the reduced or absent caloric responses are not an artifact of poor alerting of the patient. Another cause could be an extraordinary Bell's phenomenon. This phenomenon involves the superior rotation of the eye as the eyelids are closed. The further the eye moves superiorly, the more the horizontal range of motion is reduced. In some individuals, this phenomenon may be sufficient (especially in combination with reduced alertness or a mild bilateral paresis) to eliminate the response to thermal irrigations. This possibility can be explored by observing the recordings from the vertical channels as the patient is

asked to close the eyes. If this problem is suspected, the caloric irrigations could be repeated with the eyes open in darkness, with opaque goggles, or while wearing Frenzel lenses.

When a directional preponderance is observed, it usually reflects either the effect of ongoing spontaneous nystagmus or is associated with a unilateral weakness. In the latter case, this finding suggests a lack of physiologic compensation within the vestibulo-ocular reflex for the paretic labyrinthine lesion (Table 4–3). However, when directional preponderance is the only finding of significance in the ENG, this implies an abnormal bias within the system, allowing for eye movements of greater amplitude in one direction versus the other. The question to be addressed is whether this ongoing bias results from incomplete static compensation for a peripheral asymmetry (as in the case of a unilateral paresis), or if the bias results from a central vestibulo-ocular pathway lesion in the presence of symmetrical peripheral function. The approach taken by the authors is similar to the guidelines that were discussed above for interpretation of spontaneous and positional nystagmus. The directional preponderance is said to suggest peripheral system involvement provided the ocular motor findings are normal and the patient's presenting history, signs, and symptoms are not suspicious of central pathway involvement. This finding does not indicate which labyrinth is pathologic, as a paretic lesion on one side (away from the direction of the directional preponderance) or an irritative lesion on the other side (the side of the beat of the preponderance) will produce the same finding. The following three examples illustrate the interpretation of the ENG findings that have been discussed above.

CASE 12

A 43-year-old male presented with sudden onset of motion and positional vertigo without a severe vestibular crisis 18 months prior to evaluation. Symptoms last for several seconds to 1 minute and occur multiple times daily. No spontaneous events are reported but nausea and a sensation of his legs "folding out from under him" are reported. Tinnitus, aural fullness, and fluctuant hearing in the right ear were noted and radiographic evaluation showed no evidence of a cerebellopontine angle lesion.

ENG: No spontaneous nystagmus, but right-beating positional nystagmus of 4–8°/sec was noted in all 8 positions tested. Four caloric irrigations showed no unilateral weakness but a significant (27%) right directional preponderance.

Ocular motor: Results were normal with mild disruptions for movements rightward explained by a prior right lateral rectus muscle injury.

These results were interpreted as indicative of peripheral system involvement, stable but uncompensated physiologically, suggestive of a possible right side irritative vestibular lesion given the associated auditory complaints. He was treated with a vestibular rehabilitation program and within three months was asymptomatic and returned to work.

This case is contrasted with the next that presents central findings.

CASE 17

A 65-year-old male presented with sudden onset of disequilibrium and nausea following heart catheterization in the fall of 1989. Brain stem stroke was suspected but neuroradiographic studies at the time were negative. Current symptoms were constant unsteadiness and lightheadedness with sudden pulling or pushing (pulsion) sensation spontaneously 2 to 3 times per week lasting several seconds. His constant symptoms were exacerbated by head movements. The patient had a past history of significant cardiac disease requiring a triple coronary artery bypass operation in 1980. Bilateral tinnitus and aural fullness were reported with a mild high-frequency, bilateral sensorineural hearing loss.

ENG: Left-beating spontaneous and positional nystagmus with slow-component eye velocity of 4–6°/sec were seen throughout the study. Bithermal, alternating caloric irrigations produced only left-beating nystagmus. However, as can be

seen in Figure 4–6, the average values for slow-component eye velocity were significantly lower than the spontaneous value for right warm and left cool (irrigations normally resulting in right beats), and increased compared to spontaneous for the right cool and left warm (those causing left beats). This results in no unilateral weakness but a significant (79%) left directional preponderance. In this case, the ocular motor result were significantly abnormal with a pattern that suggested a left lateral medullary infarct.

The evidence for this brain stem lesion will be illustrated later in this chapter when discussing Interpretation Dilemmas. This patient also was treated with a vestibular rehabilitation program that will be reviewed in Chapters 7 and 10.

The next case shows a strong directional preponderance of peripheral origin, together with caloric indications of bilateral peripheral system paresis.

CASE 18

A 52-year-old female complained of recurrent episodes of severe unsteadiness with nausea and emesis. vertigo and lightheadedness were denied. She had been hospitalized twice, once in 1986 and once in 1990. She had been treated with multiple medications without relief. Her symptoms became worse with head movement. She had been treated for depression and headaches with no effect on her spells of unsteadiness. An audiogram showed a mild left sensorineural hearing loss in the mid and high frequencies, with normal hearing on the right and 100% discrimination bilaterally. She reported the loss to be progressive over many years. A CT scan from 1990 was reportedly negative.

ENG: Persistent spontaneous and positional right-beating nystagmus with slow-component eye velocity of 2–5°/sec throughout the study. Unlike Case 17, warm, cool, and ice water calorics had no effect on the spontaneous nystagmus, resulting in a 2% unilateral weakness and a 214% right directional preponderance. When

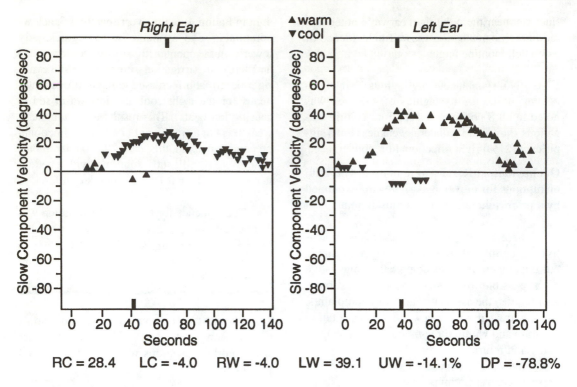

FIGURE 4–6. See Figure 4–4 legend. In this figure the maximum, average slow-component velocity values are given at the bottom of the figure, and the rectangle showing the 10-second interval used for the average has been omitted for clarity in the figure. RC, right cool; LC, left cool; RW, right warm; LW, left warm; UW, unilateral weakness (14.1% in the right ear); DP, directional preponderance (78.8% to the left).

calculating directional preponderance, if the sign of those irrigation results that are in the incorrect direction are taken and maintained as negative, directional preponderance can result in a value greater than 100%. For example, in this case the values of the responses for the four irrigations in °/sec were right warm = 4.9, right cool = –2.4 (sign indicates incorrect direction), left warm = –0.4, and left cool = 2.8. If these values, with the signs maintained, are put into the formula in Table 4–6, the above values of unilateral weakness and directional preponderance result.

Ocular motor: Normal findings for all subtests were noted.

A bilateral peripheral vestibular paresis possibly worse on the left (given the right beating spontaneous nystagmus and hearing loss on the left) was suspected from these results. Rotational chair was attempted to further evaluate the extent of the bilateral lesion; however, the patient would

not submit to the rotations of lowest frequency. She showed normal responses to the two higher frequency acceleration tests (0.32 and 0.64 Hz). This result, together with normal findings on postural control assessment, indicate that the bilateral involvement was mild, probably involving only the low-frequency responses. An MRI with contrast enhancement was obtained showing bilateral cerebellopontine angle masses leading to a presumptive diagnosis of bilateral acoustic neuromas and neurofibromatosis type II. The mass on the right was small and primarily extracanalicular, while the one on the left demonstrated more lateral extension into the internal auditory canal. It was hypothesized that the lesion on the left was likely to produce more effect upon the VIIIth nerve by compression within the bony confines of the internal canal, potentially explaining the hearing loss on the left and the right-beating nystagmus. Suboccipital resection of the mass on the right side was performed, and the mass was found to be arising from the dura at the porus acousticus. Because the VIIIth nerve was not directly invaded by the tumor, it was able to be preserved, allowing for continuation of hearing and vestibular function in the right ear. The pathology report confirmed the intraoperative impression that the lesion was a meningioma instead of a schwannoma. Postoperatively the patient's balance improved subjectively and her responses to caloric irrigations on the right became normal. She declined resection of the small left sided lesion and has been lost to further follow-up.

SOURCES OF ERROR IN ELECTONYSTAGMOGRAPHY EVALUATION

Many sources of artifact, both physiologic and nonphysiologic, may influence ENG findings. These artifacts along with several specific interpretation dilemmas primarily impact the interpretation of spontaneous nystagmus, positional nystagmus, and caloric responses. A summary of the sources of error in ENG evaluation is given in Table 4–7. Many of these will be presented here, with others discussed in association with ocular motor tests.

Nonphysiologic Artifacts

Electrical artifacts disrupt all aspects of ENG testing. Schematized examples of several types are shown in Figure 4–7. Electrode impedance less than 25k ohms is preferable for ENG recordings, although any value under 40k ohms may work unless there is a difference between electrodes that exceeds 10k ohms. The best way to avoid an unstable junction potential at the interface between the silver chloride electrode surface

TABLE 4–7. Sources of Error in ENG Evaluation

  I. Nonphysiologic Artifacts
     A. Electrical
        1. General amplifier noise or poor common mode rejection by differential amplifiers
        2. Electrode lead movement
        3. Electrode impedance
        4. Unstable junction potential
     B. Improper electrode placement
        1. Horizontal or vertical electrodes not aligned
        2. Electrodes too close to the lateral canthus or lower lid interfering with eye comfort
     C. Uncooperative patient
        1. Volitional and nonvolitional compliance with testing instructions (eyes open, eyes closed, head movement, etc.)
     D. Stimulus control—caloric temperature, flow rate of water or air, and duration of irrigation
 II. Physiologic Artifacts
     A. Eye blinks
     B. Facial/neck muscle activation
     C. Alertness—hyper or hypo
     D. Noncompliance with pretest instructions
        1. Stoppage of specified medications
        2. Consumption of alcohol
     E. Prosthetic eye
     F. Corrective lenses
     G. Novelty of ocular motor and caloric tests
III. Interpretation Dilemmas
     A. Ocular control abnormalities
        1. Congenital nystagmus
        2. Esotropia/exotropia
        3. Ocular-lateral pulsion
        4. Restriction syndrome (range of eye motion)
     B. Blindness—adventitious vs. congenital
     C. Direction-changing positional nystagmus with classically positive Hallpike maneuver(s)
     D. Canal paresis with irritative status
     E. Age-related normative data

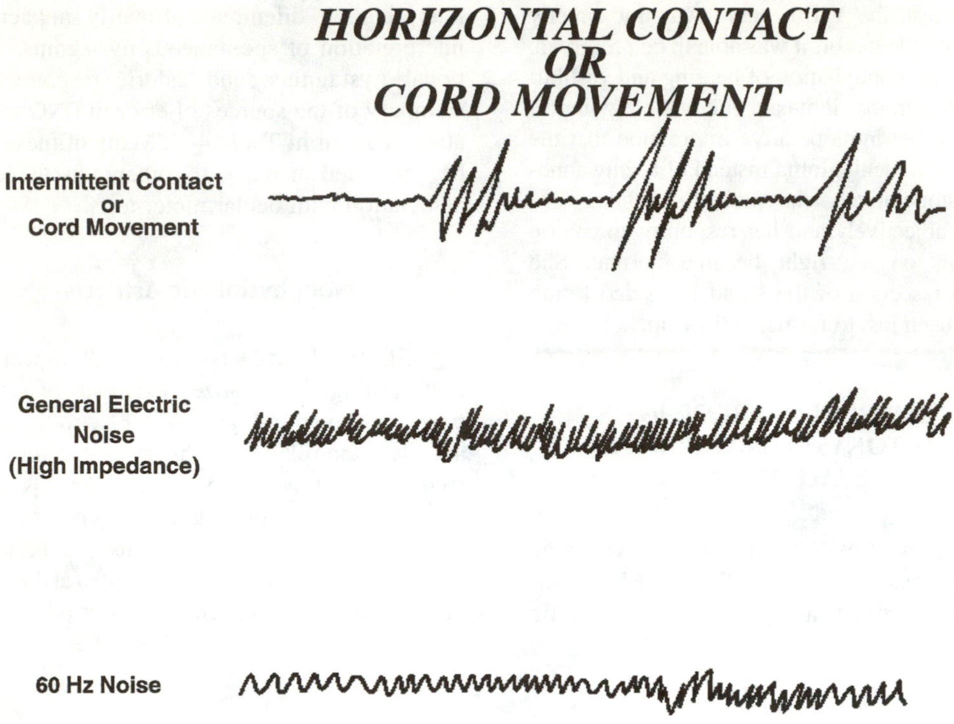

HORIZONTAL CONTACT
OR
CORD MOVEMENT

**Intermittent Contact
or
Cord Movement**

**General Electric
Noise
(High Impedance)**

60 Hz Noise

FIGURE 4–7. Drawings of horizontal eye position as a function of time illustrating different types of electrical artifact.

and the skin is to wait 5–10 minutes after application before making any recordings. This time can be used to begin the neurotologic history and to clinically evaluate ocular range of motion, conjugate eye movement, and gaze-evoked nystagmus. Two findings suggest improper alignment of horizontal recording electrodes. The first is a reduction of horizontal sensitivity, wherein a higher than normal gain of the amplifier is required for calibration eye movements. The second is excessive activity on the horizontal channel when the patient is performing directed vertical eye movements. Analogous problems are noted for misalignment in the vertical electrodes.

If findings noted during performance of the ENG seem to be inconsistent, it does not automatically follow that the patient is not cooperating and volitionally disrupting the results. Usually, the difficult patient is one who struggles to follow instructions secondary to cognitive problems such as low intellectual function, senility, or head trauma. There also may be difficulty due to

significant nausea, uncontrollable head movements associated with congenital or acquired neurological conditions, or simply failure to understand instructions. These conditions can be subtle at times, and close attention to performance during the testing is needed. As mentioned above (Figure 4–1), room arrangement can be helpful in focusing the examiner's attention to possible confounding factors. An example of a problem that may arise from a simple misinstruction or in patients with restricted lateral range of eye motion is shown in Figure 4–8. In this case, the patient was asked to perform saccades of a fixed subtended arc (fixed distance) from center position. Yet each time the target moved, although the patient performed the saccade correctly, he then followed the eye movement with a head turn toward the target. Thus the eye returned smoothly to the center of the orbit, giving the impression of an inability to sustain lateral gaze. The examiner was able to recognize the problem by watching the patient and target

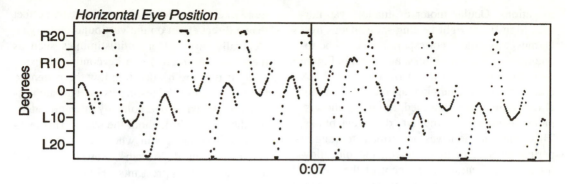

FIGURE 4–8. Compare Figure 2–1B, and see text for further details. Plot of horizontal eye position as a function of time; however, in this figure it is a problematic recording.

simultaneously, while observing the resultant eye movement tracing. The problem was eliminated simply by reinstructing the patient. Issues of patient instruction are common since many of the tests represent novel tasks, especially the ocular-motor battery. Multiple repetitions may be needed to obtain optimal test performance. In other instances, recognition of the problem may not eliminate the disruption, but should be noted to assist in proper interpretation.

Although significant attention is paid to calibration of instruments used for assessment of auditory function, examiners tend to be less concerned about calibration for balance function evaluations. However, using the appropriate distances from the subject to the target to produce eye movements of a known subtended arc is critical for ocular motor testing. This distance needs to be verified in all laboratories, whether computerized or not. The parameters of caloric testing such as flow rate, time of irrigation, and temperature of the water or air need to be verified frequently.

Physiologic Artifacts

The dominant physiologic artifact in vestibular testing is eye blinking. If the rate of orbicularis oculi contraction is excessive (typically greater than 20 episodes per minute), it is referred to as *blepharospasm*. The major problem is the detection of blink activity by the horizontal recording channel. This may produce a response that appears to be horizontal jerk nys-

tagmus. Occasionally, gentle pressure on the lid with the eye closed will reduce the impact of the orbicularis oculi muscle activity. It is ideal to use two-channel recordings of eye movements during the ENG in order to identify excessive blink artifacts, as they are easily detected on the vertical channel. When the large blink artifacts on the vertical channel are noted with apparent jerk nystagmus on the horizontal channel, the detection of actual nystagmus is difficult at best. Two criteria may be used to verify that horizontal nystagmus is not an artifact of the eye blinks: (a) If the nystagmus is direction-changing; or (b) If at least 5 seconds of recorded eye movements can be found where there is no correspondence between the eye blinks and the nystagmus (nystagmus without eye blinks or eye blinks without nystagmus). An example of the first criteria is shown with the following case.

CASE 40

A 47-year-old female presented for evaluation one year after a motor vehicle accident. There was temporary loss of consciousness at the scene of the accident. She complained of vertigo and unsteadiness provoked by head movement. Her spells lasted several seconds and occurred daily. Constant unsteadiness when walking also was reported. Her ENG showed a 90% left unilateral weakness, and a 41% right directional preponderance with warm (44°C) and cool (30°C) water calorics, with 40-second irrigations. Ocular motor evaluation was normal. Significant right-beating spontaneous nystagmus was noted, corresponding in a one-to-one fashion with eye blinks, as shown in Figure 4–9. Yet, as demonstrated by Figure 4–10 A and B, direction-changing, ageotropic positional nystagmus was identified, removing the suspicion that the nystagmus was due to eye blinks. This determination was not critical to suggest peripheral system involvement, but did allow for a more accurate assessment of the lack of static compensation, documented by the spontaneous nystagmus.

The example shown in the next case did not meet either of the above criteria and, therefore, the question of peripheral involvement was still undetermined after the ENG.

CASE 24

A 34-year-old female experienced a sudden onset of lightheadedness with hearing loss on the right three years prior to her evaluation. Spontaneous attacks of significant lightheadedness were occurring multiple times per month. She reported five spells of true vertigo with nausea and vomiting lasting 1 hour. She also had tinnitus, aural fullness, and documented fluctuant low-frequency sensorineural hearing loss on the right.

ENG showed possible spontaneous and positional left-beating nystagmus; however, blepharospasm made firm determination of nystagmus and, therefore, documentation of peripheral system involvement impossible. A sample of these tracings are shown in Figure 4–11. The nystagmus and eye blinks were associated one-to-one throughout the study, with no change in direction of the suspected nystagmus. Without other investigative tools that are not influenced by the eye blinks, or other eye movement recording techniques such as an infrared video camera, this study cannot be conclusive.

The primary concern regarding use of traditional vestibular suppressants prior to testing is that nystagmus might be suppressed. This is more likely to be due to a central sedative effect than a direct effect on the vestibular end-organ. Generally, the milder antihistiminics such as meclizine (Antivert®) can be continued, especially if they are needed to allow the patient to tolerate travel or the testing itself. The suppressive effects can be overcome by diligently alerting the patient throughout the study. This technique is less successful when benzodiazepines (such as Valium®, Ativan®, Xanax®) are used as vestibular suppressants. However, if the patient has been taking such a medication for longer than 2 months, it is unwise to stop the medication prior to testing due to withdrawal symptoms. Seizure medications should never be interrupted, but testing should be performed only after stabilization of the dose to minimize the effect of drowsiness, usually requiring a minimum of 8 weeks. Interpretation of test results for patients taking antiepileptics or other centrally acting medications should be cautious, especially if the results suggest bilateral caloric weakness or abnormalities of ocular-motor function. Repeat testing when patients are off the medication or better adjusted to their new dosage would be advised for confirmation (Cass & Furman, 1993).

The principal effect of a single prosthetic eye is to reduce the signal-to-noise ratio by approximately 50%. This obviously produces a noisier trace, yet typically one that is adequate for testing. An ocular range-of-motion evaluation or simply asking the patient about eye movement is often needed to identify a glass eye. Many patients will not think to mention it to the examiner, as they do not understand the use of eye movement recordings to assess vestibular function. As a result, much time could be wasted investigating a noisy trace when the explanation is obvious.

Use of the patient's corrective eyeglasses can be helpful during the ocular motor evaluation, but is usually not necessary. Accurate visual acuity is not needed to perform the tests discussed in Chapter 5 as long as good contrast is achieved between the background lighting and the target. A more important issue with glasses is calibration of eye movement. Corrective lenses (as opposed to contact lenses) modi-

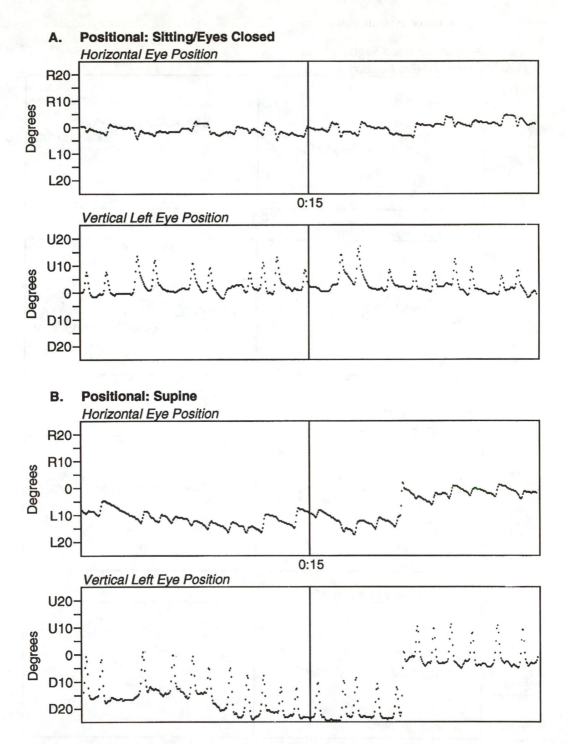

FIGURE 4–9. Plots of horizontal and vertical eye position in degrees as a function of time as recorded during electronystagmography. **A.** Sitting position, head straight, eyes closed. **B.** Supine position, eyes closed. Left-beating nystagmus is seen for either position. The number on the time axis indicates the total elapsed time for that position, not trace length in time. The trace in each plot is 14 seconds long. Note eye blinks on the vertical traces.

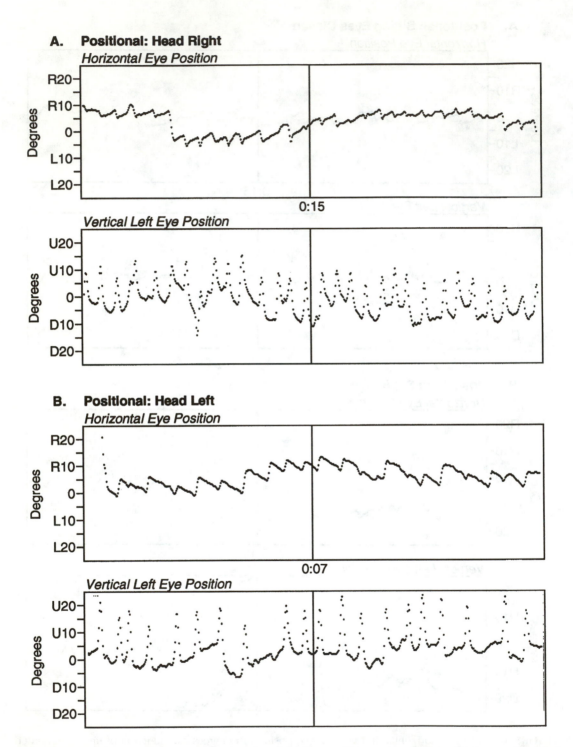

FIGURE 4–10. Plots of horizontal and vertical eye position in degrees as a function of time as recorded during electronystagmography. **A.** Supine with head turned right, eyes closed, left-beating nystagmus. **B.** Supine with head turned left, eyes closed, right-beating nystagmus. Note eye blinks on the vertical traces.

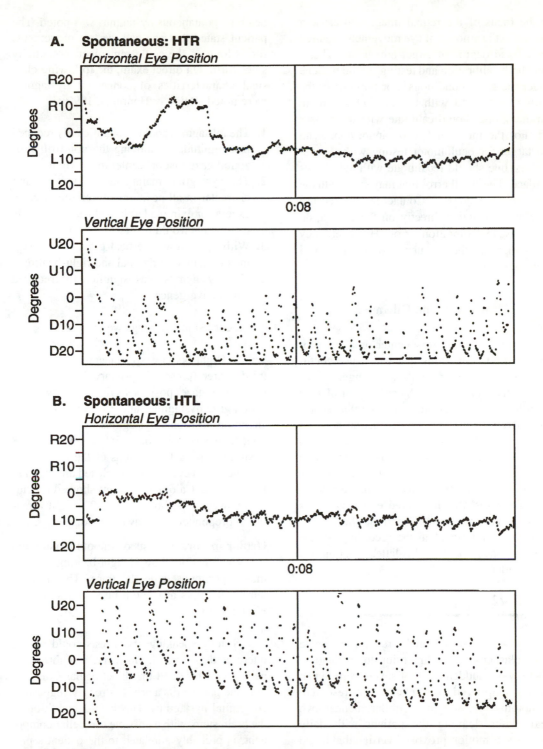

FIGURE 4–11. Plots of horizontal and vertical eye position in degrees as a function of time as recorded during electronystagmography. **A.** Sitting position, eyes closed, head turned right, apparent left-beating nystagmus. **B.** Sitting, eyes closed, head turned left, apparent left-beating nystamgus. Note eye blinks on the vertical traces.

fy the focus of the retinal image and cause a change in the amount of eye movement required for a fixed degree of target movement. Therefore, both calibration and testing should be done under the same conditions. For portions of the testing performed with the eyes closed or in darkness, one should calibrate with the glasses off. For the individual who cannot apprehend the target for oculomotor testing without eyeglasses, one should recalibrate with the glasses in place. The small error that may exist with the eyes closed is ignored. Contact lenses, because they are positioned directly on the cornea, do not cause a calibration error. However, they often increase the frequency of blinking and therefore blink artifacts.

Interpretation Dilemmas

Discussion will now center on a series of less common situations that can cause confusion in ENG interpretation. Congenital or acquired abnormalities of ocular control may significantly alter an otherwise normal recording, thereby confusing the distinction between peripheral and central pathway involvement. In some cases, the eye movement disorder may be causing the expressed symptoms (as already illustrated by Case 17; further discussed below). In other cases, the disordered eye movements are incidental and simply increase the "noise" (any irrelevant signal in the recording) of the eye movement tracing. This latter situation will be considered first.

CASE 42

A 45-year-old female reports an acute vestibular crisis 5 years prior to evaluation. There was a sudden onset of severe vertigo that slowly improved and eventually resolved. Symptoms relapsed in a similar manner two years later, leaving the patient with daily episodes of motion-provoked vertigo that lasted 1–2 minutes following a provocative head movement. There were no auditory complaints and the patient was otherwise healthy. Upon visual inspection of the eyes, persistent right-

beating spontaneous nystagmus was noted. The patient stated that she had the eye movements for as long as she could remember, potentially since birth. On direct exam, the following classical characteristics of congenital nystagmus were noted (Baloh & Honrubia, 1990):

1. The nystagmus could be significantly reduced in magnitude by moving the point of horizontal gaze just off center to the right.
2. The nystagmus maintained its right-beating character in all positions of horizontal gaze, except for extreme left lateral gaze where the nystagmus would reverse to left beats.
3. With up or down vertical gaze, the nystagmus remained horizontal and right-beating.
4. The nystagmus was significantly reduced with convergence.

The recorded test findings were:

ENG: Right-beating spontaneous nystagmus, third degree (present in primary, right, and left horizontal gaze positions) right-beating horizontal gaze nystagmus, and geotropic direction-changing positional nystagmus with slow-component eye velocity of 2–5°/second in 6 of 8 positions tested. Illustrations of the nystagmus recorded with eyes open and closed are given in Figure 4–12. Caloric irrigations showed no unilateral weakness; however, a 30% right directional preponderance was obtained.

Ocular motor: All tests of smooth pursuit and saccade function showed right-beating nystagmus superimposed on the trace. This finding during attempts at smooth pursuit is shown in Figure 4–13.

Strictly speaking, these tests could not be interpreted as normal. However, in light of the patient's history and the direct ocular examination, the pattern fits a profile strongly suggesting congenital nystagmus. This benign condition of the brain stem, with a possible cerebellar component, is probably unrelated to the patient's presenting complaints. Yet, the persistent nystagmus confounds the interpretation of the ENG, and it is impossible to incriminate peripheral versus central system involvement based on the

Congenital Nystagmus

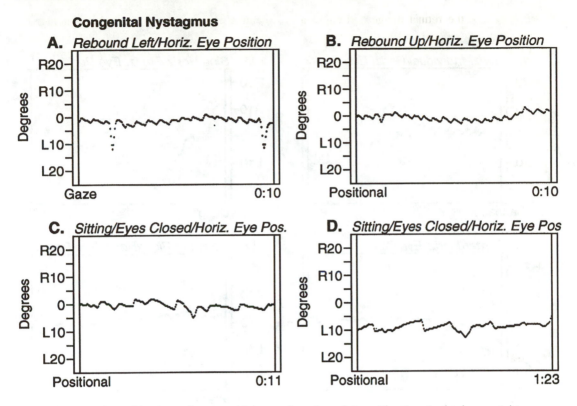

FIGURE 4–12. Plots of horizontal eye position as a function of time. The time in the lower right corner of each panel is the total elapse time in seconds for that recording, not the total time shown. Each panel represents 7 seconds of tracing. **A.** Gazing left by 37°, eyes open. **B.** Gazing up by 37°, eyes open. **C.** Sitting, head straight, eyes closed. **D.** Continuation of the trace in C.

recordings alone. The direction-changing positional nystagmus could easily be a result of the congenital nystagmus, as could the right directional preponderance. Recognition of the congenital nystagmus by history and exam allows the ENG and ocular motor results to be interpreted as principally a peripheral system problem with no significant indications of central system involvement, other than that explainable by the congenital nystagmus. This interpretation was reinforced by abnormal phase lead from rotational chair testing, a finding that would not be expected to result from congenital nystagmus.

Misalignment of the eyes, generally referred to as *strabismus,* may cause some disruption predominantly in smooth pursuit and individual eye saccade recordings. An illustration of the most common forms of misalignment that

effect the eye tracings is given in Figure 4–14. The Figure depicts these conditions at the extreme, with milder forms being more typical. Suspicion of interference from strabismus should be entertained when an abnormal tracing is noted for large and/or rapid target movements laterally on the side with esotropia and medially on the side with exotropia. When questionable abnormalities on the pursuit and saccade tracings are noted in the patient with known strabismus, a diagnosis of central ocular-motor control abnormalities should be made cautiously.

Figure 4–15 demonstrates a condition called ocular-lateral pulsion, a key finding in Wallenberg's syndrome (Waespe & Wichmann, 1990). Shown are the traces obtained with the eyes open, when fixation was removed by turning the lights on and off. In both the upper and lower panels of horizontal eye movement, deviation to the left when visual fixation was

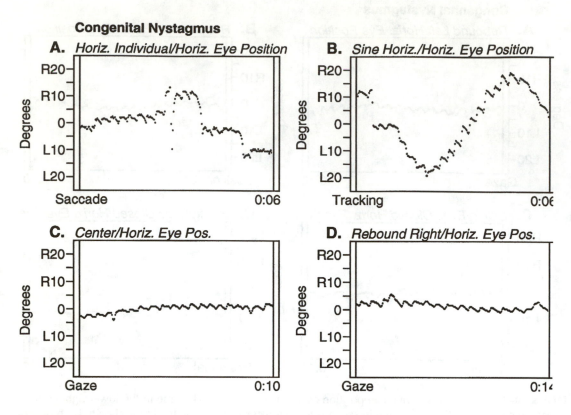

Congenital Nystagmus

A. *Horiz. Individual/Horiz. Eye Position*

Saccade   0:06

B. *Sine Horiz./Horiz. Eye Position*

Tracking   0:06

C. *Center/Horiz. Eye Pos.*

Gaze   0:10

D. *Rebound Right/Horiz. Eye Pos.*

Gaze   0:14

FIGURE 4–13. Plots of horizontal eye position in degrees as a function of time. The time in the lower right corner of each panel is the total elapse time in seconds for that recording, not the total time shown. Each panel represents 7 seconds of tracing. **A.** Sample of eye movements during individual eye saccade testing (right eye; see Chapter 5 for further information on test). **B.** Sample of trace during sinusoidal pursuit tracking task, conjugately recorded eye movements (see Chapter 5 for test details). **C.** Center gaze, eyes open. **D.** Gaze right by 37°, eyes open.

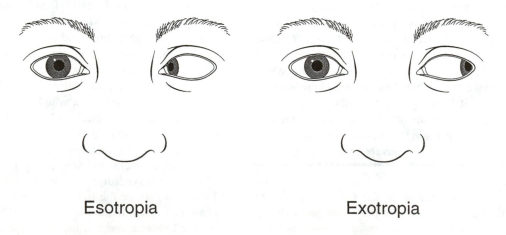

Esotropia   Exotropia

FIGURE 4–14. Two abnormal eye alignment conditions.

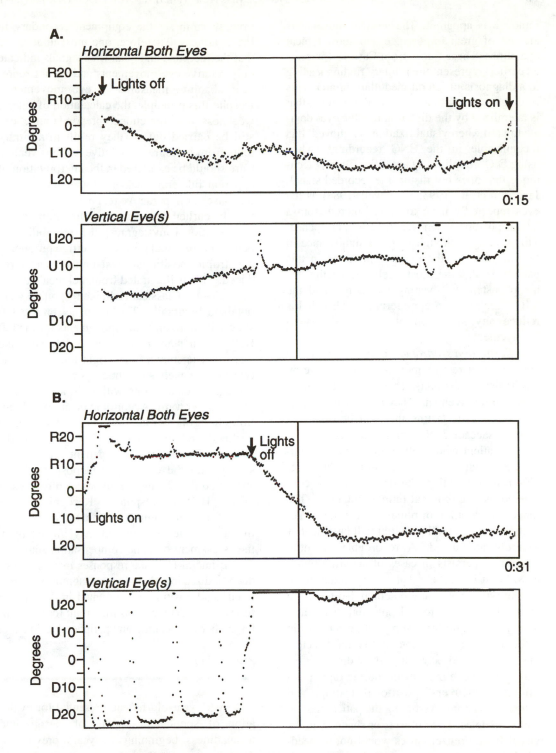

FIGURE 4–15. Plots of horizontal and vertical eye positions as a function of time. For both A and B, eyes are open and the arrows indicate times of lighted and darkened room. Part B is a continuation of the trace in part A. For both A and B, the patient is sitting, head straight.

removed is apparent. The vertical movements are not of great importance and show typical eye blinks. These traces from Case 17 (presented earlier) represent the primary finding leading to a diagnosis of lateral medullary infarct. This finding occurs with a lesion in the medulla that is lateralized by the direction that the eyes deviate toward when visual fixation is removed. It is recognizable in the ENG recordings (when using D.C. coupling, an amplifier filtering technique that does not distort the recorded signal; Jacobson et al., 1993; Stockwell, 1983) as the eyes repeatedly have to be recentered from a lateral position whenever the eyes are opened. This finding, although of great significance in the diagnosis of the brain stem lesion in this patient, is also the most likely explanation for his persistent left-beating nystagmus and the left directional preponderance. This helps reduce any suspicion of peripheral system involvement.

Restriction syndromes (Leigh & Zee, 1991) are those that restrict movements of the eye by mechanical constraints, as opposed to neuromuscular involvement. They produce abnormalities on saccade testing that will be discussed with the saccade evaluation in Chapter 5.

A patient who is blind often can be evaluated, even when there is little or no light recognition. In this setting, the first issue to be considered is the corneal-retinal potential. The longer the duration of blindness, the more likely the corneal-retinal potential will be absent or severely attenuated. A recordable potential sometimes persists in cases of acquired blindness, but it is unlikely that a congenitally blind patient will display any potential. To test for a recordable corneal-retinal potential, the examiner should begin the testing with electrodes in place. If a recordable potential is not detected, the patient could be evaluated by direct observation of the eye movements during rapid positioning maneuvers, positional testing, and caloric irrigations. Assuming the patient has no ability to detect large objects or shadows in the visual field, Frenzel lenses would not be needed. This is a situation where alternative recording techniques, such as video recording with an infrared camera system, could be most helpful. One additional problem is the inability to appro-

priately calibrate the equipment secondary to the blindness. Therefore, one must understand that the recorded and quantified signals indicate only relative eye movements and do not represent absolute measures of eye movements. Despite this principle, the calculation of caloric weakness and directional preponderance can still be carried out, as they result in arbitrary units from measures of relative responsiveness. Care should be exercised in the interpretation of apparent bilateral weakness (other than absent response) or hyperactive responses.

In earlier discussions of direction-changing positional nystagmus, the possibility of benign paroxysmal positional vertigo producing ageotropic positional nystagmus was introduced. This is illustrated from a clinical case in Figure 4–16. Classical Hallpike responses were obtained bilaterally. The top panel on the left shows the horizontal eye movements for the left Hallpike maneuver. The repeat left Hallpike maneuver is shown in the right top panel. The two lower panels show tracings recorded from static positional testing with right and left ears placed downward. Ageotropic positional direction-changing nystagmus is noted, which declined and disappeared within 30 seconds. Despite the fact that the patient was moved slowly into the ear-dependent positions, it is suspected that the nystagmus was a direct result of the Hallpike responses. Recognizing this cause for the nystagmus will not affect the identification of lesion site, but may impact upon the assessment of static compensation status.

Bilateral Hallpike responses may also produce a direction-changing nystagmus within a fixed head position, as presented in the case to follow. This distinction is important for differentiation between central and peripheral lesion site.

CASE 41

A 67-year-old female presented for evaluation of spontaneous spells of vertigo and unsteadiness beginning 12 years previously. They were currently occurring once per week, lasting 3 to 4 hours. She also reported daily motion-provoked symptoms, lasting several seconds after a rapid head movement.

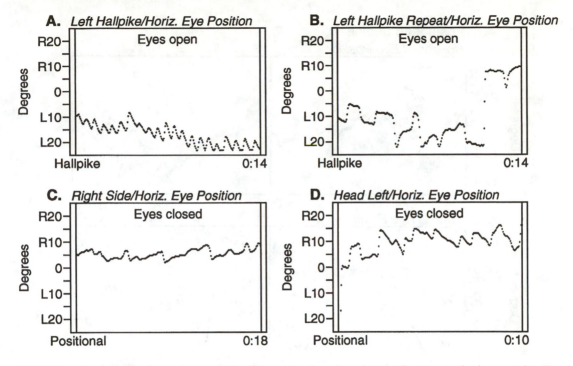

FIGURE 4–16. A–D. Horizontal eye position, plotted as function of time. The time in the lower right corner of each panel is the total elapse time in seconds for that recording, not the total time shown. Each panel represents 7 seconds of tracing. **A.** Sample of recording made during left Hallpike manuever, patient already in down position, eyes open. **B.** Repeat left Hallpike, eyes open. **C.** Right side laying (right decubitus position), eyes closed. **D.** Supine with head turned left, eyes closed.

ENG: Right-beating spontaneous nystagmus with slow-component eye velocity of 3–5°/sec and bilateral classic Hallpike responses were noted. The right-beating spontaneous nystagmus was apparent throughout the study; however, direction-changing nystagmus was noted in 3 positions, all without changes in the head position relative to gravity. Figure 4–17 shows an example of the right-beating spontaneous nystagmus in the supine position. Figure 4–18 demonstrates the direction-changing nystagmus, starting as left-beating, then changing to persistent right–beating within 6 seconds. This was also noted in the right lateral position and head hanging right position. There was no significant unilateral weakness, but a 38% right directional preponderance was obtained by caloric testing. Rotational chair results were suggestive of peripheral system involvement with a normal postural control assessment.

Ocular motor: The results were within the age-level normative data, not suggestive of central system involvement.

The interpretation dilemma for this patient involves the suggestion for a central system abnormality secondary to the direction-changing nystagmus within a given head position. The alert examiner will recognize that the direction-changing nystagmus might be explained by the positive Hallpike result with the right ear dependent, and that the response reduced in amplitude each time the patient was moved into the provocative positions. The left beats at the start of each trace resulted from the transient response to the right Hallpike position, followed by a return to the baseline right-beating nystagmus. This might have happened with the left ear dependent positions; however, it may not be as apparent, as the nystagmus would be consistently right-beating.

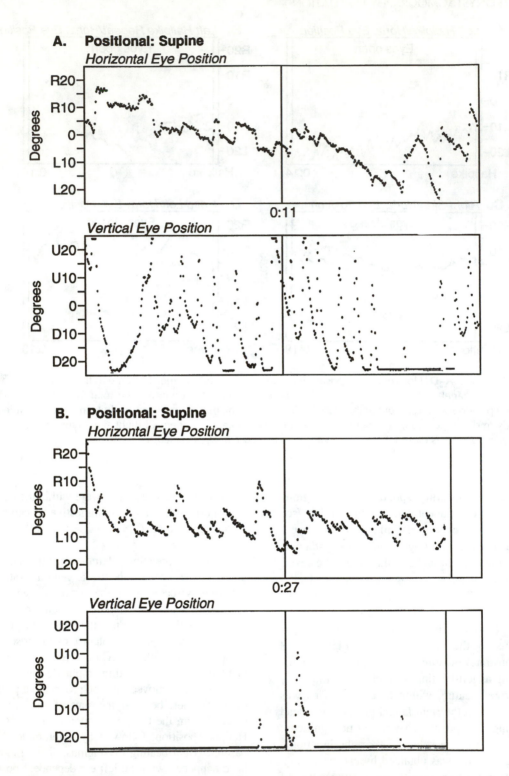

FIGURE 4–17. Plots of horizontal and vertical eye position as a function of time. In both A and B, patient is in the supine position, eyes closed. Part B is a continuation of trace from A.

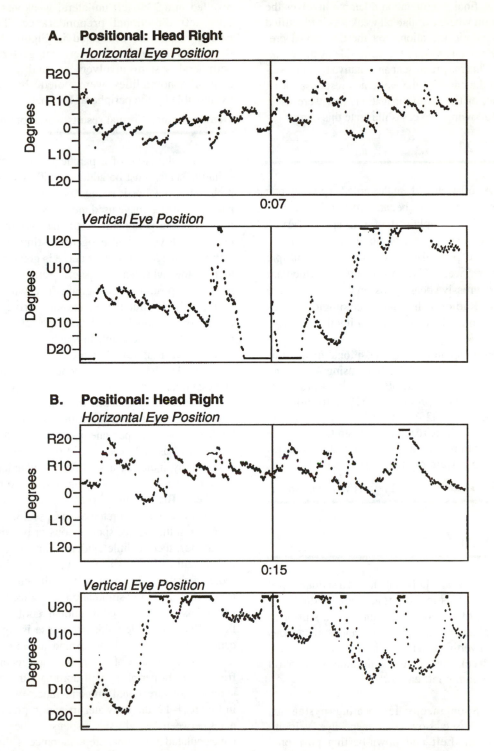

FIGURE 4–18. See Figure 4–17. Same patient with eyes closed throughout and in the supine position with head turned to the right. Part B is a continuation of part A.

A final interpretation dilemma involves the situation where a unilateral weakness is identified from caloric irrigations, yet the directional preponderance is toward the same side as the weakness. This may represent an irritative baseline status in the ear with the weakened response, or an artifact of the caloric irrigations that were used. The following two cases illustrate this contrast.

CASE 22

A 60-year-old male noted spontaneous spells of vertigo that began 4 years prior to evaluation. He complained of one spell every 6 months, lasting several hours. Brief motion-provoked spells also were experienced multiple times per week. Tinnitus, along with fluctuant and progressive hearing loss in the left ear, were noted. Radiographic and audiologic studies showed no evidence of central involvement.

ENG: No spontaneous or positional nystagmus was noted. Caloric irrigations using 40-second warm irrigations and 50 cc of ice water over 10–15 seconds, produced a 51% left unilateral weakness and 32% left directional preponderance. The caloric results are illustrated in Figure 4–19. Both rotational chair and postural control evaluations were normal.

Ocular Motor: Normal results were obtained.

CASE 23

A 55-year-old female noted a sudden onset of hearing loss in the left ear with gradual progression of the loss beginning 5 years prior to her evaluation. She reported recent, spontaneous spells of vertigo and nausea lasting 1 minute every 1 to 2 weeks, associated with tinnitus and aural fullness in the left ear.

ENG: Spontaneous left-beating nystagmus with 2–3°/sec slow-component eye velocity was noted. Left and down-beating positional nystagmus in 9 of 11 positions with 2–12°/sec slow-component eye velocity was also seen. Caloric irrigations using warm and ice water resulted in a 73% left unilateral weakness and 73% left directional preponderance. These caloric results are illustrated in Figure 4–20. Rotational chair results were suggestive of peripheral system involvement, and postural control abnormalities were noted that were explainable by the peripheral lesion.

Ocular motor: Normal results were obtained.

First, the issue of a paretic lesion with an irritative status must be addressed. This was the preliminary diagnostic suggestion in both of these patients. The language used indicates, in Case 23, that when the peripheral vestibular systems are not being driven by an exogenous stimulus, the activity of the left vestibular nerve is greater than that on the right, hence the left-beating spontaneous and positional nystagmus. Yet, when the peripheral vestibular systems are driven by caloric or rotational stimulation, the left is less responsive than the right, in spite of the higher tonic neural firing rate. In Case 23, this situation is reflected both by the spontaneous and positional nystagmus and by the directional preponderance obtained during caloric irrigation, showing a bias for left-beating nystagmus. On the other hand, there was no spontaneous or positional nystagmus in Case 22. The caloric result from that case clearly indicates a significant reduction in responsiveness for the left compared to the right periphery. The directional preponderance would, at face value, be interpreted as in Case 23. However, given the lack of spontaneous or positional nystagmus, there is little evidence for a true irritative status. Thus, an alternative explanation is more plausible. This results from the choice of asymmetrical caloric stimulation, using ice water irrigations instead of conventional cool irrigations. Because the left-sided response is significantly blunted for both warm and ice temperatures, the amplitude of the nystagmus recorded from the right periphery will dominate the measurement of directional preponderance. As seen in Figure 4–19, the ice water irrigation predominates between the right-side responses. Therefore, the calculated directional preponderance is almost certainly an artifact of the unequal temperatures selected for caloric stimulation. Certainly, this effect is also operative in Case 23, but a portion of

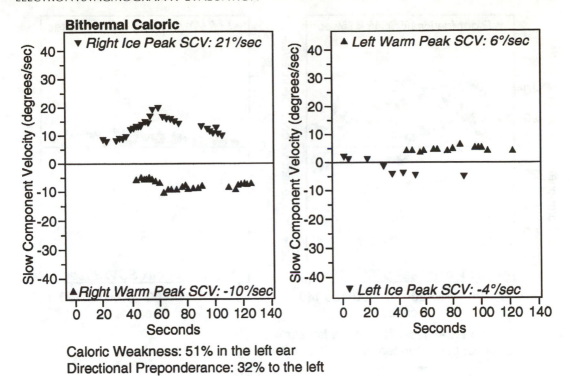

Caloric Weakness: 51% in the left ear
Directional Preponderance: 32% to the left

FIGURE 4–19. Caloric results from Case 22. Plots of slow-component eye velocity (SCV) from nystagmus provoked by open-loop water irrigations as a function of time. Each triangle represents one slow-component velocity movement of the eye from the nystagmus trace. Responses for the right ear are shown on the left, those for the left ear on the right. The orientation of the triangles represent either cool (30°C), ▼, or warm (44°C), ▲, irrigations. The plots are arranged so that right-beating nystagmus slow-component velocities are on the bottom (right warm, left cool) and left-beating nystagmus slow-component velocities are on the top (right cool, left warm). The velocity values given in top or bottom of each plot represents the average maximum slow-component velocity calculated for the nystagmus beats within the rectangle shown on each plot. These maximum, average slow-component velocity values were used to calculate the caloric weakness and directional preponderance values shown at the bottom of the figure. For purposes of calculations, rightward slow-component velocities are assigned a negative number, leftward are assigned a positive number.

the directional preponderance probably results from the irritative status. This is especially true given the response observed on the left, showing essentially only left-beating nystagmus for both warm and ice water. It is possible to estimate the effect of the unequal irrigation temperatures on the directional preponderance calculation in Case 23 by subtracting out the magnitude of the spontaneous left-beating nystagmus from the left warm and right ice water responses and adding it to the left ice and right warm responses. The amount to be subtracted and added can be derived from the left irrigation pods in Figure 4–20, suggesting the general level of left-beating nystagmus

during the caloric irrigations, approximately 8°/sec in this case. When the directional preponderance is recalculated, a value of 9% representing the effect of the unequal irrigation is left. Therefore, the majority of the directional preponderance for Case 23 is due to the ongoing spontaneous and positional left-beating nystagmus produced by the irritative status of the lesion, instead of the decision to use ice water stimulation. When the vestibular peripheries have equivalent responses within the normal range, the effect of unequal caloric irrigations is counterbalanced. This is not the case when one side is significantly weaker.

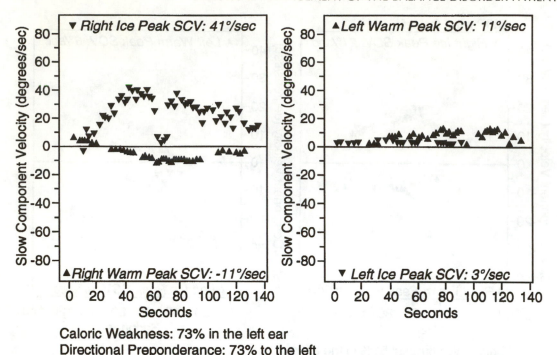

Caloric Weakness: 73% in the left ear
Directional Preponderance: 73% to the left

FIGURE 4–20. Caloric results from Case 23. Plots of slow-component eye velocity (SCV) from nystagmus provoked by open-loop water irrigations as a function of time. Each triangle represents one slow-component velocity movement of the eye from the nystagmus trace. Responses for the right ear are shown on the left, those for the left ear on the right. The orientation of the triangles represent either cool (30°C), ▼, or warm (44°C), ▲, irrigations. The plots are arranged so that right-beating nystagmus slow-component velocities are on the bottom (right warm, left cool) and left-beating nystagmus slow-component velocities are on the top (right cool, left warm). The velocity values given in top or bottom of each plot represents the average maximum slow-component velocity calculated for the nystagmus beats within the rectangle shown on each plot. These maximum, average slow-component velocity values were used to calculate the caloric weakness and directional preponderance values shown at the bottom of the figure. For purposes of calculations, rightward slow-component velocities are assigned a negative number, leftward are assigned a positive number.

CONCLUSIONS

Issues related to performance and interpretation of the ENG evaluation have been discussed to enhance the clinical utility of this study. Further examples of ENG results will be given in discussions of ocular-motor, rotary chair, and postural control assessment in the following chapters. The ENG, along with the ocular-motor evaluation, continues to be the mainstay of the laboratory evaluation of the chronic balance disorder patient. When performed carefully and interpreted with proper consideration given to the patient's clinical presentation, significant insights into the extent and site-of-lesion can be obtained. Although, this test itself does not result in a firm diagnostic conclusion, the findings can be of significant assistance in confirming a suspected diagnosis. In combination with rotational chair evaluation, a reasonably thorough assessment of the peripheral vestibular system can be accomplished.

■ OCULAR-MOTOR EVALUATION

*J*ust as the eyes serve as the window for investigating the function of the peripheral vestibular system, they provide a means to investigate the ocular-motor pathways in the brain stem and cerebellum that are required for the function of the vestibulo-ocular reflex. Eye movement studies also can be performed to examine the pathways that are involved with higher level function of saccades and initiation (within the first 100 msec) of smooth pursuit activities. A variety of testing paradigms can assist in identifying abnormalities in the central ocular-motor control system that may produce the patient's complaints. This portion of the evaluation is greatly enhanced by the use of computerized eye movement evaluation systems. The computerized systems allow for consistently repeatable stimuli and quantitative analysis of the output that would be difficult or impossible using a manual strip chart recorder. Use of a computerized evaluation system opens the opportunity to routinely use differing paradigms within a class of functional test activities such as saccades or pursuit tracking. With the enhanced evaluation ability comes an increased need for quantification of normative data for each of the various paradigms, as given in the discussion of age effects in Chapter 2 (see Figure 2–5). The principal reason to compare patient results with normative data is to reduce the number of false positive indications of central pathway involvement. The routine use of normative data and multiple test paradigms allows for a thorough investigation of the central pathways and the ability to improve the interpretation of results. This may permit stronger diagnostic conclusions regarding findings that in isolation are nonlocalizing regarding site of lesion, such as spontaneous and positional nystagmus.

What is the anatomical distinction between the central and peripheral vestibular system? Traditionally, structures lateral to the brain stem, specifically the VIIIth cranial nerve and the labyrinth, have been said to constitute the peripheral portion of the system. As was shown in Case 17 from Chapter 4, a brain stem lesion might produce findings identical to those produced by labyrinthine pathology. In that example, other disruptions in the ocular-motor function were noted, allowing the interpretation of central system involvement. This may not always be the case. Recognition that a brain stem or cerebellar lesion can produce results similar to labyrinthine lesions adds to the need for a thorough central ocular-motor evaluation (Francis, Bronstein, Rudge, & du Boulay, 1992; Magnusson & Norrving, 1993). Normal ocular-motor results, especially when coupled with signs or symptoms related to the auditory system, provide a strong case for pathology originating from the labyrinth.

The interested reader is referred to other sources for general methods of test administration and interpretation (Baloh & Honrubia, 1990; Barber & Stockwell, 1980; Hain, 1993a, 1993b; Leigh & Zee, 1991). This chapter will focus on the interpretation of the results from various test paradigms, the test options, and their usefulness. The information to be provided originates primarily from Hain (1993b), Baloh and Honrubia (1990), and Leigh and Zee (1993) together with work from our own laboratory.

The clinical utility of the oculomotor tests is improved by exploiting the redundancy in the diagnostic tools. An example would be the case where smooth pursuit tracking abnormalities suggest cerebellar involvement. This impression may be supported by abnormalities in the accuracy of saccade movements, also a suggestion of cerebellar involvement. Although this type of finding may be quite helpful, the complexity and redundancy of central system pathways makes definitive localization with any single test or combination of evaluations difficult. Therefore, any lesion sites suggested by abnormalities on different ocular-motor tests are just that, suggestions.

A general principle in the administration of the ocular-motor test battery is to repeat trials for a given test until maximum performance is achieved from the patient. The rationale for this suggestion results from the fact that the tasks required in these tests are novel, and repeated attempts may bring performance from an abnormal range to a normal level. This is especially true for the tests of smooth pursuit. When using a computerized system, the tests for smooth pursuit are more difficult than with a manual swinging target, because the target frequency and peak velocity are typically increased as part of the paradigm. Figure 5–1 demonstrates the improvement in performance in a 44-year-old female. The smooth pursuit analysis in Figure 5–1A suggests abnormal performance with a target frequency above 0.5 Hz for leftward eye movements. However, upon reinstruction and repeat testing, the patient was able to improve performance into the normal range for her age (Figure 5–1B).

VISUAL FIXATION

Paradigm

Typically the patient is asked to visualize a stationary target 1–1.5 meters away, and attempt to maintain fixed gaze. The target is initially in the primary position and then moved into horizontally and vertically eccentric locations. The eccentric gazes should be performed between a 35 and 40° subtended arc. In general, the eyes are observed for 20–30 seconds for the presence of nystagmus during the task. The test paradigm and analysis are essentially the same whether using a manual or computerized recording system.

Analysis

The analysis can be as simple as noting whether nystagmus is present or absent. Measurement of the slow-component velocity of the nystagmus could certainly be performed, but is not usually included in the formal analysis. It is not unusual to see nystagmus at the beginning of a lateral gaze trial that dies away within a 5-second interval. This is physiologic end-point nystagmus, a normal phenomenon as the eye settles in an extreme position of gaze. The key to its recognition is that it does not persist. In a case with persistent gaze nystagmus, the nature of the slow-component eye velocity trace can be important, but difficult to recognize. In such a case, one wishes to determine whether the slow-component eye velocity is linear versus exponentially increasing or decreasing. To make such a judgment from the slow-component trace requires a DC-coupled recording system as opposed to an AC-coupled system. DC coupling is more easily achieved with a computerized system. The distortion of the trace in Figure 5–2A, derived from an AC-coupled system, makes the detailed description of slow-component velocity difficult. Figure 5–2B shows the superior quality eye trace for deviation to the right using a DC-coupled system. In an AC-coupled system, the examiner must make a distinction between a linear decline in the slow-

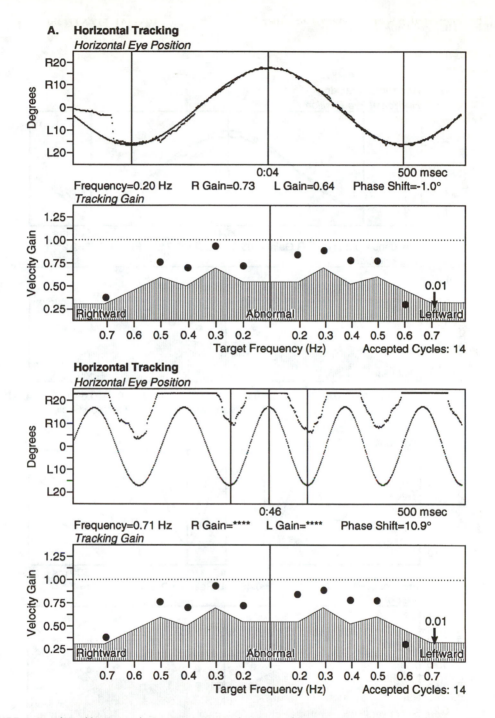

FIGURE 5–1. Plot of horizontal eye position as a function of time (500 msec time mark shown) for sinusoidal tracking (dotted trace). In the same plot (smooth line) the target position in degrees as a function of time is given. The panel below the eye and target position plots gives the value of velocity gain as a function of frequency of target movement. The shaded region represents abnormal performance. For both A and B the traces at the top are for a target frequency of 0.2Hz and at the bottom for 0.71 Hz. Part A represents the first attempt at the testing, with part B a retest. *(continued)*

FIGURE 5–1B. *(continued)*

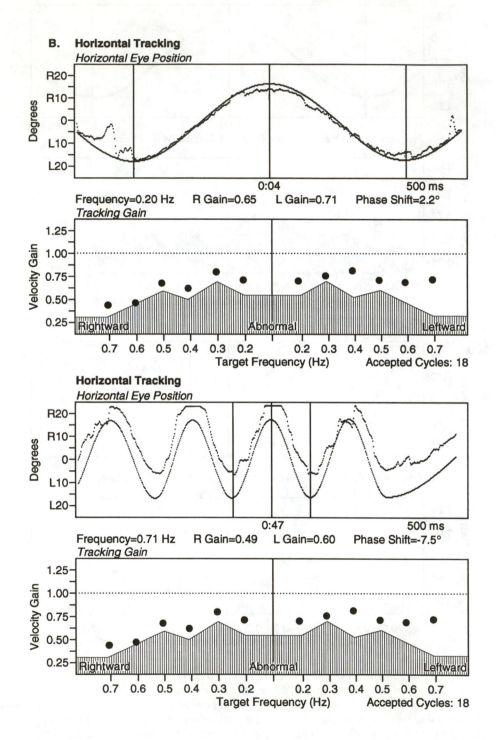

B. **Horizontal Tracking**

Horizontal Eye Position

Frequency=0.20 Hz   R Gain=0.65   L Gain=0.71   Phase Shift=2.2°

Tracking Gain

Target Frequency (Hz)   Accepted Cycles: 18

Horizontal Tracking

Horizontal Eye Position

Frequency=0.71 Hz   R Gain=0.49   L Gain=0.60   Phase Shift=-7.5°

Tracking Gain

Target Frequency (Hz)   Accepted Cycles: 18

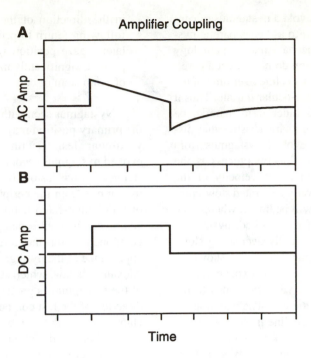

FIGURE 5–2. Schematic of horizontal eye position with amplitude of movement (amp) in degrees as a function of time. **A.** Shows the effect of AC amplifier coupling for a fixed gaze to the right. **B.** Shows the gaze to the right with a DC amplifier coupling.

component eye velocity from the recording system (Figure 5–2A) and one that shows a pathologic decreasing (Figure 3–2A, Chapter 3) or increasing velocity (Figure 4–13, Chapter 4). Further, if the change in slow-component eye velocity is linear (straight line), the distinction between a rate of change (slope of the line) accounted for by the AC coupling versus a true abnormality of eye drift is required. The two conditions that would most likely produce exponential changes in the slow-component velocity shown in Figures 3–2A and 4–13 are gaze-evoked nystagmus of central origin and congenital nystagmus, respectively. In congenital nystagmus, the slow-component velocity shows the increasing velocity pattern illustrated in Figure 4–13 (upper left panel). This helps to distinguish this disorder from other pathological processes that produce gaze-evoked nystagmus of central or peripheral origin. Although congenital nystagmus may originate in the brain stem, it can be thought of as "noise" that inter-

feres with the evaluation of a balance disorder patient, especially during the examination of ocular motor function. Several distinct characteristics suggest a congenital basis for gaze nystagmus. These features include:

1. A history of other individuals noticing persistent eye movements throughout the patient's life
2. Horizontal nystagmus only, in all positions of horizontal or vertical gaze
3. Ability to identify a point that is a few degrees eccentric to primary gaze position where the nystagmus is significantly reduced or completely suppressed
4. The nystagmus is suppressed or reduced with convergence movement of the eyes.

Gaze-evoked nystagmus can be either central or peripheral in origin. It usually signals a central lesion, but the possibility of peripheral involvement should not be overlooked. In the older literature, gaze-evoked nystagmus of central origin was referred to as "gaze paretic nystagmus." Yet, the mechanisms of pathology underlying this condition do not reflect a paretic process, but instead a decline over time of the neural signal to the extra-ocular muscle. Thus it is suggested that this older term, paretic, be abandoned. One of the characteristics that distinguish central gaze-evoked nystagmus from that generated by a peripheral process is the form of the slow-component velocity of the nystagmus. A peripherally generated slow-component velocity trace will be linear, whereas the centrally generated gaze evoked nystagmus often shows an exponentially decreasing slow-component velocity trace, like that shown in Figure 3–2A, in Chapter 3. The explanation for this slowing of the eye velocity relates to the ballistic properties of the eye. The pathological process causes a slow decline in the neural signal being delivered to the extra-ocular muscles of the eye that are holding the eyes in their eccentric position. As the strength of the neural signal is reduced, the strength of the muscle contraction is proportionally diminished. This allows the elastic forces from the connective tissues that stabilize the globe in the orbit to pull the eyes back toward their neutral (primary) position. As with a rubber band, the magnitude of these elastic forces is greatest when the eyes are at their most eccentric position, and they decrease as the eyes move closer to the primary position. This results in an exponential decrease in slow-component velocity. The other characteristics that help distinguish between gaze-evoked nystagmus of central versus peripheral origin are:

1. It is less likely that gaze-evoked nystagmus of central origin will be noted in primary position
2. Nystagmus of central origin demonstrates greater or equal slow-component velocity with visual fixation compared to a nonfixation condition, whereas the velocity is significantly reduced with visual fixation in gaze evoked nystagmus of peripheral origin
3. The presence of rebound nystagmus (transient nystagmus where the fast component is

in the direction of the last eye movement) following return to primary position from a lateral gaze position where nystagmus was present, significantly increases the likelihood of brain stem or cerebellar involvement.

Nystagmus seen with eccentric gaze and in the primary position may be due to a peripheral vestibular lesion with superimposed gaze-evoked nystagmus secondary to a primary brain stem/cerebellar lesion. It is most likely that the nystagmus from the peripheral lesion would be of a direction-fixed nature whereas that of the central origin would change direction of the fast component with the direction of gaze. The appearance of the nystagmus would then follow Alexander's law, which states that the intensity of the nystagmus is greatest when gazing in the direction of the fast component (Robinson, Zee, Hain, Holmes, & Rosenberg, 1986). This would occur when the direction of the fast component from the peripheral lesion was the same as that from the central lesion. It may be possible to recognize decreasing slow-component eye velocity with the eccentric gaze, yet not in the primary position or in the position gazing away from the fast component of the peripheral lesion. When the nystagmus is direction-fixed (always beating in the same direction), it may be characterized as either 1st, 2nd, or 3rd degree. If seen only in one position of lateral gaze then it is called 1st degree; if seen in lateral gaze and in primary position, then it is called 2nd degree; and if seen in primary and both lateral gaze positions, it is called 3rd degree. If 2nd or 3rd degree nystagmus is present and it follows Alexander's law, the examiner must be suspicious of possible mixed peripheral and central origins. An example could be a peripheral vestibular lesion from an acute insult, most probably on the side away from the fast component, together with gaze-evoked nystagmus that could be of central origin, especially if other characteristics listed above are noted. This could occur with a large (greater than 2 cm) cerebellar-pontine angle mass lesion like a vestibular schwannoma. The compression effect on the brain stem would be responsible for the gaze-evoked nystagmus of central origin, while the resulting insult to the labyrinth would cause the direction-fixed nystagmus of peripheral origin. If this lesion was on the right side, then left-beating nystagmus may be present from the peripheral component, with left beating on gaze left and right beating on gaze right from the brain stem component. Therefore, when the patient was in primary gaze, left-beating nystagmus is seen; and in gaze left, a stronger left-beating nystagmus would be noted. On gaze right, right beating could be observed if the centrally generated nystagmus was stronger than the peripherally generated component, second degree left beating. The opposite could also be seen if the peripherally generated component was the stronger, third degree left beat.

Saccade intrusions are another type of eye movements that can suggest central vestibular system involvement. They may be noted during fixation in the primary position or eccentric positions of gaze. These and other gaze nystagmus abnormalities are summarized in Table 5–1. The significance of the saccade intrusions must be tempered by acknowledgment of the age of the patient, as with many other oculomotor results. Guidelines for the number of intrusions per minute that would be clinically significant are given in Table 5–1 (Leigh & Zee, 1991). The different types of saccade intrusions listed in the table have implications for possible sites of pathology. Experience suggests that square-wave jerks are those seen most frequently. They have been strongly associated with a well-defined degenerative disorder of the cerebellum, Friedreich's Ataxia (see Figure 5–3). The other forms are less common and less specific.

TABLE 5–1. Abnormalities of Fixation

■ Lack of visual suppression of nystagmus generated by caloric irrigation or rotational stimulation. Associated with smooth pursuit abnormalities—suggestive of brain stem/cerebellar involvement.

■ Congenital nystagmus—while of brain stem/cerebellar origin, it represents a "noise" interference in analysis of ENG and rotational chair evaluations.

■ Gaze-Evoked Nystagmus

 ■ Central origin—suggestive of brain stem/cerebellar involvement.

 ■ Peripheral origin—(a) when an acute labyrinthine or vestibular nerve lesion produces nystagmus of such strength that visual fixation suppression is unable to eliminate it until central compensation progresses; (b) in a patient with a fluctuating peripheral lesion during or shortly following a spell of vertigo; (c) combination of peripheral and central lesion, causing failure of fixation suppression; or (d) presence of torsional nystagmus in a complete peripheral lesion with incomplete compensation.

■ Rebound Nystagmus—Increases the likelihood of brain stem/cerebellar involvement suggested by gaze-evoked nystagmus.

■ Saccade Intrusions

 ■ Square-wave jerks—0.5–5° subtended arc movement in one direction away from point of fixation, with intersaccade intervals. Abnormal if: (a) > 5/min for those under 50 years of age; (b) > 25–30/min for those over 65 years of age. Suggestive of cerebellar involvement.

 ■ Macro square-wave jerks—5–15° subtended arc movement in one direction away from the point of fixation, with intersaccade intervals. Suggestive of brain stem/cerebellar involvement.

 ■ Macro saccadic oscillations—eyes moving in both directions around a fixation point with intersaccade interval. Suggestive of cerebellar involvement (dorsal vermis and fastigial nucleus).

 ■ Ocular flutter—bursts (typically 2–5 seconds in length) of eye movement in horizontal or horizontal and vertical dimensions, in both directions away from the point of fixation without intersaccade intervals. Suggestive of brain stem involvement.

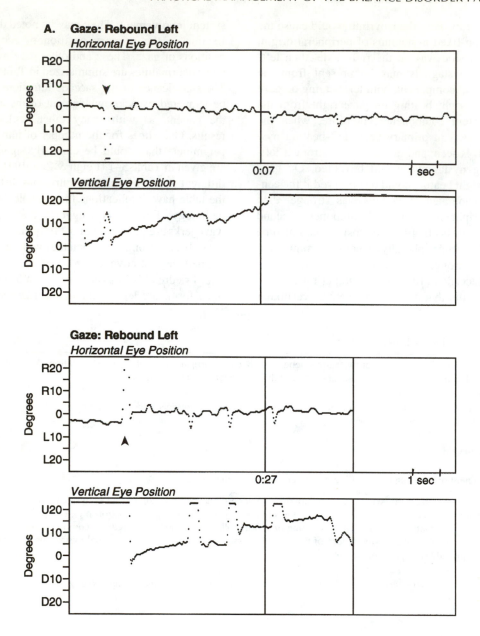

FIGURE 5–3. Plots of horizontal and vertical eye position in degrees as a function of time. **A.** Patient gazes left by 37° (at first arrow) and holds that eye position, returning to the center at the second arrow. The trace is electronically recentered for ease in viewing. **B.** Same patient now gazing to the right by 37° and then back to the center at the arrows.

Recognition of saccade intrusions with eyes open is the important finding in identifying central pathology. Saccade intrusions noted only when the eyes are closed usually indicates a high level of anxiety about the test conditions.

The characteristics of nystagmus observed by direct visualization of the eyes is important in determining the structures involved in producing the abnormal eye movements. Purely torsional or vertical nystagmus would be rarely,

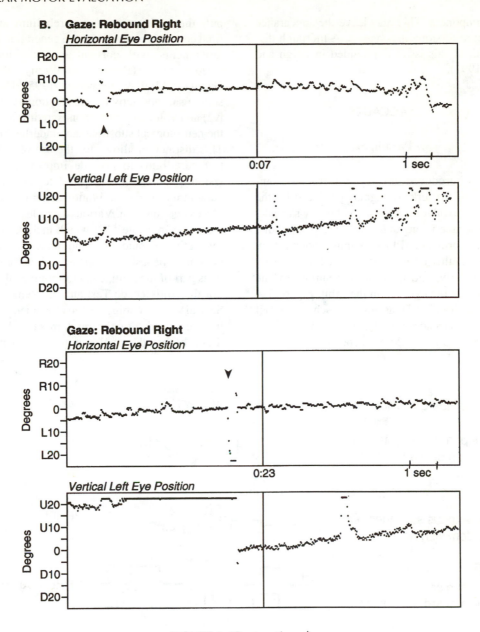

FIGURE 5–3B. *(continued)*

if ever, caused by peripheral system abnormalities alone. Although theoretically possible, such a finding would require extremely unusual lesions, such as damage to both superior canals to produce pure vertical down-beating nystagmus. Pure counterclockwise nystagmus would require a lesion in both the superior and posterior semicircular canals in the right ear, with the horizontal canal spared. One exception is that a pure torsional situation may occasionally be seen after a unilateral lesion affecting the entire vestibular periphery. Although these lesions would typically produce a nystagmus with both horizontal and torsional components, as central compensation proceeds, visual suppression of the nystagmus is far more effective for the linear component. This may leave the appearance of a pure torsional nystagmus. A thorough discussion of this issue is provided in Leigh and Zee (1991).

SACCADES

Paradigms

As introduced in Chapter 1, the fast component of the jerk nystagmus produced by the vestibulo-ocular reflex is a reactionary saccade. This saccade is engendered by the parapontine reticular formation (PPRF) within the brain stem. However, this is only the lowest level of saccade activity, and is stimulated simply by the position of the eye within the orbit. Figure 5–4 shows a simplified classification scheme for all levels of saccade activity. Note that although the first two levels do not depend on visual in-

put, the brain stem and cerebellum are the final common pathway for the generation of eye movements, with cortical areas dividing the various tasks (Pierrot-Deseilligny, Rivaud, Gaymard, Muri, & Vermersch, 1995). The division of saccade activity into reactionary (reflexive) and voluntary corresponds to differences in the neurological substrate that underlie the task. This distinction allows for the use of differing test paradigms to provide improved site-of-lesion information, compared to the standard paradigm of using calibration activities as a test of saccade function. Various saccade paradigms are given in Table 5–2, which includes entries for both computerized and noncomputerized systems. The last three are used in our laboratory as part of the routine oculo-motor evaluation. For the Antisaccade Test and the Remembered Saccade Tests, conjugate eye movement recordings are used. For the random saccade paradigm, both individual eye and conjugate eye

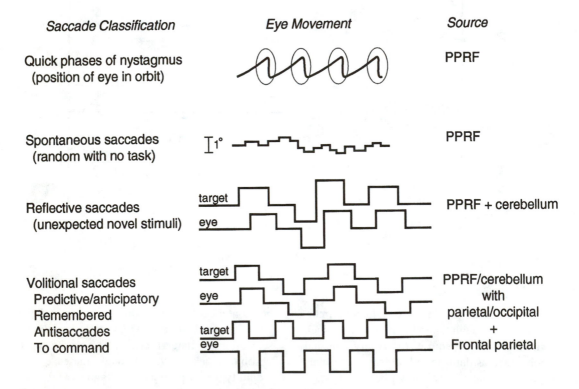

Saccade Classification	Eye Movement	Source
Quick phases of nystagmus (position of eye in orbit)		PPRF
Spontaneous saccades (random with no task)		PPRF
Reflective saccades (unexpected novel stimuli)	target / eye	PPRF + cerebellum
Volitional saccades / Predictive/anticipatory / Remembered / Antisaccades / To command	target / eye / target / eye	PPRF/cerebellum with parietal/occipital + Frontal parietal

FIGURE 5–4. Saccade organization chart showing the classification of the saccade, a sample of the eye position as a function of time plot, and the suggested primary source of origin in the central nervous system.

TABLE 5–2. Saccade Paradigms

■ Calibration Test
For use with noncomputerized systems

- Volitional/predictive saccades of 10–20° jump to right and left of center

- Analysis by accuracy

■ Random Saccade Test

- For use with computerized systems

- Typically, position of target randomized from 0–30° to the right or left of center—time of movement may also be randomized

- Reactionary saccades—analysis by accuracy, latency and velocity

■ Antisaccade Test
For use with either computerized or noncomputerized system

- Volitional/predictable 10–20° jump to the right and left of center

- Analysis by the ability to have eyes go in direction opposite the target suppressing the reactionary saccade

■ Remembered Saccade

- For use with computerized or noncomputerized system

- Volitional/predictable 10–20° jump to the right and left of center

- Analysis by ability to continue saccades for 3–5 eye movements after target is extinguished

---

movement recordings are made. Some commercially available computerized systems allow for the recording of individual eye movements using the standard lateral canthi electrodes and a center common electrode, instead of medial and lateral canthus electrodes for each eye. Although this electronic separation of the eyes does allow for individual eye recordings, it may introduce a bias in the recordings that will require obtaining normative data using the specific piece of equipment and the test paradigm in use to permit accurate interpretation of patient results (Smith-Wheelock et al., submitted). Clinically, the use of individual eye recordings allows for identification of eye muscle palsies and the specific condition of internuclear ophthalmoplegia. These conditions would be missed with only conjugate eye movement recordings. Although the prevalence of these disorders in the balance disorder population is small, it is important to recognize. The decision

to use individual eye recordings depends both on the equipment available and the nature of the referral population. Since normative data is so important for performing individual eye saccade testing, Table 5–3 provides these data for saccade velocity, latency, and accuracy. This data was collected using a paradigm that randomized the location of the target, with a fixed timing of the movement (Charter software; ICS, Inc.). Age did not seem to make a clinical difference in performance, even though there were statistical effects. Details of the data collection and the statistical analysis are given in the work by Smith-Wheelock et al. (submitted).

Analysis

When computerized evaluation is available, the analysis of saccade data from the Random Saccade Test involves three parameters that assist

TABLE 5–3. Normative Data for Individual Eye Saccade Recordings

Velocity in deg/sec for Use in a Main Sequence Plot

	10° amp.	15° amp.	20° amp.	25° amp.	30°amp.
Right eye Adduction	n = 64 373 204–540	n = 74 448 254–642	n = 24 493 312–672	n = 19 515 377–653	n = 6 546 323–767
Right eye Abduction	n = 73 294 174–414	n = 65 352 210–494	n = 35 380 210–550	n = 21 424 258–590	n = 6 448 294–602
Left eye Adduction	n = 61 369 201–537	n = 42 457 276–636	n = 35 459 273–645	n = 30 527 343–711	n = 13 578 406–750
Left eye Abduction	n = 99 284 150–418	n = 52 352 256–448	n = 24 378 236–520	n = 10 403 283–523	n = 7 435 294–574

The following data were developed from the ICS, Corp., Charter system. Shown in each cell is the number of saccade observations used, the mean and the 2 standard deviation range about the mean. All ages are grouped together for these data, as no significant effects of age were noted. For this task only the target position was randomized with timing fixed.

Accuracy in % with Latency in Milliseconds

	Accuracy	Latency
Right eye Adduction	n = 857 99 60–116	n = 1645 180 74–296
Right eye Abduction	n = 800 87 51–103	n = 1645 180 74–296
Left eye Adduction	n = 869 100 63–129	n = 1656 181 71–291
Left eye Abduction	n = 772 90 52–128	n = 1656 181 71–291

in localizing the lesion site. Figure 5–5 schematically illustrates the parameters of (a) saccade velocity ("main sequence plot," i.e., velocity as a function of eye displacement); (b) saccade accuracy; and (c) latency to onset of the saccade movement. For reactionary saccade tasks, like that performed by randomizing the target position, accuracy is felt to be determined by the posterior vermis region of the cerebellum, while velocity and latency are dominantly controlled by the parapontine reticular formation in the brain stem. If a noncomputerized system is used, only accuracy can be easily analyzed. Determining saccade velocity and latency without a computerized system requires exceptionally fast paper speed and extremely laborious calculations.

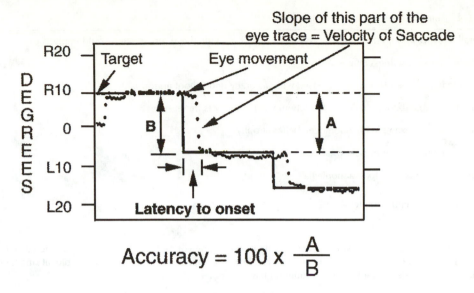

$$\text{Accuracy} = 100 \times \frac{A}{B}$$

FIGURE 5–5. Schematic of eye and target position in degrees, as a function of time demonstrating the calculations of velocity, latency, and accuracy of the saccade eye movement for analysis.

Abnormalities along with suggested lesion sites for the three parameters of the Random Saccade paradigm are listed in Tables 5–4 through 5–6. For the Remembered Saccade paradigm, the first 3–5 eye movements after extinguishing the light should approximate the eye movements seen when the predictable target was present. The result is abnormal, suggesting frontal/parietal (occipital) cortex pathology if the amplitude for the first few attempts is less than 50% of the expected value. The antisaccade paradigm is abnormal when the patient is unable to suppress the reactionary saccade and produce an eye movement in the opposite direction. This suggests frontal/parietal cortex pathology.

It has recently been determined that age and gender do not significantly impact the development of normative data for individual and conjugately recorded saccades using a randomized position paradigm (Smith-Wheelock et al., submitted). Figures 5–6, 5–7, and 5–8 show the normal data for individual and conjugate eye recordings for normal subjects ranging in age from 20–80 years, with approximately 10 subjects per decade.

SMOOTH PURSUIT

Paradigms

The two major paradigms for testing smooth pursuit involve stimuli that have either predictable or unpredictable trajectory. The use of a stimulus with an unpredictable trajectory may be helpful in evaluating various cortical areas involved in the "open loop response" of the tracking mechanism. This activity is limited to the first 100–150 msec following an unpredictable movement of the target. Software for the production and analysis of this paradigm is not, at present, commercially available and has to be developed by the local laboratory. Thus, clinical use of this test methodology is rare. The interested reader is referred to Leigh and Zee (1991) for details of this paradigm.

Most clinical testing of smooth pursuit uses a target with a predictable trajectory and analyzes performance in the "closed loop" format. In the closed loop format, there is an efference copy (an internal mapping of the target movement to occur based on past immediate movements of the eyes following the target) of

TABLE 5–4. Abnormalities of Saccade Velocity

■ Overall slowing in both directions by conjugate and/or individual eye recordings—could imply:

   ■ Medications/drowsiness/fatigue

   ■ Basal ganglia when latency is increased with accuracy undershoot abnormality

   ■ Brain stem (parapontine reticular formation) when latency is increased

   ■ Cerebellar, for example olivopontocerebellar atrophy

   ■ Oculomotor nerve or muscle weakness

   ■ Bilateral internuclear ophthalmoplegia

■ Abnormally fast—could imply:

   ■ Calibration errors

   ■ Restriction syndromes (mechanical condition limiting the range of motion of the eye but not the velocity; therefore, fast velocities for movements larger than can be made appear on the main sequence plot at smaller eye displacements where slower velocities would normally be noted)

■ Asymmetrical velocity—could imply:

   ■ Restriction syndromes

   ■ Internuclear ophthalmoplegia

---

the target movement that allows for the prediction of the target movement. If computerized equipment is used, the target is presented using an oscillatory movement on a light bar, with either a sinusoidal or fixed velocity pattern. When a sinusoidal pattern is presented, target frequency is typically the stimulus parameter that is varied, while the excursion distance of the target is consistent and the peak velocity changes as a consequence of the frequency selected. The frequency is typically varied from 0.2 Hz up to 1 Hz, depending on the manufacturer or the individual laboratory's program. This range of testing frequencies challenges the smooth pursuit system across a reasonable range of physiologic performance. Even though target frequency is used as the independent variable under study, the performance of this task is limited by the acceleration of the target. Therefore, the study is referred to as an acceleration limited paradigm. Alternatively, smooth pursuit testing may be performed with a target that moves at a fixed velocity. In fixed velocity paradigms, the target velocity is sequentially increased, varying from 20 to 100°/sec. The analysis is similar for both of these paradigms.

When noncomputerized equipment is used, one may employ either a manual pendulum producing a damped sinusoidal movement or a light bar with a target moving in a sinusoidal manner. Analysis options for these paradigms is quite limited. As discussed in Chapter 2, smooth pursuit is quite sensitive to the effects of advancing age. Normative data must be developed for comparison across age ranges, whether using computerized or noncomputerized equipment. This is certainly easier with computerized analysis, as most manufacturers provide some normative data with their smooth pursuit paradigms. It is wise to know the details of how that normative data was collected so that the user can realize the limits to its application. The data used for Figure 2–5 showing the effects of age and frequency on velocity gain and phase (Smith-Wheelock et al., submitted) are detailed for use as a normative data set in Table 5–7. The target frequencies, excursion, and associated peak velocities are also given in the table. This was again collected using the ICS, Inc. equipment and the Charter software (version 5.60).

TABLE 5–5. Abnormalities of Saccade Accuracy

■ Overshoot dysmetria—could imply:

- Cerebellar pontine angle pathological process (ipsilateral eye movements)

- Cerebellar (bilateral eye movements)

- Internuclear ophthalmoplegia (ipsilateral to medial longitudinal fasiculus lesion)

- Visual field deficits

■ Undershoot dysmetria—could imply:

- Cerebellar (bilateral eye movements)

- Basal ganglia when velocity is slowed and latency is increased

■ Glissades (eye velocity slows just prior to reaching the target and the eye gradually assumes the target position or steps with a small additional saccade)—could imply:

- Cerebellar (unilateral or bilateral)

- Muscle or nerve weakness

■ Ocular-lateral pulsion—could imply:

- Posterior inferior cerebellar artery (PICA) distribution involvement (ipsilateral-medullary syndrome)

■ Antisaccade abnormality—could imply:

- Frontoparietal cortex

■ Remembered saccade abnormality—could imply:

- Dominantly frontal (secondary parietal) cortex

TABLE 5–6. Abnormalities of Saccade Latency

■ Overall increased latency—could imply:

- Inattention/medication/drowsiness

- Basal ganglia when velocity is slowed and ocular dysmetria with undershoots present

- Brain stem (parapontine reticular formation) when velocity is reduced

- Seen with Parkinson's disease for volitional saccade tasks not reactionary

■ Asymmetrical latency—could imply:

- Parietal or occipital lobe involvement—for example with cerebral vascular accidents

Analysis

When analyzing data from a predictable trajectory paradigm, removal of the saccades prior to calculation of outcome measures is important, regardless of whether the target is in fixed velocity or sinusoidal motion. This allows for the outcome measures to represent smooth pursuit tracking performance and not total tracking performance, which includes the catch-up saccades needed to stay with the target. This principle applies to both computerized and noncomputer-

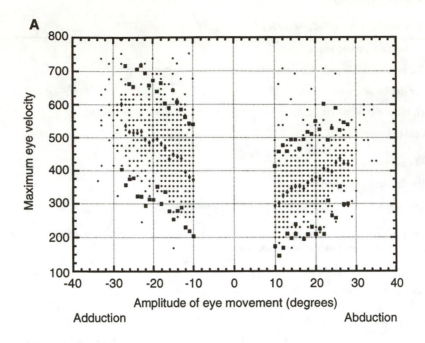

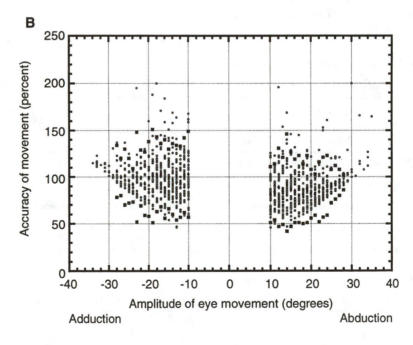

FIGURE 5–6. Scatterplot with means (◆) and 2 standard deviation limits (■) for normal subject performance on a random saccade task, horizontal eye movements. This is for the individually recorded right eye, using a lateral canthus electrode referenced to an electrode placed between the eyebrows. Each saccade parameter is plotted as a function of amplitude of eye movement. The number of saccades that made up the mean and standard deviations are given in Table 5–3. **A.** Saccade velocity plot. **B.** Saccade accuracy plot. **C.** Saccade latency plot.

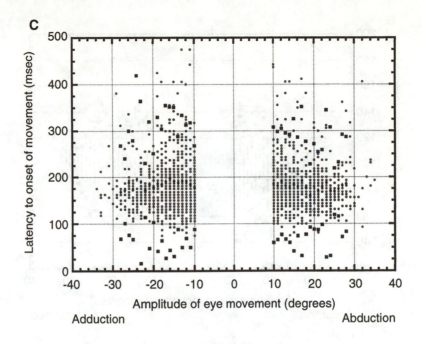

FIGURE 5–6C. *(continued)*

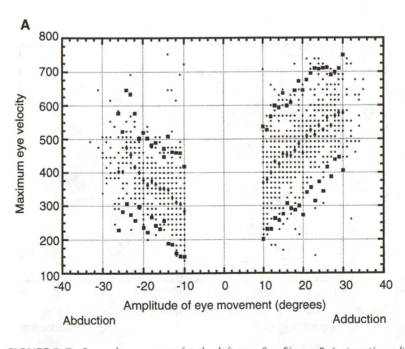

FIGURE 5–7. Saccade measures for the left eye. See Figure 5–6. *(continued)*

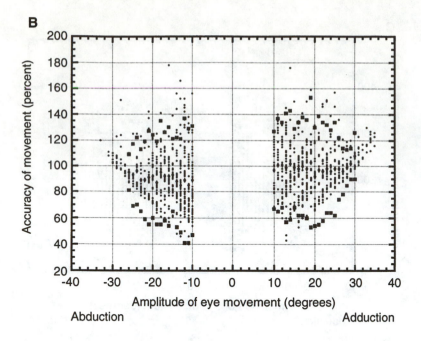

FIGURE 5–7B. *(continued)*

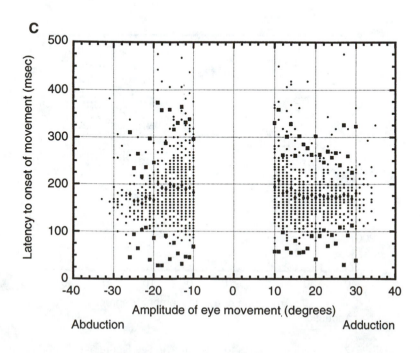

FIGURE 5–7C. *(continued)*

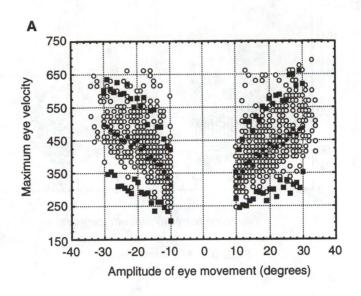

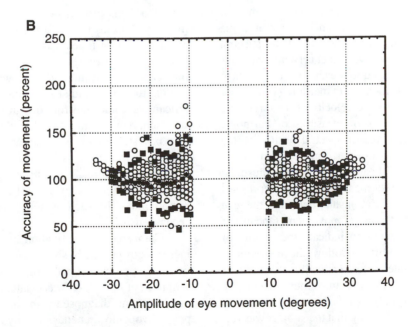

FIGURE 5–8. Saccade measures for conjugate eye recordings. See Figure 5–6. *(continued)*

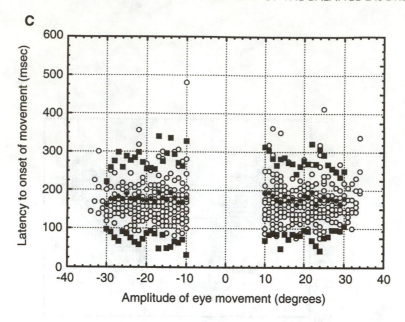

FIGURE 5–8C. *(continued)*

ized test systems. Computerized schemes of analysis allow easier assessment of the outcome parameters, utilizing a measure of the spectral purity of the eye movement (with saccades removed) referenced to the target. This can take the form of a velocity gain measure (velocity of the eye divided by the velocity of the target at a specific frequency), or measures of harmonic distortion. Measures of spectral purity are the principal indicators of performance for identification of potential pathology. For the sinusoidal paradigms, another measure is *phase*, representing the timing relationship between the eye movement and the target movement. One use of this measurement is to indicate the quality of the patient's ability to follow the instructions for the appointed task. Typically, it would be anticipated that the eye movement would lag behind the target (*phase lag*, usually a negative phase value), indicating that the subject was following the target as instructed. When subjects anticipate the target movement, which can degrade their performance, then a *phase lead* is noted. If the value of the phase lead or lag becomes too large, the patient is not performing the task appropriately and the data should not be analyzed. This problem can be overcome in a majority of cases by repeating instructions and retesting several times, assuming that the optimum performance best represents the patient's true capability. Some patients will persist in leading the target and simultaneously have significant saccadic interruptions in spite of reinstruction. Our opinion is that this represents their best strategy for tracking the target, as they perform extremely poorly if they attempt only to follow the target. This is probably not volitional, but a subconscious event controlling the performance. In such patients, analysis proceeds as usual.

Compared to gaze fixation and saccade testing, smooth pursuit is significantly more sensitive to the presence of pathology. Sensitivity performance of these tests was evaluated in a group of 134 patients diagnosed with multisystem atrophy, olivopontocerebellar atrophy, Friedreich's ataxia or multiple sclerosis. All had clearly defined brain stem/cerebellar lesions on MRI. Eighty-seven percent had evidence for central vestibulo-ocular pathway dysfunction on oculomotor testing, as indicated by abnormal performance on any single or combined test of gaze

TABLE 5–7. Normative Data for Conjugately Recorded Pursuit Tracking

Frequency	Peak Amplitude °	Velocity °/sec	Acceleration °/sec2
0.2	17.5	21.9	27.6
0.3	17.5	32.9	62.7
0.4	17.5	43.9	110.5
0.5	17.5	54.9	172.7
0.6	17.5	67.1	257.1
0.7	17.5	78.1	348.3

For the normative data shown below, the excursion of the stimulus remains constant across the frequencies tested. The subject is 4 feet from the light bar and the peak to peak excursion of the stimulus is 29 inches = 35° subtended arc movement. The parameters for amplitude, velocity, and acceleration of the target are given in each cell above.

Age 20–49 Years

	0.2	0.3	0.4	0.5	0.61	0.71
Gain L	0.82	0.84	0.82	0.83	0.72	0.71
	0.42–1.22	0.64–1.04	0.62–1.02	0.63–1.03	0.32–1.12	0.37–0.95
Gain R	0.85	0.84	0.87	0.82	0.78	0.73
	0.45–1.25	0.58–1.1	0.67–1.07	0.62–1.02	0.52–1.04	0.39–0.97
Phase	−0.36	−0.13	−0.25	−1.85	−2.36	−4.72
	−6.36–5.64	−4.13–3.87	−4.25–3.75	−7.85–4.15	−8.36–3.64	−12.72–3.2

Age 50–69 years

	0.2	0.3	0.4	0.5	0.61	0.71
Gain L	0.86	0.82	0.82	0.78	0.69	0.61
	0.56–1.16	0.60–1.04	0.58–1.06	0.50–1.06	0.39–0.99	0.27–0.95
Gain R	0.83	0.84	0.80	0.76	0.73	0.66
	0.53–1.13	0.56–1.12	0.56–1.04	0.40–1.12	0.43–1.03	0.32–1.00
Phase	−0.4	−0.79	−0.89	−2.38	−5.06	−7.89
	−6.40–5.60	−4.79–3.21	−4.89–3.11	−8.38–3.62	−13.06–2.9	−17.89–2.1

(continued)

fixation, saccades, and smooth pursuit measures. Smooth pursuit measures alone identified central system involvement in 73% of these cases, independent of results on saccade and fixation testing, compared with only 40% identified by saccade testing alone and 47% for fixation testing.

TABLE 5–7. (*continued*)

Age 70–79 years

	0.2	0.3	0.4	0.5	0.61	0.71
Gain L	0.90	0.82	0.75	0.7	0.63	0.48
	0.68–1.12	0.60–1.04	0.45–1.05	0.34–1.06	0.27–0.99	0.08–0.88
Gain R	0.87	0.85	0.8	0.7	0.68	0.5
	0.59–1.15	0.65–1.05	0.6–1.00	0.4–1.00	0.46–0.9	0.24–0.76
Phase	0.13	−0.01	−1.4	−2.32	−4.2	−3.7
	−3.87–4.13	−3.81–3.79	−6.8–4.0	−10.3–5.7	−11.4–3.0	−12.7–5.3

Age 80–89 years

	0.2	0.3	0.4	0.5	0.61	0.71
Gain L	0.77	0.81	0.76	0.7	0.61	0.6
	0.49–1.05	0.61–1.01	0.54–0.97	0.54–0.96	0.27–0.95	0.38–0.82
Gain R	0.83	0.8	0.71	0.61	0.63	0.6
	0.57–1.09	0.5–1.1	0.39–1.03	0.31–0.91	0.29–0.97	0.23–0.87
Phase	−0.49	−2.64	−2.3	−4.07	−7.8	−8.9
	−4.29–3.31	−12–6.8	−6.3–1.7	−14.1–5.9	−15.8–0.2	−20.9–3.1

Note: Each cell shows the mean and 2 standard deviation range for the frequency of test by age group for Velocity Gain for **L**eftward and **R**ightward eye movements and Phase. The age groupings were developed from statistical analysis showing differences in mean performance at the p < .05 level.

These tools also can suggest central nervous system involvement in patients without obvious structural abnormalities identified by MRI. As it is possible to have abnormal central system function without structural changes on neuroradiographic studies, it is difficult to provide overall sensitivity figures. Statistically, as normal values are typically based on two standard deviations from the mean performance, a small percentage of those with suspected central involvement will be false positives.

The data given above suggest a fairly reliable ability to identify brain stem and cerebellar lesions for the specific pathological processes listed. However, these 134 patients only represent 2% of over 6000 patients tested during the same 8-year period. The rate of suspicion for central system involvement using the three ocular-motor tests is significantly greater than 2% in our testing facility. In a review of 2266 patients seen over a 32-month period, 14% had abnormalities suggesting brain stem and/or cerebellar involvement without any indications for peripheral system involvement. The percentage of those suspect for central system involvement increased to 21% when combinations of peripheral and central system abnormalities were included. Therefore, since exact sensitivity and specificity performance figures cannot be determined, it seems best to employ test protocols that may reduce the false positive rate (increase specificity), yet without decreasing test sensitivity. The three crucial principles to assist in these goals are: (a) the use of computerized, quantitative analysis; (b) application of age-appropriate normative data comparisons;

and (c) repetition of initially abnormal test measures to obtain optimal performance.

Anatomic localization of a lesion identified by smooth pursuit testing is more difficult than with saccade testing. This results from the complexity and redundancy of the neurological substrates within the brain stem and cerebellar structures that comprise the smooth pursuit system. Therefore, once age, inattentiveness, central-acting medications, and congenital nystagmus have been ruled out as possible causes for disruptions to smooth pursuit, nonspecific dysfunction within the brain stem or cerebellum is implied, with more emphasis placed on vestibulo-cerebellar lesion site. In addition, it has been suggested that those patients with posterior cortical lesions, Alzheimer's disease, or schizophrenia perform more poorly on the acceleration-limited (sinusoidal) paradigms than on the velocity-limited (fixed velocity) paradigms.

OPTOKINETIC NYSTAGMUS

Paradigms

Optokinetic nystagmus is an involuntary oculomotor response to continuous motion in the visual field, as might be seen when observing the eyes of a child who is looking out the window of a moving train. Approximately 90% of the visual field must be filled with the target in order to achieve adequate retinal stimulation to produce true optokinetic nystagmus. Stimulation of the retinal fovea alone is insufficient. Therefore, testing of optokinetic nystagmus by use of a light bar or hand-held rotating drum does not provide true optokinetic stimulation and is really a smooth pursuit task. The eye movements that are achieved with the use of light bars resemble optokinetic nystagmus obtained with full field stimulation, but the nystagmus is obtained because of the rapid, repetitive nature of the target. Although stripes are the traditional stimulus, any repeating pattern that fills the visual field will produce the desired effect. The stimulus can be driven with a constant velocity both clockwise and counterclockwise, or it can be presented with a repeating sinusoidal pattern. Although the optokinetic response of nystagmus can be stimu-

lated with fixed or sinusoidal target speeds up to 100°/sec, the more effective comparisons of clockwise versus counterclockwise responses for fixed velocity stimulation fall between 20 and 60°/sec. In this range, a change in speed of the target typically will produce a similar change in the slow-component velocity of the nystagmus. Thus, the resulting calculated *gain* (velocity of the eye divided by the velocity of the target) remains nearly constant. Once target speeds exceed 60°/sec, the gain begins to deteriorate as target speed increases. This indicates that while the visual system is still responding, the increase in slow-component velocity of the eye is less than that of the target velocity. Only the fixed velocity target movement can be used to generate optokinetic afternystagmus (to be discussed in Chapter 6).

Of all the ocular-motor tasks discussed, this test can be affected most significantly by instructions. Ideally, the patient is gazing straight ahead and the targets are passing by, producing a small amplitude excursion of the eye. This is referred to as *stare nystagmus* and is felt to be produced by use of both retinal and foveal visual pathways. On the other hand, if a subject repeatedly fixates on a specific target and follows it to the limit of the eye excursion, then resets the eyes to mid position (a saccade movement), the task is a smooth pursuit activity. In this case, only the foveal system is stimulated, even though the visual field may be filled with the stimuli. This has been called *look nystagmus*. The ability to produce both types of nystagmus during optokinetic testing implies that the patient can selectively use either the optokinetic system (fovea plus retina) or just the foveal input system (smooth pursuit). This can be evaluated by alternating instructions to the patient. If the optokinetic system is to be evaluated, it is best to have the patients try to achieve stare nystagmus. For further discussion of this issue, the reader is referred to Stockwell (1983) and Honrubia et al. (1968).

Analysis

The current standard for analysis is to compare the gain of the optokinetic nystagmus for fixed velocity or sinusoidal target to the velocity gain from fixed or sinusoidal velocity smooth pursuit tasks, respectively. Assuming similar velocities of target movement, and the same frequency and peak velocity in the case of a sinusoidal target, the gains should be similar. Normative data should be developed by the individual laboratory for this comparison, given the variations on the paradigms and instructions that could be used.

The sensitivity of the optokinetic task for identifying central vestibulo-ocular pathway involvement is poorer than for pursuit testing. This loss of sensitivity probably results from the fact that true optokinetic tasks are a combination of both foveal and retinal system stimulation. The task is not nearly as sensitive as smooth pursuit testing to inattention, medication, or age. The examiner must remember that optokinetic testing results are influenced by the instructions provided and that the stimulus itself can be quite provocative with regard to nausea and vomiting. Therefore, fixed velocity optokinetic nystagmus testing is performed only if we are going to study optokinetic afternystagmus.

Optokinetic nystagmus can be used as a cross-check when a very poor smooth pursuit result is identified. In general, disordered smooth pursuit should be associated with reduced optokinetic gain as well. There are, however, situations where optokinetic nystagmus gain may be reduced symmetrically despite normal smooth pursuit function. One example is retinal disorders that may diminish the effectiveness of extra-foveal stimulation, such as retinitis pigmentosa. Disorders that slow saccade velocity without affecting smooth pursuit function will show a corresponding decrease in optokinetic gain. This finding may be seen in progressive supernuclear palsy, a degenerative disorder that involves saccade pathways prior to smooth pursuit. There is little clinical utility for the routine use of this test on all patients in its present form for site-of-lesion testing since the situations indicated above would typically be recognized via other abnormalities. It may be useful in a cross-check manner on a limited grouping of patients with other saccade and pursuit combinations such as that indicated above. Ongoing investigations into the actual production of optokinetic nystagmus may lead to other paradigms with either a site-of-lesion or functional application in the future.

CONCLUSIONS

In summary, it seems that proper identification of central vestibulo-ocular and ocular-motor pathway lesions requires integrated interpretation of multiple tests. These tests must be repeated often to ensure optimal performance for the individual patient to avoid false positive results. In addition, carefully developed normative data are required to distinguish normal from abnormal performance. When performed in a thorough and careful manner, oculomotor studies may allow for improved interpretation of abnormal findings produced by either peripheral or central vestibular system lesions.

6

■ ROTATIONAL CHAIR TESTING

CLINICAL UTILITY

As discussed in the first two chapters, the peripheral vestibular system functions across a range of intensity (acceleration) and frequency. Our ability to evaluate the range of physiologic function using an electronystagmography (ENG) evaluation is limited, given that the use of caloric irrigations stimulates the system in a manner equivalent to a frequency between 0.002 and 0.004 Hz and accelerations of less than $10°/sec^2$. These values are well below the level within which the vestibulo-ocular reflex generally functions in daily activities. Therefore, as discussed in Chapter 4, absent caloric responses should not be taken to imply completely absent peripheral vestibular function. An ENG also may demonstrate the presence of spontaneous and/or positional nystagmus, with caloric irrigations being well within normal limits. This finding typically indicates pathology within the peripheral system, as long as a thorough ocular-motor evaluation is normal. However, it is useful to have additional physiologic measures of peripheral system function that may add objective indications of normal or abnormal function, as well as expanding the ability to investigate the peripheral system beyond the very low frequency region. Lastly, because of the limitations intrinsic in ENG

testing, it is not surprising that a certain percentage of patients with symptoms of peripheral involvement have completely normal studies. Therefore, rotary chair testing has been used to expand the evaluation of the peripheral vestibular system. The utility of this test modality will be highlighted by presenting cases that illustrate each of the potential shortcomings of ENG as discussed above.

CASE 47

A 35-year-old female experienced a gradual onset of unsteadiness lasting for one month in 1989. An ENG had suggested bilateral mildly reduced responses to caloric irrigations, with slow-component velocities below 10°/sec for warm and cool stimuli. Her symptoms resolved spontaneously. A second similar event of unsteadiness lasting one month occurred in 1991. A repeat ENG showed the same findings with further reduction in caloric responses. A third event took place in the fall of 1994, yet the unsteadiness did not resolve as previously. An ENG at that time suggested caloric responses at 5°/sec for warm and cool irrigations. No ice water testing had been performed. Oscillopsia slowly began to progress by February 1995. At that time, all direct examinations, including neuro-ophthalmologic consultation, were normal. Testing in May 1995 documented unresponsiveness to warm, cool, or ice water irrigations. Rotational chair testing demonstrated no response for frequencies up to 0.16 Hz, with functional response returning to borderline normal range by 1.28 Hz. This finding, together with the ice water caloric testing, helped to document a severe bilateral peripheral system paresis. The results over time indicate a progressive bilateral loss of function, with discrete points of significant change. The use of rotational chair allowed for assessment of the extent of the paresis, which directly affected the vestibular rehabilitation program that was designed. It also sets a baseline to monitor for continued progression. No etiology has been identified for the bilateral loss of peripheral function. Use of chair testing from the onset may have provided better insight as to the progressive nature of this disorder and is appropriate in any situation suggesting bilaterally weak caloric responses.

CASE 20

This case was introduced in Chapter 4. The patient had a history and ENG suggestive of peripheral system involvement. The positive findings on the ENG were direction-fixed, right-beating positional nystagmus. Although clinically positive by the criteria discussed in Chapter 4, the positional nystagmus was seen in only a few positions and the slow-component velocity was modest. This finding alone would be considered only mildly positive for peripheral involvement. The patient's rotary chair results were strongly positive, with an abnormal time constant and asymmetry (both discussed in detail below). This finding, along with the positional nystagmus, provided a strong and consistent case for peripheral vestibular system involvement.

CASES 45 and 46

In both of these cases, the individuals had normal ocular-motor results with no indications of spontaneous or positional nystagmus.

Case 45: A 77-year-old female had symptoms of unsteadiness that began with an acute

vestibular crisis lasting continuously for 12 hours. The initially continuous unsteadiness resolved into intermittent bouts of unsteadiness provoked by head movement. She had been bothered by this symptom for several years. Audiometric testing indicated bilateral high-frequency sensorineural hearing loss, worse on the right than the left, with excellent speech discrimination bilaterally. She presented to the ENG with ventilation tubes with long shafts in place bilaterally, preventing use of closed-loop irrigation. (Air calorics could have been used.) The remainder of her ENG was normal.

Case 46: The symptoms of this 34-year-old female consisted of an initial spontaneous event of vertigo and nausea lasting five minutes, followed by several hours of persistent nausea in 1986. A second similar spontaneous event took place in 1988, this time lasting over four hours. In the 2 years prior to testing, she had experienced an additional 6–8 spontaneous events of vertigo with nausea lasting several hours. She was also experiencing motion-provoked vertigo lasting several seconds between her spontaneous events. Tinnitus and aural fullness were reported bilaterally, significantly worse on the left. She had normal hearing on the right, a high-frequency sensorineural hearing loss on the left, and 100% speech discrimination bilaterally. An auditory brainstem response test was normal. She was able to undergo caloric irrigations and responses were well within normal limits. She had a subjectively positive left Hallpike response, but no objective nystagmus and no spontaneous or positional nystagmus was appreciated.

Rotary chair findings: For both patients, the results of the ENG could neither support nor refute dysfunction within the peripheral vestibular system suggested by the presenting histories and normal ocular-motor findings. In both cases, rotary chair results gave strong indications of peripheral system involvement, with abnormal time constants and asymmetrical responses to the rotational stimuli. These objective findings supporting peripheral system involvement demonstrate the usefulness of the information obtained from rotary chair evaluation.

The review of 2266 patients introduced in Chapter 5 was also used to investigate the clinical utility of rotary chair testing in the evaluation of the peripheral vestibular system. Among this group of patients, 16% had completely normal ENG studies. Another 20% showed positional nystagmus as the sole ENG abnormality, suggesting peripheral system involvement. Additionally, 4% of the group had absent or severely reduced caloric responses using ice water irrigations. Among those with normal ENG results, rotary chair testing indicated abnormalities suggesting peripheral system pathology in 80% of the cases, 35% by phase abnormalities and 45% by asymmetry findings. Obviously, failure to test these patients with rotary chair would have led to an erroneous impression of normal vestibular function in a vast majority of symptomatic patients with normal ENG findings. When the patients with positional nystagmus alone were reviewed, greater than 80% again had abnormalities from rotary chair, supportive of peripheral system involvement, giving further evidence for peripheral dysfunction. In all cases of bilateral caloric weakness, the chair findings confirmed the bilateral reduction in peripheral system function. The test further defined the extent of the lesion as mild in half of these patients, and moderate to severe in the other half. This additional information plays an important role in designing a vestibular rehabilitation program for these patients. There are also patients who for reasons other than vestibular dysfunction (discussed in Chapter 4) have mildly reduced caloric responses. Of these patients, greater than 90% have normal rotary chair responses.

The figures provided thus far give the incidence of abnormal chair findings in a population of patients for whom the laboratory evaluations suggest peripheral system involvement. These values do not constitute performance measures of test sensitivity. As with the identification of central system involvement (see Chapter 5), an independent means of recognizing peripheral system involvement is needed to serve as the standard against which to evaluate test performance. Patients diagnosed by clinical presentation and hearing test results, independent of balance function test results, with Ménière's disease, labyrinthitis, or vestibular neuritis numbered 311 during the period of this study. Of this group, ENG was abnormal in 90%, suggesting a test sensitivity of this value. Rotary chair had a sensitivity suggesting peripheral system involvement of only 66%. However, it is important to note that the 66% of patients identified by chair testing did not completely overlap with those identified by ENG, as the combination of ENG and chair had a sensitivity of 100% in this group. Since there is no objective gold standard for identification of balance system lesions, there is currently no way to develop specificity figures, that is, the percentage of patients who do not have peripheral or central system abnormalities who will have normal test results.

From the above discussion, there appears to be good support for obtaining the adjunctive information available from total body, low-frequency rotary chair testing in the investigation of peripheral vestibular system function. Let us now turn our attention to the protocols used to perform this testing, and the means of analysis and interpretation.

PARADIGMS

Historical

The reader is referred to other literature for details of the routine paradigms (Baloh & Honrubia, 1990; Jacobson et al., 1993). The general format for the test paradigms will be briefly reviewed, along with special protocols for variations of the typical rotational chair evaluation.

It must be remembered that with total body rotational testing, the stimulus is being delivered to the head via movement of the whole body. Thus, the head must be secured to the chair with a restraint system. To make analysis as simple as possible, it is assumed that whenever the chair moves, the head is also making the same movement. Because of the potential for movement of the skin relative to the skull, this assumption becomes faulty at frequencies of 1 Hz or greater. Therefore, unless special restraint systems such as bite bars (not practical for routine clinical use), or systems for measuring the head movement independent of the chair are used, testing above 1 Hz will provide erroneous results. Because of this most commercial systems and clinical research have restricted test frequencies to 1 Hz or less.

Historically, a variety of stimuli have been used for total body rotation testing. In all cases, an attempt is made to provide frequency-specific information in a practical protocol that is comfortable for the patient. Attempts in the early 1900s used an impulse stimulus by sudden stoppage of the chair (Barany, 1907) to produce post-rotary nystagmus for characterizing the horizontal canal system. Expansions and im-provements on this stimulus system were eventually termed "cupulometry" (Van Egmond, Groen, & Jongkees, 1948). It was assumed that the plot of decay of post-rotary nystagmus as a function of time represented the activity of the cupula. As presented in the discussions in Chapters 1 and 2, the velocity storage integrator makes this assumption erroneous. A test popularized in France used a damped sinusoidal stimulus at a single frequency where the intensity of the stimulus was determined by the characteristic of the spring and the weight of the subject; this was called the "torsion swing test" (Van de Calseyde, Ampe, & Depondt, 1974). Over the years, the use of single frequency stimuli has continued and has been reported by some investigators to be the stimulus of choice (Cramer, Dowd, & Helms, 1963; Mathog, 1972). One drawback to the use of sinusoidal stimuli is the time it takes to test 4–6 individual frequencies. This is especially true when frequencies in the 0.01–0.08 Hz range are used, given the long time required to undergo a single cycle of movement. For example, at 0.01 Hz the period is 100 seconds. Therefore, attempts to shorten the testing time have involved rotating the patient with multiple frequencies, and then separating the responses associated with each of those frequencies by mathematical analysis following the testing. For this to be reliable, the system under study (peripheral vestibular system inputs, with central connections to eye movements as output) is assumed to be a linear, time invariant system.

This assumption is fairly valid if the frequency range and the speed of the chair are kept within certain constraints. The two most popular paradigms for this were the pseudo-random impulse testing and the sum of sines evaluation. The pseudorandom impulse paradigm used an impulse acceleration, rotating the patient to the right or the left for a fixed interval, then suddenly changing the direction as well as the level and duration of the acceleration. As with any impulse stimulus, the duration of the impulse governs the frequency content of the stimulus. Theoretically, this method was sound and allowed for a very short test, yet from a practical standpoint it was difficult to use, given the amount of noise in the human system (Wall, Black, & O'Leary, 1978). The sum of sines method used the sum of the sinusoidal stimuli, at the specific frequencies desired for testing (e.g., 0.01 + 0.02 + 0.04 + 0.08 + 0.16 + 0.32 Hz) (R. J. Peterka, personal communication, 1985) to produce the waveform that was used to drive the chair system. Again, mathematical analysis was used to separate the responses of the patient to the various frequencies applied. This method provided for less noise interference and a more gentle ride, as well as a short test. Although this method enjoyed more success, it has not been adopted by the manufacturers, possibly because of the complexity of the analysis. Therefore, this methodology has not been used except in clinics with the individual expertise to develop the necessary software. Out of the developmental work performed on the rotary chair, two paradigms have found repeated use in most clinical situations. These are the use of single sinusoidal testing at multiple frequencies and the use of step testing, a variation on the impulse response. For both of these paradigms, a main goal is to extract information that will allow for characterization of the peripheral system's time constant, overall responsiveness (gain), and any biases in the response.

Sinusoidal Protocol

The patient is seated in a chair driven by an electric torque motor under computer control. Typically the chair is within an enclosure that places the patient in total darkness, with no visual input even after adapting to the darkness (see Figure 6–1). This allows for testing of the vestibulo-ocular reflex where the influence of lid closure is removed. Recording of the eye movement is then performed indirectly via the electro-oculographic methods described in Chapter 4, or through the use of infrared camera

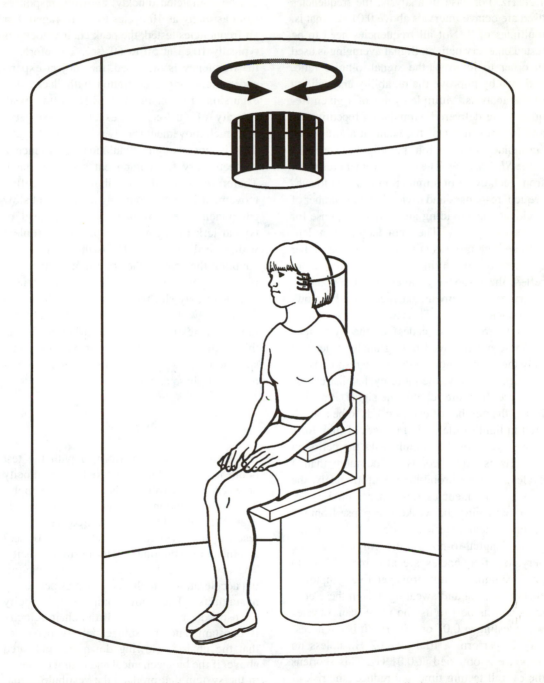

FIGURE 6–1. Generic rotational chair setup. The chair is on a comupter-controlled motor within an enclosure and can be rotated in either direction. A device for holding the head to the chair is shown. A means for producing optokinetic stimulation is shown as the drum in the ceiling.

or scleral coil eye movement recording techniques. Typically, starting with the lower frequencies, the chair is stimulated with sinusoidal wave forms at a specific frequency from 0.01 to 1.28 Hz. For ease in analysis, the frequencies used are octave intervals above 0.01 Hz, that is, multiples of 2. Not all frequencies need to be tested on every patient. Signal averaging is used in order to improve the signal-to-noise ratio, and thereby improve the reliability and validity of the analysis. Multiple cycles of a given frequency are delivered, stimulating repetitive to-and-fro movement of the chair in a *Sinusoidal Harmonic Acceleration* paradigm, hence the name *SHA testing*. The eye movement response from each cycle of stimulation is added to subsequent responses and divided by the number of cycles used, providing an average response for the test frequency. The frequency is then doubled and the process is repeated. As with other evaluations involving the vestibulo-ocular reflex, the response of interest is the compensatory eye movement, characterized by slow-component velocity. Therefore, the fast components (corrective saccades) of the nystagmus response are removed during analysis, leaving only the slow-component velocity responses for averaging. Ideally, the more cycles that can be averaged the more reliable the signal. Pragmatically, the number of cycles needs to be considered in light of the period (length of time for a single cycle) of the stimulus. As the period at 0.01 Hz is 100 seconds, to do more than 3 cycles becomes prohibitive. Unfortunately, the very low frequencies (less than 0.08 Hz) are those producing the weakest response from the vestibulo-ocular reflex system, therefore the poorest signal-to-noise ratio. In general, the very low frequencies are also most likely to produce unpleasant neurovegetative symptoms, such as nausea and sweating. Given these constraints, it is best to use no more than 3 cycles when testing at 0.01 or 0.02 Hz. It is not necessary to perform a trial at 0.02 Hz unless no response is obtained at 0.01 Hz. This shortens the overall testing time and reduces the risk of significant nausea. Our protocol actually begins with 0.08 Hz, then the frequency is reduced in octave steps to 0.01 Hz. Testing then proceeds

from 0.16 Hz up to 1.28 Hz. Using such a protocol produces better responses and significantly reduces the stimulation of unpleasant symptoms. The frequencies from 0.16 Hz and above can be completed quickly, allowing responses from as many as 10 cycles to be averaged. For all frequencies tested, the peak chair velocity is typically fixed at 50 to 60°/sec. Therefore, as the frequency is increased, the subject experiences increasing acceleration with decreasing excursion of the chair. At 1.28 Hz, with a peak velocity of 50°/sec, the excursion associated with each movement is only 6.2° per half cycle. This is not enough stimulation to produce a compensatory fast-component eye movement. Therefore, only the vestibulo-ocular reflex movement is seen, producing a sinusoidal slow component eye movement pattern instead of typical jerk nystagmus. The principal problem with recording at 1.28 Hz is the difficulty in coupling the head to the chair in a manner that is stable yet still comfortable for the patient. The head may slip relative to the chair due to the intensity of the movements produced by the rapid changes in chair motion when testing at this frequency. This problem can be detected by specific response patterns in the outcome parameters of phase and gain.

Step Test

This protocol is performed with the test booth in total darkness. A fixed chair velocity between 60 and 180°/sec is achieved by applying an acceleration impulse with a magnitude near 100°/sec². Once the desired velocity is reached, the acceleration is returned to 0°/sec² and the patient continues at the desired velocity. The vestibulo-ocular reflex response to the initial acceleration stimulus is known as per-rotary nystagmus. The slow-component velocity intensity decays over time if the chair velocity is constant, and the subject falsely perceives that the chair is slowing down. As indicated above, if the biomechanical and neural elements in the system that produce the vestibulo-ocular reflex were linear and time-invariant, the response to an acceleration impulse would give all the information needed to completely characterize the system. Although such linear, time-invariant assumptions are not completely accurate, they do approximate how the system functions. This allows us to utilize the decay in slow-component eye velocity over time to estimate the system's time constant, as defined in Chapter 2. After 45–60 seconds of fixed velocity rotation, a second impulse is applied to the chair. This is a deceleration step, usually of equal magnitude to the initial acceleration, bringing the chair to a rapid stop. Although the chair is now stationary, the subject will perceive motion in the opposite direction. The vestibulo-ocular reflex response will produce nystagmus beating in the direction opposite to that produced by the initial acceleration, known as post-rotary nystagmus. The decay of the slow-component eye velocity over time should be similar to that seen after the acceleration impulse and, ideally, both should give the same estimate of the system's time constant. The entire procedure is then repeated with the initial rotation in the opposite direction.

Although both ears are involved in responses to rotary stimuli, the right periphery (horizontal semicircular canal and superior vestibular nerve) is primarily responsible for responding to accelerations to the right or decelerations from fixed velocity rotation leftward. The reverse is true for the left labyrinth. Therefore, per- and post-rotary step tests also allow comparison of the time constant for dominant stimulation to one peripheral system.

The subject's alertness at the time of the impulses may significantly influence the magnitude of vestibulo-ocular reflex response. Averaging the data from multiple measures of per- or post-rotary slow-component velocity would improve test reliability by reducing the impact from anxiety or drowsiness during a single trial. Although this is a desirable goal, it would significantly lengthen the time required for the test. Occasionally, this test also produces symptoms of nausea and repeated impulses would significantly increase this unwanted effect.

Sinusoidal and step protocols can be used in the same patient to increase the utility of rotary chair testing. The discussion has centered on time constant estimates from the step test, but this protocol also gives some information about overall system responsiveness (gain) and bias (asymmetry) of the eye movement response. The step test data may thus help provide a cross check for test reliability between the two protocols, although no frequency-specific information can be acquired.

Other Protocols

A variety of other tests may be performed with the use of a rotary chair. These will be briefly defined before turning attention to analysis and interpretation of the sinusoidal and step tests.

Visual-Vestibular Interaction

The evaluation of visual-vestibular interaction usually consists of two subtests (Mizukoshi, Kobayashi, Ohashi, Shojaku, & Watanabe, 1985). The first tests the patient's ability to *suppress* the vestibulo-ocular reflex using a stationary visual input (relative to chair movement). The subject is rotated at a frequency between 0.08 and 0.32 Hz and is instructed to stare at an object approximately 2–3 feet away that is moving with the subject. This could be a projected light, such as a laser light in an otherwise dark environment, or a small incandescent light that is attached to and moves with the chair. The subject could even stare at his or her raised thumb or some other object in a fully lighted environment. The best situation is a single light in a dark environment, as a lighted environment presents some opportunity for unwanted optokinetic stimulation. The higher the frequency of rotation selected, the poorer the suppression of the vestibulo-ocular reflex will become.

The second test involves attempting to *enhance* the vestibulo-ocular reflex by sinusoidally rotating the subject at 0.04–0.16 Hz while simultaneously presenting a stationary (relative to the booth) optokinetic stimulus. In this case, the vestibulo-ocular reflex and the optokinetic nystagmus response are additive and produce an enhanced nystagmus response. Normative data should be developed for the particular protocols used in each laboratory.

Both of these tests primarily evaluate the function of the central vestibulo-ocular pathways. Failure of vestibulo-ocular reflex suppression using visual input usually correlates with gaze fixation and pursuit deficits suggestive of brain stem and/or cerebellar abnormalities. These subtests are not used in our facility as the primary source for documenting central system involvement, but can be a helpful cross check.

Optokinetic-Afternystagmus

When a motionless subject is provided with a full field optokinetic stimulus for approximately 1 minute, the optokinetic nystagmus should continue at a significantly reduced magnitude after the stimulus is extinguished if the subject remains in darkness. This persisting eye movement is called optokinetic-afternystagmus, and is a highly variable response (Fletcher, Hain, & Zee, 1990; Hain & Zee, 1991; Hain et al., 1994; Tijssen, Straathof, Hain, & Zee, 1989). It has been noted to show significant asymmetrical responses or severely reduced responses for clockwise and counterclockwise optokinetic stimuli in the presence of a significant unilateral or bilateral weakness, respectively. Another clinical implication is the suggested alteration of optokinetic-afternystagmus (significant increase in response to both clockwise and counterclockwise optokinetic stimuli) seen in individuals with mal de debarquement (disembarkment syndrome) (Hain, 1993b). This disorder is diagnosed when an individual returns to land after a sea voyage and continues to perceive the sensation of rocking or linear motion experienced on board ship for periods longer than several days (Brown & Baloh, 1987; Gordon, Spitzer, Doweck, Melaned, & Shupak, 1995; Murphy, 1993). This may persist for several weeks or months after the trip. Typically, other vestibular testing is negative.

High-Velocity Sinusoidal Testing

Following the principles of Ewald's second law, each semicircular canal displays a much greater range of response to stimulation versus inhibition. An increase in the peak chair (head) velocity to near 300°/sec may reveal an asymmetry in response that would be masked at a lower peak velocity due to adequate central

compensation for a peripheral lesion (Paige, 1989). It is this same theory that leads to use of the head-shaking nystagmus test and head-shaking Fukuda stepping test that were discussed in Chapter 3 as useful office procedures.

Off-Vertical-Axis-Rotation (OVAR)/Centrifuge Testing

Rotation of the subject in a manner that stimulates the otolithic organs independent of the semicircular canals may be used as a test of otolith function. OVAR is performed with the chair rotating at a constant velocity to eliminate eye movements from stimulation of the horizontal canal. The chair is then tilted so that the subject is as much as 30° off the earth-vertical axis. The axis of rotation remains along the long axis of the body, but that axis is no longer perpendicular to the pull of gravity. Thus, gravity has a variable effect on the otolith organs throughout each cycle of rotation. The nystagmus from this protocol has characteristics that are different from earth-vertical axis rotation, but the test paradigms can be quite provocative for nausea (Furman, 1993; Furman, Schor, & Kamerer, 1993; Zimberg, Shepard, Boismier, & Telian, 1991). Investigational work in normal subjects has been completed, but clinical test batteries that can be tolerated by patients with vestibular disorders are difficult to develop. The use of a centrifuge for stimulation, where the patient is seated at the end of a radius arm and rotated around a center point, also provides for well-controlled forces directed to the otolithic organs (Halmagyi, Curthoys, & Dai, 1993). The equipment required for these procedures is expensive and the clinical utility may prove to be limited. However, a clinically acceptable test protocol for otolithic function could help to define abnormalities in a subset of patients that cannot be diagnosed using current clinical techniques (Furman & Baloh, 1992).

Head on Body Rotation Testing

In an effort to expand our ability to evaluate the vestibulo-ocular reflex in its physiologic range of function above 1 Hz, techniques have been developed using head on body rotation, instead of total body rotation (Goebel, Hanson,

Langhofer, & Fishel, 1995; Hoffman, O'Leary, & Munjack, 1994; Matthew, Davis, & O'Leary, 1993). This technique has the patient sit in a stationary body position while moving the head in the horizontal or vertical plane. The head movements typically are performed by having an auditory signal to follow in order to stimulate the movements in the desired frequency range. The patient moves their head in a sinusoidal manner with increasing frequency. A body of literature that investigating the 2–6 Hz region may have clinical utility beyond that of low-frequency, total body rotation. Yet, a study comparing the results of low-frequency total body rotation to head on body rotation in the same patient population, with full ENG, oculomotor studies, and clinical examination, has not been reported. Therefore, the incremental clinical utility of the head on body protocols awaits the outcome of studies in progress.

ANALYSIS AND INTERPRETATION

Sinusoidal Protocol

Three parameters are measured during rotational chair testing to characterize the function of the vestibulo-ocular reflex, and thereby evaluate the function of the peripheral vestibular system. These parameters are phase, gain, and asymmetry. Figure 6–2 shows a schematized version of an averaged slow-component velocity response from multiple cycles of stimulation at a single frequency. The chair velocity is also shown, which correlates exactly to head velocity, assuming the head is properly stabilized. The parameters that characterize vestibulo-ocular reflex function are developed by comparing the slow-component eye velocity profile to the head velocity profile.

Phase

This parameter of the vestibulo-ocular re-flex (VOR) is the least intuitive of the three, but has the greatest clinical significance in its ability to document peripheral system dysfunction. *Phase* measurements objectify the timing relationship between head movement and reflex eye movement. Figure 6–2 illustrates findings expected from a normally functioning vestibulo-ocular reflex system at test frequencies below 0.16 Hz. When the head is moving with a given velocity to the right, the eyes are moving at a specific velocity to the left. Yet the eye

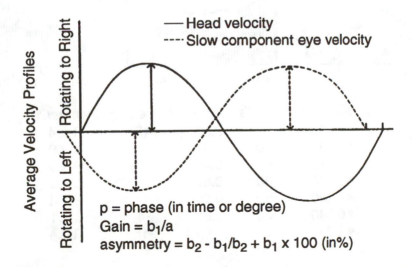

p = phase (in time or degree)

Gain = b_1/a

asymmetry = $b_2 - b_1/b_2 + b_1 \times 100$ (in %)

FIGURE 6–2. Averaged head and eye velocity plotted as a function of time or degrees is shown with indications for the development of the three parameters used to characterize performance with chair stimulation by sinusoids. b_1, the maximum excursion of the slow-component eye velocity trace for rotating to the right; a, the maximum excursion of the head velocity trace for rotating to the right; b_2, the maximum excursion of the slow-component eye velocity trace for rotating to the left.

movements are not exactly opposite to the head movement; in other words, they are not exactly 180° out of phase, as one might expect. Why is this the case? When a low-frequency sinusoidal rotation stimulus is used, if it is assumed to have been ongoing for some time before sampling of the eye movements began, a special condition exists. Under these circumstances, the compensatory eye movements can *lead* the head movement, as shown in the Figure. This would not be the case for any sudden single movement of the head, where the reflex eye movement would obviously have to lag slightly behind the unanticipated head movement. Examining Figure 6–2 carefully, one can see that the eye movement tracing is displaced to the left of the head movement tracing, indicating that the eye movement is indeed slightly ahead of (leading) the head movement. The

amount of this *phase lead* is called the *phase angle* and is typically measured in degrees. The center panel of Figure 6–3 shows a plot of phase angle versus frequency of rotation in a patient with normal rotary chair findings. The phase results can be used to calculate the system time constant from any frequency tested; however, assumptions can be applied that significantly simplify the calculations if the frequencies are restricted to 0.04 Hz and below (Baloh & Honrubia, 1990). Using the lowest frequency in this restricted range for which phase angle data is available, the following formula can be applied:

$$T = 1 \div \omega \tan \Theta \quad (\omega = 2\pi f)$$

where: T = time constant

ω = angular frequency of rotation in radians/sec

π = 3.1416

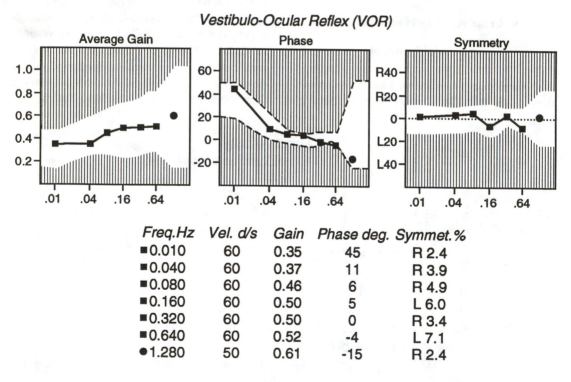

Freq.Hz	Vel. d/s	Gain	Phase deg.	Symmet.%
■0.010	60	0.35	45	R 2.4
■0.040	60	0.37	11	R 3.9
■0.080	60	0.46	6	R 4.9
■0.160	60	0.50	5	L 6.0
■0.320	60	0.50	0	R 3.4
■0.640	60	0.52	-4	L 7.1
●1.280	50	0.61	-15	R 2.4

FIGURE 6–3. Normal rotary chair results from a patient. The plot on the left shows gain (eye velocity divided by head velocity) as a function of frequency of chair sinusoidal stimulation. The center plot shows phase angle in degrees as a function of frequency, and the plot to the right gives symmetry data in percent as a function of frequency. The shaded areas represent abnormal and the individual values for gain; phase and symmetry are given in the table at the bottom of the figure. Normal ranges are a two-standard deviation range about the mean.

f = frequency of rotation in Hz

Θ = phase angle in degrees

Note, that at Θ = 45°, the tan Θ = 1. Therefore, by inserting the frequency of rotation in Hz (f), at the phase angle of 45°, the formula for the time constant reduces to:

$$T = 1 \div 2\pi f$$

In the example shown in Figure 6–3, the frequency of rotation at a phase angle of 45° is f = 0.01 Hz, and the time constant is calculated at T = 15.9 sec. Therefore, as the phase angle increases, time constant decreases. Time constant, as used here and as discussed in Chapters 1 and 2, is a an alternative measure to phase angle for characterizing the timing relationship between the head and eye movement. One measure, time constant or phase angle may be more easily derived for a specific protocol, such as velocity step tests versus sinusoidal rotation. For all practical considerations, their use can be considered equivalent, yet the more common manner in which this timing issue is discussed is by using time constant. As seen in the center panel of Figure 6–3, the normal range for phase (based on two standard deviations above and below the mean) is indicated by the shaded areas. An increase in the phase lead outside this range implies an abnormally low time constant. From experimental studies of the velocity storage integrator that regulates the vestibulo-ocular reflex system time constant (see Chapters 1 and 2), we know that damage to the labyrinth or the vestibular portion of the VIIIth cranial nerve causes a decrease in the time constant. Hence, increased phase lead, implying an abnormally low time constant, strongly suggests pathology in the peripheral system. One caution in this interpretation: damage in the vestibular nuclei within the brain stem may also result in an abnormally low time constant. Therefore, other clinical information is needed to help localize the lesion to the labyrinth or VIIIth nerve. Figures 6–4, 6–5 and 6–6 show the rotary chair results for Cases 20, 45, and 46, respectively. In each case, the abnormal phase lead provided reliable and objective evidence of peripheral system involvement when interpreted alongside the presenting history and other test results. The significance of an abnormally *low* phase lead is still not known with certainty, but may suggest a lesion in the nodulus region of the cerebellum, an area that influences the velocity storage integrator in the brain stem (Waespe et al., 1985).

Gain

The second parameter of the VOR measured in rotary chair testing is *gain*. Classically, this is calculated by dividing the slow-component velocity of the eye by the velocity of the head (measured by chair velocity). Gain measures give an indication of the overall responsiveness of the system. This variable is influenced by alertness, mechanical or neurological restrictions of eye movement (see Chapter 5), or other reductions in the range of eye motion like that in Case 17 (see Chapters 4 and 5), where the eyes deviated severely to the left in darkness. These situations can cause the measured gain of the system to be reduced; however, they should be suspected as the cause by careful observation, history, and a clinical eye movement examination for range of motion and nystagmus (see Chapter 3). Unilateral peripheral weaknesses can cause a mild reduction in gain, especially at the lowest frequencies (Honrubia, Jenkin, Baloh, Yee, & Lau, 1984). However, the principle clinical use of gain measures is to define the extent of a bilateral reduction in peripheral system responsiveness. The gain value helps verify that severely reduced or absent responses to caloric irrigations accurately reflect a bilateral weakness and did not result from an artifact of alertness or some other test pitfall (see Chapter 4). The panel on the left in Figure 6–3 shows normal results for gain as a function of sinusoidal frequency stimulation. The results from Case 47 described above are given in Figure 6–7. As seen in this figure, the gain values are significantly reduced from 0.01 to 0.32 Hz and mildly reduced at 0.64 Hz. The values below 0.16 Hz represent an absent vestibulo-ocular reflex, with nothing but random noise recorded in the eye movement trace. These findings indicate a severe loss of function, and one can predict that the patient will experience significant oscillopsia and balance

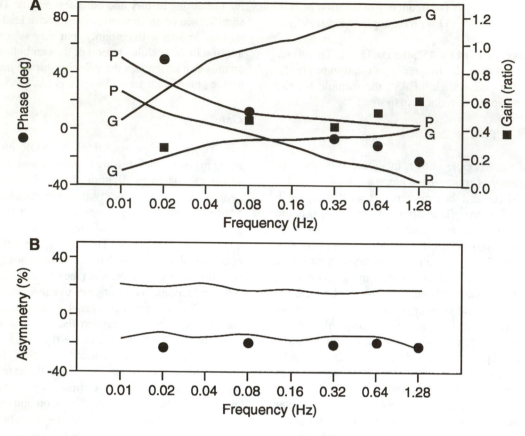

FIGURE 6–4. Chair results for Case 20. Phase and gain are plotted as a function of frequency in the top with symmetry in the bottom. The lines labelled P and G give the two standard deviation normal range for phase and gain respectively. The lines in the bottom plot also represent the two standard deviation range for normal.

problems, especially when visual and foot support surface cues are disrupted. These results would be used to shape the counseling and activities that would be emphasized in a vestibular rehabilitation therapy program involving the expected ability with postural control when residual vestibular function inputs are all that are available (see Chapter 10). It is important to realize that if the gain is quite low (0.1 or less), the signal-to-noise ratio is too low to reliably calculate values for phase and asymmetry. Therefore, these values should be ignored whenever gain values are below 0.1, and should be interpreted cautiously until the gain value exceeds 0.15.

Two additional situations arise that may produce clinical confusion. The first is when

normal gains are documented by rotary chair testing, but mildly reduced caloric responses (< 10°/sec with warm and cool irrigations) are obtained bilaterally. When this finding is encountered, a mild, very low-frequency reduction in bilateral peripheral system function is a real possibility. This assumes that artifactual reasons for a reduction in caloric responses have been ruled out. The second area of confusion arises when the patient is found to have normal caloric irrigation responses but reduced gain on the rotary chair. This is less likely to represent a truly pathologic condition. More often than not, the reduced chair gain is due to reduced alertness during the rotational testing. Given the relatively gentle nature of the low-frequency stimuli, along with the absolute dark-

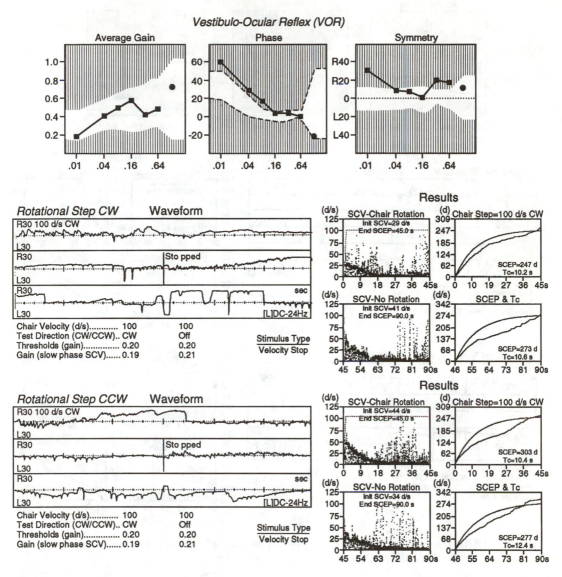

FIGURE 6–5. Chair results for Case 45. The top of the figure gives the results for sinusoidal stimulation; see legend of Figure 6–3 for details. The bottom of the figure gives the results for rotational step test clockwise (CW) and counterclockwise (CCW). The plots on the left in the middle and bottom give the raw nystagmus trace showing eye position as a function of time for per- and post-rotary step stimulations. The extracted slow-component velocities (SCV) from the nystagmus are plotted as a function of time in the center section of graphs. The plots on the far right give the slow cummulative eye position (SCEP) and our estimate of the time constant T_C. Time constant was calculated from the SCV decay plots by finding the length of time required for the slow-component velocity to decay from its originating value at the step stimulus, to a value of 37% of the original. There are proposed methods for using SCEP to calculate the time constant from step chair tests; however, this was not done.

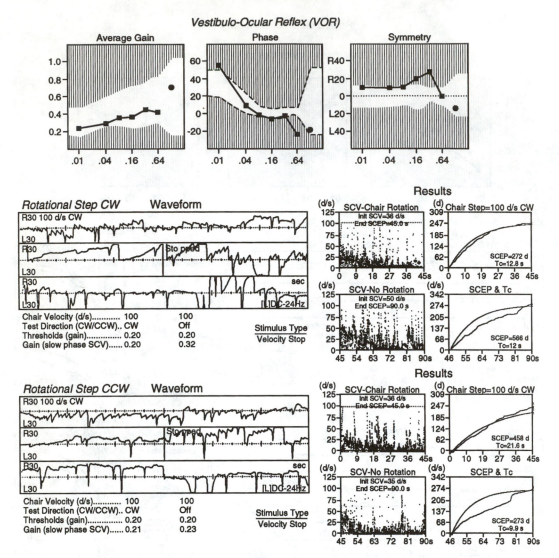

FIGURE 6–6. Chair results for Case 46. See legend of Figure 6–5 for explanation.

ness in the quiet test room, drowsiness is likely. Another possible problem is leakage of light into the booth, allowing gaze fixation and suppression of the nystagmus. These situations can be prevented by maintaining constant conversation during testing to improve alertness, and simply asking if the patient can see anything inside the booth. One last artifact source would be eliminated by making sure that the chair is traveling at the peak velocity and frequency that

has been programmed. This is done by calibration of the equipment and direct measurement of chair peak speed and frequency with the chair loaded and unloaded. With heavier patients, it becomes difficult to achieve the acceleration needed to get to the peak velocity required at the higher test frequencies. Rarely, degenerative conditions of the brain stem and cerebellum will result in reduction of gain values from chair testing without reduction in

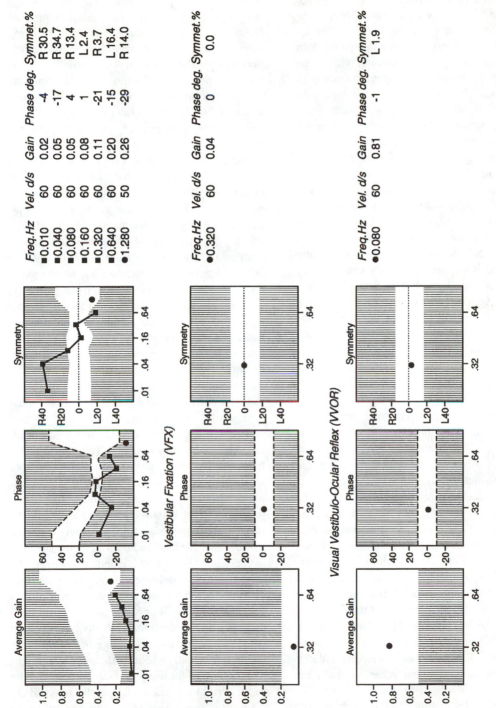

Freq.Hz	Vel. d/s	Gain	Phase deg.	Symmet.%
■ 0.010	60	0.02	-4	R 30.5
■ 0.040	60	0.05	-17	R 34.7
■ 0.080	60	0.05	4	R 13.4
■ 0.160	60	0.08	1	L 2.4
■ 0.320	60	0.11	-21	R 3.7
■ 0.640	60	0.20	-15	L 16.4
● 1.280	50	0.26	-29	R 14.0

Vestibular Fixation (VFX)

Freq.Hz	Vel. d/s	Gain	Phase deg.	Symmet.%
● 0.320	60	0.04	0	0.0

Visual Vestibulo-Ocular Reflex (VVOR)

Freq.Hz	Vel. d/s	Gain	Phase deg.	Symmet.%
● 0.080	60	0.81	-1	L 1.9

FIGURE 6–7. Chair results for Case 47. See legend of Figure 6–5 for explanation of top three plots. The middle panels give the results from the test for fixation suppression and the bottom three for vestibulo-ocular reflex enhancement. Only the gain values are of clinical interest. For this patient, the fixation test is a cross check; as she shows no vestibulo-ocular reflex in the dark with rotation, we would not expect any with failure of fixation.

caloric irrigation responses. In a series of 90 patients studied in our facility who have a clinical diagnosis of Friedreich's ataxia or olivopontocerebellar atrophy, approximately 20% demonstrate bilateral reductions in vestibuloocular reflex responses as documented by both caloric and rotary chair results. However, approximately 5% show consistent reduction in chair gains with normal caloric responses. As the caloric irrigation is a nonphysiologic stimulus, it may actually elicit a response when the more natural rotational stimuli fail. The explanation could also relate to frequency-specific reductions in the VOR response due to selective degeneration in the brain stem region. One should be careful not to generalize these unique observations from highly specific disorders. An isolated reduction in chair gains without a reduction in caloric responses is most likely due to testing artifact, and the rotary chair testing should be repeated. Such a finding should not be interpreted to suggest central nervous system pathology unless substantial ocular-motor findings or other clinical evidence supports brain stem or cerebellar involvement.

Asymmetry

In Figure 6–2, the schematic representation of asymmetry involves a comparison between the slow-component eye velocity to the right (positive values) compared to the left (negative values). It is important to recognize that these values are calculated and *named* by the direction of the eye movement that is produced by the VOR, that is, the slow-component. The situation is reversed when discussing directional preponderance from caloric irrigations. Directional preponderance values are calculated by slow-component velocity but, by convention, are *named* by the direction of the fast component of the nystagmus. Therefore a patient who exhibits a *right-beating* directional preponderance (left slow-component velocity greater than right slow-component velocity) could be expected to show a *left* asymmetry on rotational chair testing. Indicating that during chair testing left slow-component velocity was greater than right slow-component velocity, consistent with the directional preponderance. Not always

will the directional preponderance and asymmetry from chair testing both be abnormal. Both directional preponderance (caloric testing) and asymmetry (rotary chair testing) give an indication of bias within the system, favoring larger slow-component velocities in one direction versus the other. A bias usually results from a peripheral lesion with incomplete dynamic compensation in the central nervous system (see Chapter 3). Less commonly, it may indicate the presence of an uncompensated lesion in the central pathways. Whenever a VOR asymmetry is noted on rotary chair testing, the finding may be due to abnormalities in either peripheral system: either a peripheral weakness on the side of the stronger slow-component velocity response or an irritative lesion on the opposite side. For example, a patient with an uncompensated *right* peripheral weakness will generally demonstrate a *right* greater than left slow-component velocity asymmetry. This is due to an ability to produce a greater rightward compensatory eye movement when rotated toward the intact left side, and a less intense leftward compensatory eye movement response produced after rotation toward the weaker right side. The right panel in Figure 6–3 shows a normal result for the asymmetry measurement. On the other hand, in Case 20 (Figure 6–4) a left greater than right slow-component velocity asymmetry is noted. This could result from either a left paresis or right irritative lesion. His ENG showed persistent right-beating positional nystagmus, also suggestive of left paretic or right irritative lesion. Therefore, the results are consistent, and together with the abnormal phase lead and normal gains, strongly suggest peripheral involvement. However, the lesion cannot be definitely localized to the right or left, since his history and auditory findings are inconclusive. For Case 45 (Figure 6–5) there is a right greater than left slow-component velocity asymmetry, suggestive of a right paresis or left irritative lesion. Because her asymmetric loss of hearing is much worse on the right, a right paresis would be the most likely diagnostic conclusion. Case 46 (Figure 6–6) also shows a right greater than left slow-component velocity asymmetry. Yet in this case, the symptoms of tinnitus and aural fullness, along with a documented loss of hearing, are on the left. We also know that the spells of vertigo are typical of Ménière's disease and that irritative lesions are more common among patients with this diagnosis. Therefore, the most logical interpretation of the rotary chair results in this case would be to suggest a left irritative lesion rather than a right paresis.

Occasionally, a right asymmetry will be noted at one or more frequencies, whereas others may show an asymmetry to the left. Assuming technical factors such as stimulus delivery or recording problems have been ruled out, this finding suggests that the pathologic peripheral system behaves in a paretic fashion at some frequencies and an irritative one at others. Regardless of the ear involved, one can clearly infer that the system is uncompensated under dynamic conditions. The patients who are most likely to demonstrate this finding are those with a hydropic inner ear condition, such as Ménière's disease or posttraumatic endolymphatic hydrops.

Before concluding the discussion of interpreting results from sinusoidal testing, we need to reconsider the issue of localizing the lesion to the vestibular "periphery," given findings such as an increased phase lead and asymmetry. As with other vestibular test findings that are often used to support peripheral system involvement, these too may result from central system lesions. Therefore, the cautious clinician always bases the interpretation of rotary chair results in light of other test data, presenting history, signs, and symptoms. This principle is illustrated by Case 17, introduced in Chapter 4 and 5. The chair results from this patient showed an abnormal phase lead and a right greater than left asymmetry, along with decreased gain. Yet in this case, all of these results are explained by a brain stem lesion (causing the abnormal phase) and the lateral ocular-pulsion eye movements (causing the decreased gain and the asymmetry). In addition, there are no peripheral auditory symptoms that could be used to support the diagnosis of a labyrinthine lesion. Therefore, when viewed in the context of the clinical information available, a posterior inferior artery distribution occlusive event is suspected and, all of the test findings support the diagnosis of a brain stem (medullary) infarct.

A summary of the principles used to interpret phase, gain and asymmetry results in order to characterize the vestibulo-ocular reflex by rotary chair testing is provided in Table 6–1.

Step Test

Although information about gain and asymmetry can be obtained from this protocol, a primary purpose of the step test is to estimate the system time constant. This is especially true if it is used along with the sinusoidal paradigm. The lower half of Figures 6–5 and 6–6 illustrates results of the step test. The actual nystagmus response is shown on the left, with a plot of slow-component eye velocity as a function of time on the right. The far right-hand box in each Case gives an estimate of the time constant. Any value less than 13 seconds is abnormal for our normative data. For Case 45, the estimates of the time constant obtained from per- and post-rotary step testing are both in the 10–12 second range. These values compare favorably to the 8-second value of the time constant estimated from the sinusoidal paradigm in this Case. The time constant values do not always agree so consistently, as shown for Case 46 in Figure 6–6. While three of the estimates are close to the 11-second value from the sinusoidal paradigm, the per-rotary time constant from the counterclockwise rotational step is over 21 seconds. This is probably because of background noise in the trace. As indicated earlier, the results are heavily influenced by the noise in the system and the arousal of the patient prior to the acceleration, as averaging is not used in this paradigm. For this paradigm, there is a decreased signal-to-noise ratio if the gain is 0.15 or less. Caution must be used in interpreting the results under these circumstances. Ideally the step test and the sinusoidal acceleration tests can be employed in parallel to increase the accuracy of estimates of the system time constant and identification of an abnormally functioning system. We use the two protocols in parallel and suggest an abnormal time contant if either the step or the sinusoidal paradigm produces an abnormal estimate of time constant.

TABLE 6–1. Rotary Chair Abnormalities

■ Abnormal Increase in Phase Lead (from low frequency, less than 0.04 Hz, sinusoidal rotations)

Implies an abnormally low system time constant suggestive of peripheral system involvement (labyrinthine, VIIIth nerve), although possible involvement at the level of the vestibular nuclei must be considered.

■ Abnormal Decrease in Phase Lead (from low frequency, less than 0.04 Hz, sinusoidal rotations)

Clinical implications not well defined; however, possible central system influences either at the level of the brain stem or the posterior cerebellar area (nodulus) need to be considered if the result is reliable.

■ Abnormally Low Gain

Implies bilateral reduction in peripheral vestibular system sensitivity.

■ Abnormally High Gain

Can be seen in cerebellar lesions; however, concomitant indications of vestibulo-cerebellar involvement should be noted from ocular-motor evaluation. This finding may occasionally be noted in patients with a suspected endolymphatic hydops condition.

■ Abnormal Asymmetry

Implies a lack of physiological compensation, suggesting a central vestibular system bias for stimulation of compensatory vestibulo-ocular reflex eye movements in one direction versus the other. If central vestibulo-ocular system involvement is not suggested by other testing, then the asymmetry is taken as an implication of possible paresis on the side of the greater slow-component velocity, or an irritative lesion on the side opposite the greater slow-component velocity (Hamid, Hughes, & O'Keefe, 1985).

Other Protocols

Optokinetic Afternystagmus (OKAN)

Our primary purpose for this test is the identification of mal de Debarquement (disembarkment syndrome) for patients whose histories suggest this condition. The classic indication of this syndrome is hyperactive OKAN following optokinetic stimuli in both directions. Complete explanations of the test protocol and normative data are presented in the works of Hain and co-workers (1991, 1994) and will not be repeated here.

Visual-Vestibular Interaction

These tests for suppression and enhancement of the VOR using visual system inputs are the only rotary chair findings that specifically suggest central vestibulo-ocular system pathology. Table 6–2 reviews the suggested interpretation of the possible combinations of abnormalities (Mizukoshi et al., 1985). As these tests

can be influenced by instructions to the patient or by nausea from the testing, they should be used only to support other indications of central system abnormalities. If all the ocular-motor studies are normal, central involvement cannot be confirmed by isolated visual-vestibular interaction abnormalities.

PEDIATRIC EVALUATIONS

Thus far no mention has been made of evaluation of children and infants via any of the methods of testing discussed (Ben-David, Podoshin, Fradis, & Faraggi, 1993; Casselbrant, Furman, Rubenstein, & Mandel, 1995; Cyr, 1983; Levens, 1988; Telischi, Rodgers, & Balkany, 1994). Children, as with adults, have symptoms and disorders related to balance and dizziness. Some of the disorders are the same as seen in adults, but less frequent (for example, Ménière's, labyrinthitis, vestibular neuritis, labyrinthine trauma, bilateral system paresis, or central brain stem/cerebellar disorders). Other

TABLE 6–2. Visual-Vestibular Interaction Abnormalities

Enhanced vestibulo-ocular reflex gain = VVOR (vestibulo-ocular reflex gain from chair rotation with stationary optokinetic stimulation present).

Regular vestibulo-ocular reflex gain = RVOR (vestibulo-ocular reflex gain from chair rotation in the dark).

Fixation vestibulo-ocular reflex gain = VFX (vestibulo-ocular reflex gain with chair rotating and a fixation target moving with the patient).

■ Abnormally high VVOR and RVOR → consider cerebellar involvement

■ Abnormally low VVOR and RVOR → consider brain stem involvement

■ Abnormally high VFX → consider cerebellar involvement

---

disorders, such as benign vertigo of childhood and possible disturbances from episodes of serous otitis media, are typically seen only in those under age of 12. Testing for ENG, ocular motor, and chair can proceed as described for adults with modifications designed to accommodate the attention span and cooperation of the child. In our facility the rotary chair is the principal instrument of investigation for any person with mental age under 10 years. Starting with the chair as the first evaluation allows for significant information gathering in a quick manner. If the child is old enough and willing, the child be seated in the chair system alone. However, given the demands of the situation, the child be seated on a parent's lap, with head restraint performed by the adult. This flexibility in testing allows for evaluations to the age of the infant, a few weeks old. If cooperation with the placement of electrodes (standard electrooculographic techniques discussed in Chapter 4) is a problem, simply using an infrared monitoring camera to qualitatively assess the vestibulo-ocular reflex with chair rotations provides the information needed to rule out significant bilateral paresis. Bilateral paresis is, in many very young children (less than 2 years of age), the major concern for those with delayed milestones of motoric development with congenital deafness or status post meningitis. If electrodes can be placed, information discussed above can be used to define the peripheral system status, for either unilateral or bilateral involvement. Whether the head of the child is restrained by a holding parent, or the standard chair device, slippage of the head, relative to

chair motion, is greater in the child than the adult. Therefore, frequencies of test are typically kept to below .32 Hz. This also reduces the time of testing. In many children fear of the dark may impede the ability to evaluate the child. If possible, having the parent who will accompany the child and be holding the child during testing practice easy oscillations in a swival chair or stool in a darkened room at home for several days prior to testing can be helpful.

For the child under age 5 or 6 years, ocular-motor evaluation needs to be abbreviated, due to attention span. Performing pursuit tracking and conjugately recorded saccade evaluation in the rotational chair booth in complete darkness increases the likelihood of the child successfully viewing the target. This technique can allow for at least pursuit testing for even the child of an age of a few weeks to a few months. Optokinetic stimulation can also be used in this environment to test pursuit or optokinetic responses, depending on the speed of the target.

The cooperative child of any age can then proceed to testing for positional nystagmus, and caloric irrigation responses. Again, these protocols are abbreviated as needed to suit the attention span of the child. Typically, in the very young child, using a situation of turning all the lights out in the examining room or holding Frenzel lenses to the face of the child is required to assess the eye movements, as the child will not volitionally maintain eyes closed for a long enough interval of time. Evaluation of postural control assessment of the child will be discussed in Chapter 7.

NORMATIVE DATA

Commercial systems typically are supplied with suggested ranges for normal. In general, parameters of phase, gain, asymmetry, and time constant from step tests are normally distributed variables, and use of a two standard deviation range around the mean is appropriate for defining normal. Knowing the number of subjects, the age distribution of the normal subjects, and the criteria for normal subjects used to define the normative values provided is important in deciding what additional efforts are needed at the individual facilities to be confident in the ranges used for each of the parameters. As with other normal ranges, decisions need to be made regarding use of normative ranges that are age-dependent. Well-controlled studies of age effects show changes in the vestibulo-ocular reflex across frequency as a function of age. Although these changes are of statistical significance, they do not appear to be of great clinical significance. Therefore, extensive normative data across a wide age range, such as

that needed for pursuit tracking, is probably not required for rotational chair. However, using data for defining the normal range from individuals all under the age of 40 would not be advisable and potentially misleading, with an increase in the false positive rate. Scrutinizing the methods used to calculate the various parameters, especially phase and time constant from rotational step tests, provides the user with information about potential sources of error in these calculations that may influence the manner in which normative data should be taken or verified. Attempts have begun in a cooperative manner between experienced users of rotational chair equipment and the various manufacturers to review some of these issues in an effort to provide for better standardization of test protocols, normal ranges, and analysis schemes to improve comparisons of patients across facilities (Goebel, Hanson, Fishel, & The Interlaboratory Rotational Chair Study Group, 1994). Until that standardization can be achieved, users are strongly advised to verify and add to normative data supplied in commercially available systems.

7

■ POSTURAL CONTROL EVALUATION

CLINICAL UTILITY

The testing discussed in earlier chapters involves those studies designed to evaluate the extent and location of pathology in the vestibular system and related oculomotor pathways. On the other hand, dynamic posturography involves a battery of tests that helps to assess the functional capacity of the balance disorder patient. Even though certain findings on the electronystamography (ENG) or rotary chair testing may reflect the status of CNS compensation, these studies often do not correlate well with measures of the patients' functional capacity or their perception of disability. This difference between these measures of balance function were recently studied experimentally (Beynon & Shepard, 1996; Gavie et al., 1994). The first study investigated the ability of balance function studies to predict balance disorder patients' performance on high-level activities of daily living. There were four tasks involving large head movements, including rising from a chair, rising from a bed, ascending and descending stairs, and walking with a 180° turn, with and without horizontal head movements. No statistically significant correlation was found between these mobility tasks and the various subtests of the ENG or parameters of the rotary chair evaluation. Statistically significant

correlations and predictive ability was demonstrated for both dynamic posturography and the Dizziness Handicap Inventory (DHI), a questionnaire instrument designed to measure the physical, functional, and psychological impact of balance and dizziness symptoms (Jacobson & Newman, 1993). The combination of the DHI and dynamic posturography accounted for 30–50% of the variability of performance in the mobility tasks (for walking and ascending stairs), as indicated by linear regression analysis. The second study further reviewed the relationship between the DHI, the various tests, and performance in vestibular rehabilitation programs. Jacobson and Newman (1993) previously had suggested that a correlation with dynamic posturography was the only significant relationship between the DHI and vestibular testing. This finding was confirmed in a series of over 200 patients, all of whom had full ENG, rotary chair, and posturographic testing. Additionally, the DHI showed a strong correlation with the various measures of functional performance used to asses the outcome of a vestibular rehabilitation program. This work further supports the contention that measures of postural control, especially those from dynamic posturography, primarily evaluate the functional ability of the patient, rather than provide information regarding extent and site-of-lesion. One possible exception where posturography may contribute to our understanding of the site-of-lesion involves expanding the postural control evaluation to include the use of electromyographic (EMG) recordings. As will be discussed later in this Chapter, this evaluation may provide very site-specific information .

The survey of 2266 consecutive balance disorder patients introduced in Chapter 6 can again be used to assess the percentage of patients with abnormalities on dynamic posturography (Equi-Test) and to study the types of patients most likely to have abnormal posturography results. This data is presented in Table 7–1. Developing sensitivity and specificity figures for a test of functional capacity is difficult at best. However, it is possible to gain some indication of the ability of this technology to recognize functional deficits in specific disorders. In Chapter 5, a group of patients with balance and gait disturbance as a primary symptom was introduced and used to derive sensitivity measures for ocular-motor studies. Many of these individuals have specific lesions involving sensory and/or motor tracts in the brain stem and spinal cord. In that select group of patients, dynamic posturography (EquiTest) was abnormal 94% of the time. Again, this figure can not be taken as a measure of general test sensitivity, but relates only to the sensitivity to detect these specific disorders. Nonetheless, it is reassuring to see such a high sensitivity figure in a group of patients who would be expected to have abnormal postural control.

The following information will review posturography results in a large series of patients and provide examples of clinical cases that illustrate the diagnostic utility of posturography. Each of the cases will be presented in a general manner, with the specific postural control results discussed later in the chapter (Interpretation section) following a review of the paradigms and analysis used in the testing.

CASE 5

This 76-year-old female reported a sudden onset of 15–30 second vertigo spells provoked by head movements occurring up to twice a day. There was no history of a clear antecedent event or vestibular crisis. She denied any spontaneous spells that were not provoked by motion. The remainder of her presenting history was negative and she had normal hearing. Her ENG showed a 27% right unilateral weakness with no other abnormalities. Rotary chair and ocular-motor evaluations were normal. Dynamic posturography was abnormal, suggesting a lack of functional compensation, despite the normal measures of static and dynamic physiologic compensation. (*Note:* the reader should review Chapter 3 if this distinction is unclear.) In the survey of 2266 patients, those with indications of isolated peripheral vestibular involvement showed lack of physiological compensation 74% of the time, lack of both physiological and functional compensation 20% of the time, and lack of functional compensation alone (as in this example) only 2% of the time. The remaining 4% had results suggesting complete physiologic and functional compensation. Therefore, as with rotary chair,

TABLE 7–1. Percentage of Patients With Abnormal Dynamic Posturography

The percentages given represent any abnormality on dynamic posturography, from either subtest (see text under Test Paradigms).

■ For all patients taken together (*N* = 2266)	35%
■ Dynamic posturography was the only abnormality (*N* = 2266)	4%
■ Those with only peripheral system involvement (*N* = 1372)	35%
■ Those with indications of central system involvement (*N* = 476)	42%

dynamic posturography can provide adjunctive information concerning compensation status.

In patients with bilateral peripheral vestibular system involvement, the functional impact on postural control also can be assessed using dynamic posturography. One can estimate the extent of bilateral involvement using dynamic posturography results and tests for oscillopsia when rotary chair testing is not available. The contrast between the following two cases illustrates this point.

CASE 3

A 72-year-old male noted constant unsteadiness following discharge from the hospital after treatment with 21 days of intravenous gentamicin for bacterial endocarditis. Additional factors that may have contributed to his complaints included peripheral neuropathy in his hands and feet, along with a left hip replacement two months prior to his evaluation. No auditory symptoms were noted. His ENG demonstrated only minimal response to ice water caloric irrigations, with clinically significant spontaneous and positional right-beating nystagmus. Rotary chair demonstrated severely reduced vestibulo-ocular reflex gain through the low and mid frequencies, returning to normal at 0.64 Hz. Oculo-motor evaluation showed mild abnormalities that could be explained by his age. His dynamic posturography evaluation demonstrated inability to use vestibular system cues for maintaining upright stance, as expected. He showed a particularly severe type of fall reaction ("free falls") under all conditions when visual and foot support surface information were disrupted. He also demonstrated abnormal posturography performance if foot support surface information was disrupted, even when provided with accurate visual information. This finding could not be explained by the bilateral peripheral system paresis nor by his peripheral neuropathy. In addition, abilities that might be adversely influenced by the peripheral neuropathy or the hip replacement were within a normal range, suggesting that these issues did not play

a significant role in his complaints. The information obtained in the postural control evaluation specifically focused his vestibular rehabilitation program in a manner that would otherwise have been overlooked. (The use of vestibular rehabilitation to address such issues will be discussed in detail in Chapter 10.)

CASE 18

This case, introduced in Chapter 4, is a good example of how dynamic posturography may provide evidence that a suspected bilateral paresis was mild in nature. She demonstrated normal performance on all conditions of quiet stance, regardless of the system input cues available. Of the 2266 patients reviewed, 4% had bilateral involvement as demonstrated by reduced or absent caloric responses and reduction in the vestibulo-ocular reflex gain on rotary chair. Half of these patients had normal dynamic posturography, while the other half had significant difficulty when forced to rely on the use of vestibular system input alone. As with Case 3, these findings help to shape the activities and prognosis of vestibular rehabilitation programs.

Table 7–1 demonstrates that a small percentage of patients have dynamic posturography findings as the only abnormality discovered in vestibular testing. The vast majority of these are older patients, typically over 65 years of age, whose principal complaint is unsteadiness when standing or walking. This is illustrated by the following case.

CASE 19

This 84-year-old man began complaining of constant unsteadiness when standing or walking approximately 1 year prior to his balance function evaluation. No symptoms were noted when sitting or recumbent, and his symptoms were not provoked or exacerbated by head movements. He had no auditory symptoms. He had a severe peripheral neuropathy with pitting edema in both ankles. ENG, rotary chair, and ocular-motor evaluations were well within normal limits, suggesting no central or peripheral vestibular component to his symptoms. Dynamic posturography demonstrated difficulty maintaining stable stance when relying on proprioceptive and somatosensory inputs or vestibular system input alone. Additionally, abnormalities were noted in his automatic responses for coordinated recovery from an unexpected perturbation in the center of mass. This case demonstrates two important aspects of the evaluation process. First, this patient's only abnormalities are extra-vestibular in nature. Although that might have been suspected from the patient's presenting history, the balance evaluation process verified this impression and directed the development of an appropriate treatment program. Second, as will be discussed in more detail in the interpretation section, this man's difficulty using vestibular system information to maintain upright stance is not due to a lesion in either the peripheral or central vestibular pathways. The explanation for this finding will be discussed below, but it is important to reemphasize that the functional evaluation performed by a postural control assessment is not related to site-of-lesion.

CASE 17

Case 17, introduced in Chapter 4 and followed through Chapters 5 and 6, presents an example of the use of dynamic posturography to help rule out significant long-loop, automatic pathway coordination problems. The presence of such abnormalities would have altered the approach to his vestibular rehabilitation program. As it stands, his abnormalities reflect balance difficulties related to a mix of sensory input system use, probably secondary to a central vestibular system lesion in the medulla.

A very different use of the combined protocols is illustrated in the following patient.

CASE 1

A 47-year-old male underwent a left retro-labyrinthine vestibular nerve section in 1980 for intractable Ménière's disease. Due to continued spells of vertigo and further deterioration of hearing, he subsequently underwent a left transmastoid labyrinthectomy in 1981 to ablate any residual vestibular function in the involved ear. By history, his postoperative course reflected good central compensation with only rare mild spells of vertigo, lasting several seconds, beginning 2–3 months following the second surgery. Since approximately the same period he had noted persistent pain and swelling in the left lower limb toward the end of each work day. This complaint had been evaluated, but no diagnostic explanation or treatment had been provided. His condition continued until the fall of 1987, 6 months prior to his balance evaluation, when he developed mild flu symptoms after having a flu shot. Two days later he had a suspected central vestibular decompensation, with relapse of vestibular symptoms similar to those experienced during recovery from his vestibular operations. These continuous symptoms resolved over several days, leaving him with vertigo provoked by head movement. No change in his left leg discomfort was noted. ENG showed a mix of spontaneous left-beating nystagmus with right-beating positional nystagmus. There was no caloric response to irrigations on the left. Ocular-motor evaluation was normal and rotary chair showed an abnormal phase lead, with no asymmetry. Dynamic posturography showed difficulty maintaining quiet stance when forced to rely on vestibular system information alone. These results suggested lack of both physiological and functional compensation. An additional result from dynamic posturography showed that he maintained a stance at rest that distributed his weight almost exclusively onto his left leg. He also used the left leg as the major source of force generated to recover from unexpected forward or backward sway. He was able to volitionally shift his weight from left to right, and had no range of motion or strength deficits in the right leg that would have required the predominant use of the left leg. His vestibular rehabilitation program was a direct outgrowth of his dynamic posturography results, together with other measures that will be discussed in Chapter 10. In this case, we speculated that his weight shift to the left was a maladaptive strategy developed following his surgery. Although this strategy may have improved his sense of security and stability initially, it was now causing constant swelling and discomfort in his left leg. His rehabilitation program reversed this process and eliminated his left leg complaints, as well as reestablished his central vestibular compensation.

One expanded use of postural assessment involves adding EMG recordings from the distal lower limbs. As previously indicated, this may provide some site-of-lesion information not available from routine posturography. A significant amount of work has defined recognizable patterns of muscle response and their association with specific lesion sites and disease classifications (Dichgans & Diener, 1987; Friedemann, Noth, Diener, & Bacher, 1987). Normative results for the paradigm described below have been developed over the age range and have been shown to have sensitivity and specificity of 68% and 87%, respectively for identifying the specific disease entities reflected by the defined patterns of abnormal responses (Fortin, Shepard, Diener, & Lawson, 1996; Lawson, Shepard, Oviatt, & Wang, 1994; Shepard, Lawson, Boismier, Oviatt, & Wang, 1994). Two cases will be discussed briefly to illustrate this evaluation tool.

CASE 35

This 22-year-old female with known multiple sclerosis was reporting episodic lightheadedness and unsteadiness, usually when standing or walking. The spells were provoked by head movements, lasted seconds to several minutes, and occurred once or twice per month. She was referred for balance function testing to investigate the possibility of peripheral vestibular system involvement. Her ENG, ocular-motor, and rotary chair results were all normal. Her dynamic posturography showed normal ability to maintain quiet stance, independent of the input systems available. She showed mild abnormalities suggestive of long-loop, automatic pathway involvement. Her Postural Evoked Responses using the EMG showed a pattern of abnormality previously shown to be associated with multiple sclerosis (Diener et al., 1984). Overall, the results showed no suggestion of peripheral or central vestibular system involvement, but simply findings consistent with long tract involvement that were attributable to her multiple sclerosis.

CASE 48

This case illustrates a different situation, with a 34-year-old female referred for evaluation of complaints of four spontaneous spells. In 1985, 1986, and twice in 1995, she had experienced true vertigo with nausea and headache lasting for 2 days. Her milder residual symptoms slowly improved over a three week interval each time. Between the events she was asymptomatic. Left ear fullness was the only auditory symptom reported. Her ENG showed marginally significant right-beating positional nystagmus and a 26% left unilateral weakness. Rotary chair results were normal except for a single right greater than left slow-component velocity asymmetry, of marginal significance. These results alone, together with the presenting history, would suggest possible left endolymphatic hydrops. Dynamic posturography results showed normal ability to maintain quiet stance, yet demonstrated an unexplained delay in the initiation of recovery from induced forward and backward sway, suggesting abnormality in the long-loop pathway. Postural Evoked Responses gave an abnormal pattern that has been associated with multiple sclerosis. As a result of these findings, she has been referred for neurological evaluation.

These examples and the population studies to date suggest that use of EMG recordings for Postural Evoked Responses may add an additional dimension for a limited set of balance disorder patients. Suggested criteria for using such evaluations will be discussed below.

Given the lack of a significant relationship between the functional capacity of the patient and the ENG, ocular-motor, and rotary chair results, the repeated use of these studies to monitor progress in treatment programs is not recommended. These tools may be useful in monitoring the results of procedures that directly impact peripheral vestibular function, such as the use of surgical procedures or ototoxic antibiotics in the treatment of Ménière's disease. Assessment of postural control may play a more formal role in the objective evaluation of patients following treatment, especially after vestibular rehabilitation programs. This use also will be limited to those with postural control abnormalities prior to treatment, and primarily involves assessment of volitional control of quiet stance with changing sensory input conditions.

TEST PARADIGMS

The functional physiology of postural control discussed in Chapter 2 sets a framework for the understanding of paradigms used to assess postural control. With the functional physiology framework in mind, a detailed discussion of dynamic posturography by EquiTest will be presented. It is beyond the scope of this text to present a detailed analysis of all currently available methods for postural control assessment. Other methods will be discussed briefly and the interested reader will be referred to other sources for details. For techniques that do not use an *actual force* plate measurement system, refer to the clinical office tests in Chapter 3. The methods below all use a force plate measurement system. Force plates are devices that allow for the measurement of changes in vertical or horizontal forces placed on the surface of the plate. Patients use the force plate as the floor support surface, and changes in their weight distribution over their feet are reflected in changes in the forces detected by the platform. These forces are referred to as *floor reaction forces*.

Approaches Other Than Dynamic Posturography by EquiTest

Static Force Plate—Nondynamic

Use of static force plate posturography or other postural assessment measures to assess volitional control of static stance (no perturbation of the center of mass) has been purposed for a number of years (Yoneda & Tokumasu, 1986). More recent work has suggested various paradigms that increase the challenge to the postural control system, attempting to increase the sensitivity of this assessment tool to more subtle abnormalities and to better differentiate between patients (Norré, 1994; Norré, 1995; Triolo, Reilley, Freedman, & Betz, 1993). These methods provide for quantitative assessment and paradigms to manipulate sensory input conditions in an inexpensive manner.

Static Force Plate—Dynamic

Methods for perturbing the body's center of mass, other than by movement of the force plate, have been used for clinical investigations. The first method involves a vibratory stimulus applied to the tricep sura muscle area (calf region) with a variety of different stimulus configurations (Eklund & Hagbarth, 1966; Johansson, Magnusson, & Ckesson 1988; Karlberg, Johansson, Magnusson, & Fransson, 1996; Magnusson & Johansson, 1993;). Recently, this method has been extended to the muscles of the neck (Karlberg, Persson, & Magnusson, 1995). In either case, the vibratory stimulus causes brief, repeated contractions of the muscle with sudden uncontrolled movement of the body's center of mass, requiring a compensatory reaction by the patient. The second method uses galvanic stimulation of the vestibular system with DC current pulses presented by electrodes applied to the mastoid region (Johansson, Magnusson, & Fransson, 1995). Although this technique is not new, its recent combination with the vibratory method has been used for investigation of patient selected for cochlear implantation (Magnusson, Petersen, Harris, & Johansson, 1995). Various other mechanical means for disturbing a patient's postural stability include calibrated abdominal pulls (not used with a force plate), and use of air jets on a head mounted device (Patla, Koyama, & Mackintosh, 1994; Wolfson, Whipple, Amerman, & Kleinberg, 1986).

Movable Force Plate—Ankle Rotation

An extensive amount of work has been reported involving force plate rotations that alter the ankle angle as a means of perturbing the patient's center of mass and stimulating the muscles of the lower limbs. Adding measures of EMG and various calculated dynamic measures of movement has provided for improvements in evaluation capabilities. These have been used to provide much information about normal functioning and information about the ability of various patient groups to provide for reactions to the perturbing stimulus (Allum & Pfaltz, 1985; Allum et al., 1994b). These types of paradigms, when combined with ones investigating volitional stance, provide for a relatively complete assessment of the system described in Chapter 2. A summary comparison between translational and rotational means of perturbing the center of mass (gravity) is given by Allum (1990).

Movable Force Plate—Translation

A body of literature also reports using anterior/posterior translations of the force plate as the mechanism to perturb the center of mass. This has been done using both unexpected transient stimuli and random or pseudo-random support surface perturbations of the patient's center of mass (gravity) (Maki, Holliday, & Fernie, 1987; Ledin, Gupta, Larsen, & Ödkvist, 1993; Ledin, Loft, Öhman, & Ödkvist, 1993; Ledin & Ödkvist, 1993). The use of the unexpected transient stimuli will be discussed in more detail below. Use of randomized translational perturbations suggests that this method

may investigate aspects of dynamic postural control not fully assessed by either rotational or transient translational methods.

Dynamic Posturography by EquiTest

Details of the technique for using EquiTest for dynamic posturography and general interpretation guidelines are summarized by Nashner (1993a, 1993b, 1993c; Voorhees, 1989, 1990), who is primarily responsible for the development of this technology. The test paradigms used with this equipment follow the lines of function that were discussed in Chapter 2. The sensory organization test gives an indication of the patient's ability to maintain volitional quiet stance as the sensory inputs available for use (vision and somatosensory/proprioception information) are manipulated. The patient's ability to react to sudden unexpected perturbations in the center of mass position is provided through the motor control test. The principal outcome measure for EquiTest, as well as many of the other techniques introduced above, is the position of the center of mass. It is important to understand that center of mass is not a directly measurable quantity. For any system such as EquiTest that gives center of mass as the outcome measure, typically the actual measure recorded is reaction force transmitted to the support surface (vertical and horizontal floor pressure). This quantity is then manipulated through mathematical relations and assumptions concerning the center of mass in an average person (from anthropometric data) to calculate the movement of the center of mass (Shepard, Schultz, Alexander, Gu, & Boismier, 1993). This relationship between these two parameters allows for prediction of center of mass from the floor reaction force in a simple manner until the frequency of sway begins to exceed approximately 1–1.2 Hz, or large relative movements in different segments of the body occur during sway. The latter condition would be seen with significant movement of the upper body compared to the lower body in a hip stategy situation. For the frequency constraint, when sway begins to exceed 1–1.2 Hz, the relationship becomes much more complex and the predictions of center of mass position from floor reaction force by the techniques typically used in clinical equipment need cautious interpretation (Gu, Shepard, Schultz, & Fassois, 1992). Fortunately, it is rare to see total body sway exceed frequencies above 1.2, Hz and the magnitude of hip strategy upper body movements are typically not excessively large.

The protocols for EquiTest assess various aspects of quiet and dynamic postural control abilities. Although certain aspects of postural control are prerequisites for gait activities, and certain abnormalities of postural control may cause ambulation problems, posturography cannot be used in isolation to evaluate gait deficits. Gait evaluation has its own complete set of parameters that must be tested under a completely different set of conditions.

Sensory Organization Test

Briefly, this test measures the ability to perform volitional, quiet stance during a series of six specific conditions (Figure 7–1). The first three provide for uninterrupted, accurate foot support surface information on a surface with adequate friction that is larger than the foot size. Condition 1 has eyes open, while in Condition 2, the eyes are closed. Under Condition 3, the visual surround moves in a pattern that is stimulated by the anterior/posterior sway movements of the patient. Conditions 1 and 2 are a modified Romberg test, as the feet are at their normal separation rather than close together. Condition 3 presents a situation of visual conflict, where visually accurate information is provided but of no significant help in maintaining quiet stance. Condition 3 presents misleading optokinetic and foveal visual cues about the position of the body in space. Conditions 4, 5, and 6 utilize the same sequence of the three visual conditions, but with the foot support surface giving misleading information. As with the movement of the visual surround in Condition 3, when testing under Conditions 4, 5, and 6, sway movements of the patient in the sagittal (anterior/posterior) plane drive the movement of the support surface in a rotational manner about an axis parallel to

the ankle joint. In this way, somatosensory and proprioceptive information is not removed in Conditions 4, 5, and 6, but is of limited use in maintaining upright stance in that there is a disrupted relationship between body position and the ankle angle (that angle made between the upper surface of the foot and the anterior portion of the lower leg). Typically, after the simpler Conditions 1 and 2, three trials are given for each of the more challenging conditions. The average performance is taken as representative of the patient's postural control ability under that sensory condition.

The equilibrium score is a percentage representing the magnitude of sway in the sagittal plane for each trial of each condition. Details of how this score is obtained will not be repeated here (Shepard, Schultz, Alexander, Gu, & Boismier, 1993). However, it is important to realize that this score is based on a normal value of 12.5° of anterior/posterior sway about the ankle joint, typically 8° forward and 4.5° backward. It is assumed that this range of sway is available to patients during the test. Some patients may not have this normal range because of physical restrictions at the ankle, or because of limits of sway patients have adopted secondary to their sense of imbalance and fear of a potential fall. It is important to recognize the patient who has a reduction in limits of sway. If the limits of sway are reduced more than 50%, interpretation of the patient's results may be inaccurate. If the reduction is not a permanent physical restriction, it can be addressed in a vestibular rehabilitation program. Therefore, we test the limits of volitional sway for each of our patients as part of the sensory organization test protocol. Prior to testing under Condition 1, patients are asked to lean as far forward onto their toes as possible without taking a step or reaching out, and then as far back on their heels as possible. This is done with the eyes open, stressing that the movements are to be done about the ankle joint rather than bending at the hip. Following this practice trial allowing the patient to explore the limits of sway, the equipment is activated under Condition 1. Rather than maintaining stable stance at first, the patient is asked to repeat the limits of sway task again during the 20-second

SENSORY ORGANIZATION PROTOCOL

Condition	Vision	Support	Patient Instructions
1	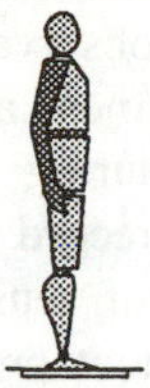 Normal	Fixed	Stand quietly with your eyes OPEN
2	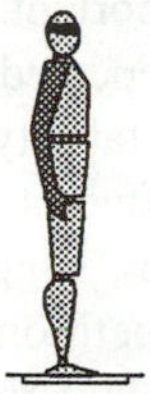 Absent	Fixed	Stand quietly with your eyes CLOSED
3	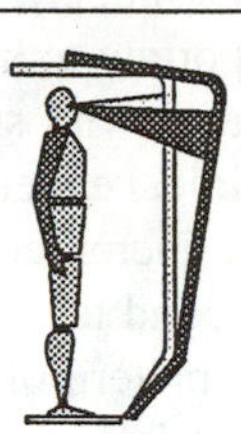 SwayRef	Fixed	Stand quietly with your eyes OPEN
4	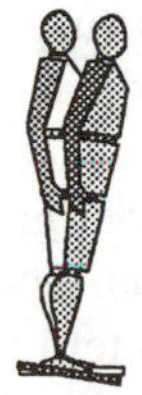 Normal	SwayRef	Stand quietly with your eyes OPEN
5	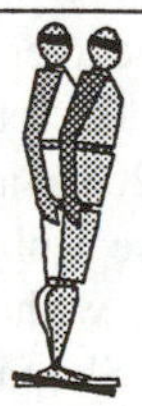 Absent	SwayRef	Stand quietly with your eyes CLOSED
6	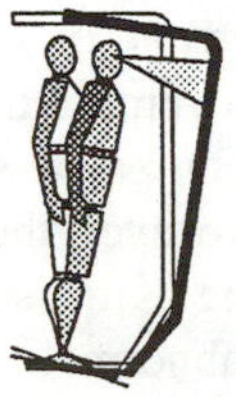 SwayRef	SwayRef	Stand quietly with your eyes OPEN

FIGURE 7–1. The six sensory organization test conditions showing which sensory input cues are available or accurate for each condition. (Reprinted with permission from NeuroCom International, Inc.)

trial. When completed, the equilibrium score on the screen can be interpreted roughly as the percent reduction in limits of sway in the sagittal plane. The authors take a score of 35% or less as no significant reduction, knowing that the range of movement only increases if repeated practice is allowed. Then, the actual Condition 1 test is repeated, so that the limits of sway test result does not enter into the calculation of the cumulative equilibrium score at the end of the test. Use of the limits of sway measurement to help explain apparent inconsistencies in performance will be discussed in the interpretation section below.

An additional measurement that also may be important in explaining results that appear to be inconsistent is that of the average position of the center of mass during each trial. Normal distribution would have the weight positioned 2–3° in front of the ankle joint. The interactive display can give the examiner an indication as to whether the patient appears to be standing with his or her weight distributed significantly over the heel of the foot. When this situation is noted during Condition 1 testing, correct patient foot placement and a normal comfortable posture should be confirmed prior to continuing.

The EquiTest force plate provides a measure of the amount of horizontal floor reaction force (shear force). This is not needed in calculations of center of mass position. This shear force between the feet and the support surface typically increases with increased upper body movement. This may be found either with low-frequency movement with large excursions, as would occur with bending about the hip joint, or with low-amplitude high-frequency movements that may occur about the ankle joint. The latter situation is seen in patients with distal lower limb peripheral neuropathy and may be seen in normals when they are experimentally deprived of appropriate cutaneous somatosensory and proprioceptive information from the foot and ankle region (Mauritz & Dietz, 1980). In a pilot study of patients with well-defined peripheral neuropathy, every patient had significant increases in shear force on Conditions 2–6. This finding was especially pronounced in Conditions 4–6, with low-amplitude movements of

the center of mass, but high frequency of sway (1–1.2 Hz). Therefore, before using shear force information to infer an abnormal use of movement about the hips or the ankles, the recorded force information must be corroborated by the examiner using visual observation during these trials. Abnormal movement about the hip can easily be discerned during the testing, and should be noted in the record.

Given serial use of sensory organization testing to monitor patient progress, test-retest reliability becomes important. Studies looking directly or indirectly (repeated tests for reasons other than testing repeatability) at this issue in normals retested on different days indicate no significant improvement, suggesting no learning effect with test repetition (Black, Pabski, Reschke, Calkins, & Shupert, 1993; Kubo & Wall, 1990). It is important to know if the same result occurs in patients who start with abnormal performance. Clinical experience suggested that patients had an increased likelihood for improvement on a second test administration if they either showed a pattern of improving performance across three trials of a given condition or if the test result was suspected to be unreliable secondary to significant anxiety noted by the examiner. A study investigating this issue prospectively showed that greater than 50% of such individuals with an abnormal test result changed to a normal pattern with repeat testing on the same day (Boismier & Shepard, 1991). To study this issue in the average balance disorder patient not suspect for retest improvement, a prospective random 20% sample of 650 consecutive patients were subjected to repeat dynamic posturography within 120 minutes of the original testing (Shepard & Boismier, 1992). The study did demonstrate statistically significant improvement in sensory organization test scores for several of the test conditions and for the overall composite score, suggesting a learning effect. However, the clinical significance of this finding is questionable, as only 10% of those with abnormal sensory organization test composite scores initially changed to a normal score with repeat testing. All of those changing to a normal score were initially outside the normal range by an amount less than the variance in normals for the conditions in question. Another study confined to elderly patients also showed statistically significant improvement, but given that all subjects had initially normal studies, and the observed changes were again within the recognized variance, the clinical significance of the findings are reduced (Ford-Smith, Wyman, Elswick, Fernandez, & Newton, 1995). Therefore, we now routinely repeat an abnormal sensory organization test on patients only if they meet one of the initial criteria from Boismier and Shepard's 1991 study (improving pattern over the three trials of a test condition; or if the test results are suspected to be unreliable secondary to significant anxiety) or if they have an abnormal composite score within 20 points of the lower limit of normal results.

The validity of assessing postural control using only information available from floor reaction force was addressed in a study comparing young and elderly normals on EquiTest to their performance using an experimental laboratory device that monitors multiple points on the body from the head to the feet (Shepard, Schultz, Alexander, Gu, & Boismier, 1993). The conclusions were that the general characterization of movements made by a platform analysis system such as EquiTest are accurate, except that the platform cannot account for head movement.

To increase the sensitivity of the sensory organization test in identifying peripheral vestibular system lesions, especially those functionally compensated, alterations in the test protocol, using changes in head position, have been attempted (Barin, Seitz, & Welling, 1992; Chandra & Shepard, 1996; Jackson & Epstein, 1991). The general result of these changes has not demonstrated significant increases in sensitivity of the sensory organization test, suggesting that not static but dynamic movements of the head will be needed during testing to disrupt compensated mechanisms on a short-term basis (Panosian & Paige, 1995).

Motor Control Test

Information about patients' ability to react to unexpected perturbations in their center of mass position is obtained with the motor control protocol. The center of mass perturbations are created by abrupt anterior or posterior horizontal translations of the support surface. Typically, three increasingly large translations in both directions are administered. The increase in size of the translations created a stimulus intensity series. The profile of the surface movement is varied for each patient based on height, so that all translations are normalized to a 6-foot tall person (Shepard, Schultz, Alex-ander, Gu, & Boismier, 1993). This allows for direct comparison of results across patients. After the three posterior and the three anterior translations, unexpected rotations about the ankle are used. Contrary to the horizontal translations, the typical muscle response that is mapped to the stimulus provoked by rotary stimuli is destabilizing. The patient must then be able to adapt to the new stimulus on repeated trials. Five randomly timed toes up or toes down rotations provide relative information about the patient's ability to adapt to this familiar but destabilizing stimulus. For this protocol, as with the sensory organization test, floor reaction force detected by the force plates in the support surface is measured. The principal output parameter is the latency to onset of active recovery from the unexpected translations. Other information obtained from the protocol includes weight distribution onto right or left leg, and a relative measure of strength as a function of the size of the perturbation (Shepard, Schultz, Alexander, Gu, & Boismier, 1993).

As with the sensory organization test, the issues of test-retest reliability and validity of the movement coordination test were addressed in the studies described above (Shepard & Boismier, 1992; Shepard, Schultz, Alexander, Gu, & Boismier, 1993). Statistically significant improvements were again noted but of minimal clinical impact. For this reason, we repeat the study at the time of the initial testing if the latencies are abnormal by no more than 50 msec.

Postural Evoked Responses

Details of the testing protocol used in our facility are given elsewhere and will only be reviewed briefly here (Lawson et al., 1994; Nashner, 1993c). Muscle activity from the distal lower extremities is stimulated by sudden toe up rotations of the support surface (the force plate platform of EquiTest). The muscle activity stimulated by this dorsiflexion movement at the ankle is recorded with surface EMG electrodes. In the paradigm used for the patients presented here, the response from the medial gastrocnemius and the anterior tibialis was recorded. To improve the signal-to-noise ratio of the evoked EMG activity, the rotation is repeated, with random interstimulus intervals and the EMG responses rectified and averaged over 15–20 responses. This allows for much clearer identification of onset and offset times of muscle contraction following the stimulus. There are three specific responses obtained as illustrated in Figure 7–2. The short (SL) and medium (ML) latency responses are seen from the contraction of the gastrocnemius shown in traces from channels 1 and 3 (CH1 and CH3) of Figure 7–2. The third response is the long latency (LL) obtained from the contraction of the anterior tibialis, shown in channels 2 and 4 (CH2 and CH4) of Figure 7–2. Note the follow-up contraction shown for the anterior tibialis on channels 2 and 4. This represents one of the difficulties in using techniques of this type: defining the true onset and offset of the muscle response. In this example, the follow-up contraction is recognized as a separate event on the tibialis and not the primary contraction by the definitions used in analyzing the traces. This and other sources of error were investigated in a two-institutional, double-blind study of the reliability of marking traces of this type. A group of recordings from our facility and from another laboratory was evaluated with each facility marking their own subjects twice and the other lab's subjects once. High values of reliability measures were noted, suggesting that the repeatability of the markings is satisfactory. The two major sources of errors were interference contractions such as that shown in Figure 7–2, multiple contractions of the gastrocnemius for the medium latency response, and inexperience on the part of the person doing the analysis (Fortin et al., 1996). Therefore, with practice and care in the recordings, repeatable valid responses can be obtained with this protocol. Interpretation of these responses will be briefly discussed below.

Platform Pressure Test

It has been suggested that posturography technology could be used as a tool for evaluating patients suspected of having a perilymphatic fistula. The premise of testing for a fistula in this way involves changing pressure in the external auditory canal and recording the effects on postural control. A similar test using eye movement recordings, like those for ENG testing, presents pressure changes to the external canal and observes for provoked nystagmus. In general, this test has estimated sensitivity and specificity that are in the 50% range, and thus has had only limited clinical use. It was postulated that because postural control involves a greater portion of the balance system and different vestibular output pathways, using this as the outcome measure may improve sensitivity. The test is performed by presenting pressure pulse changes to the external canal and assessing the change in the anterior/posterior or lateral sway compared to a no-pressure condition. Estimates of sensitivity using this test have been as high as the 90% range. At present the major problem with this testing, or any other evaluation for perilymphatic fistula, is that there is no definitive manner to document that the condition is actually present. Surgical observation is too variable and subject to bias, given the extremely small quantities of fluid involved and the presence of fluids other than perilymph in the middle ear during exploratory surgery for fistula. Thus, until a gold standard for the diagnosis of this disorder is available, it is impossible to obtain accurate positive or negative predictive values for this or any other preoperative test for fistula. A full discussion of this issue and a complete description of the testing techniques is provided elsewhere (Shepard, Telian, Niparko, Kemink, & Fujita, 1992).

INTERPRETATION

Sensory Organization Test

As with the overall balance system evaluation, this study is also interpreted using pattern

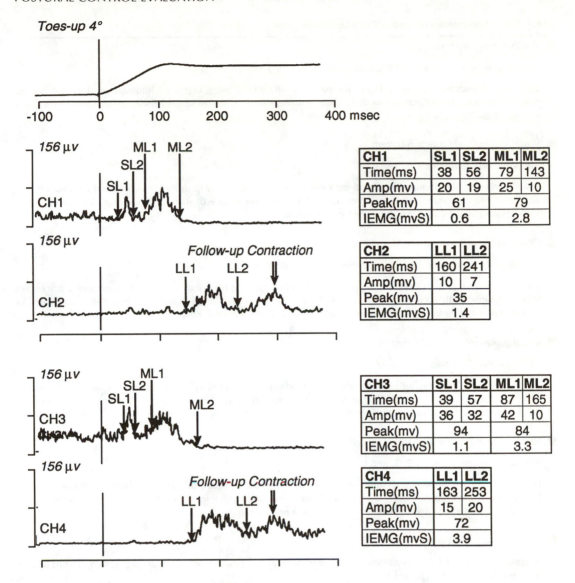

FIGURE 7–2. Postural Evoked Response results for a normal subject. The plot at the top shows the position profile of the rotation of the surface the subject is standing on, as a function of time. Deflection upward indicated toe up rotation. The four plots on the left give the averaged, rectified surface electromyographic responses in amplitude of contraction (in microvolts) as a function of time. Channels 1 and 3 (CH1 and 3) are results from the left and right gastrocnemius muscles, respectively. Channels 2 and 4 (CH2 and 4) are the results from the left and right anterior tibialis muscles, respectively. The short (SL), medium (ML), and long latency (LL) responses are indicated at onset with a number 1, and offset with a 2. The tables at the right give the numerical values for each response, indicating onset and offset times and amplitudes, peak amplitude contraction, and integrated amplitude (IEMG).

recognition. The combination of the six conditions that are abnormal are used to define a pattern of abnormality that can then be func-

tionally interpreted. Table 7–2 presents the most common patterns and the related nomenclature. By far the most common pattern is the vestibu-

TABLE 7–2. Abnormalities of Sensory Organization Testing

■ Vestibular dysfunction pattern

Abnormal on Conditions 5 and 6 (alternatively Condition 5 alone).

Vestibular dysfunction pattern indicates the patient's difficulty in using vestibular information alone for mainte-nance of stance. When provided with accurate visual and/or foot somatosensory information, stance is within a normal range.

■ Visual vestibular dysfunction pattern

Abnormal on Conditions 4, 5, and 6.

Visual and vestibular dysfunction pattern indicates the patient's difficulty in using accurate visual information with vestibular information, or vestibular information alone for maintenance of stance. When provided with accurate foot support surface cues, stance is within a normal range.

■ Visual preference pattern

Abnormal on Conditions 3 and 6 (alternatively, Condition 6 alone).

Visual preference pattern indicates the patient's abnormal reliance on visual information, even when inaccurate. When provided with accurate foot support surface information together with accurate or absent visual cues, or absent vision and vestibular information alone, stance is within a normal range.

■ Visual preference/vestibular dysfunction pattern

Abnormal on Conditions 3, 5, and 6.

Visual preference and vestibular dysfunction pattern indicates the patient's difficulty in using vestibular information alone and the patient's abnormal reliance on visual information, even when inaccurate. When provided with accu-rate foot support surface information together with accurate or absent visual cues, stance is within a normal range.

■ Somatosensory/vestibular dysfunction pattern

Abnormal on Conditions 2, 3, 5, and 6.

Somatosensory and vestibular dysfunction pattern indicates the patient's difficulty in using foot support surface information with vestibular information, or vestibular information alone for maintenance of stance. When provid-ed with accurate visual information, stance is within a normal range.

■ Severe dysfunction pattern

Abnormal on four or more conditions not covered in the above descriptions, for example, 3, 4, 5, and 6; or 2, 3, 4, 5, and 6; or 1, 2, 3, 4, 5, and 6.

Severe dysfuction pattern indicates the patient's difficulty with stance independent of the sensory information (vestibular, visual, and/or somatosensory) provided. Note that these situations many times involve a dominant fea-ture such as significantly abnormal Conditions 5 and 6, or they may involve equally distributed difficulties on all conditions affected.

■ Inconsistent pattern

Abnormal on Conditions 1, 2, 3, 4, or any combination and normal on Conditions 5 and 6.

Inconsistent pattern indicates that performance of the patient is difficult to explain with normal or typical patho-physiologic conditions and could imply volitional or nonvolitional exaggerated results.

---

lar dysfunction pattern, comprising approxi-mately 45% of all abnormalities on this test in our facility. Figure 7–3 shows the results from

Case 5 on the sensory organization test. For this and subsequent figures that show sensory orga-nization tests, a single bar will be used to show

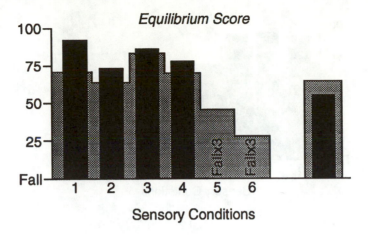

FIGURE 7–3. Sensory organization test results for Case 5. The plot gives the equilibrium score in percent for each of the six test conditions and the weighted composite score as the bar on the far right.

the average performance of the multiple trials within each condition unless there were significant differences between the trials; then individual trial results are shown. Case 5 represents the common vestibular dysfunction pattern, with fall reactions on the six trials for Conditions 5 and 6. The interpretation is that this patient is unable to adequately use isolated vestibular system information to maintain quiet, upright stance. This brings us to the most important aspect of interpretation for the sensory organization test. It provides information as to which input system cues the patient is unable to utilize for performing the task of maintaining postural control. This in no way implies that there is a central or peripheral vestibular system lesion, nor does it imply central or peripheral pathway lesions in the visual or somatosensory/proprioceptive systems. The information should be interpreted only to reflect which input information the patient is able to use for the task at hand. We will revisit this issue repeatedly with the next several cases. In Case 5, as with many of the other cases, there is evidence from the other extent and site-of-lesion studies to suggest peripheral vestibular system involvement that may explain why this patient has a vestibular dysfunction pattern. Overall, this result now suggests that, even though the Case 5 patient was compensated physiologically, functional

compensation has not been achieved. In the recent survey of patients in our facility discussed in the last several chapters, this lack of functional compensation with apparent physiological compensation occurs only 2–4% of the time with peripheral lesions. More commonly, the patients with peripheral lesions are uncompensated physiologically (74%), or there is a combination of poor physiological and functional compensation (20%). A vestibular rehabilitation program in this patient's case was able to bring sensory organization test results completely within a normal range and significantly reduce the patient's complaints of motion-provoked symptoms.

For patients with significant bilateral peripheral vestibular system paresis, such as in Case 3, the sensory organization test result would be expected to include disruption in performance of Conditions 5 and 6 (Herdman, Borello-France, & Whitney, 1994). Figure 7–4 shows the sensory organization test results from Case 3. As anticipated this patient shows fall reactions on all six trials of Conditions 5 and 6. In addition, we see inconsistent performance on Condition 4, with two fall reactions and one trial with abnormal, but reasonable stance. This is an example of the visual-vestibular dysfunction pattern, the second most common pattern noted in our patients. Although the results on

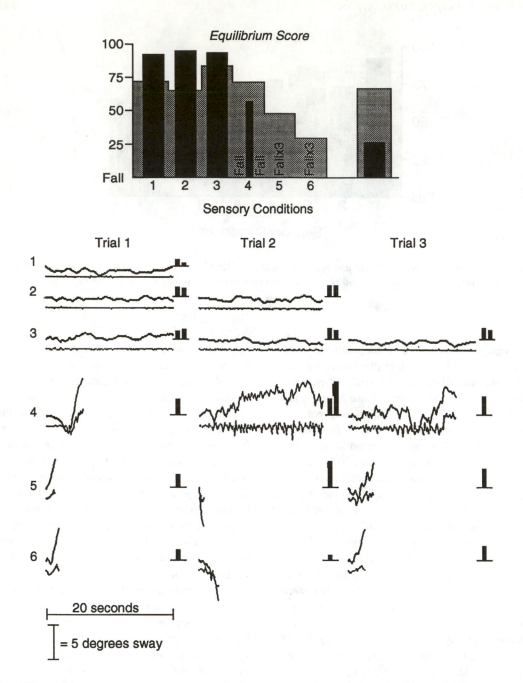

FIGURE 7–4. Sensory organization test results for Case 3. Included below the bar graph are the individual traces of calculated center of mass (gravity; top line in each plot) for each of the three trial for each of the six conditions. The lower trace in each plot gives the shear (horizontal) force response during each of the 20-second trials. The small bars to the right of each pair of traces give the initial alignment (position of the center of mass relative to the ideal, the line under the bars) and the second bar is the average of the last 17 seconds of the trial. If the small bars are above the line on which they sit, the patient is leaning forward, as is the case for this individual. If no bar is shown, the center of mass (gravity) position is at the theoretically ideal position.

Conditions 5 and 6 look similar to those in the last case (Case 5), they were significantly different. To appreciate this difference, the examiner must review the raw data tracings. In general, this is something that should *always* be done when interpreting vestibular function tests, not just dynamic posturography. The calculated center of mass tracing for each of the three trials of the six sensory conditions are shown in the bottom of Figure 7–4 for Case 3. While there were six falls on Conditions 5 and 6, the character of the falls is one that is commonly seen with significant bilateral paresis. Specifically, it can be easily appreciated that no attempts were made to correct the center of mass position on any of the trials for Conditions 5 and 6. The patient simply underwent a free fall in the anterior or posterior direction. The patient did not perceive that he was falling until he was stopped by the examiner. Given the severity of his bilateral involvement, with disrupted somatosensory/proprioceptive input and absent or disrupted vision, he had no significant sensory input available to inform him of the impending fall. On the other hand, the woman in Case 5 demonstrated falls like those seen here on Condition 4, where attempts were made to correct the position of the center of mass. However, even after multiple corrections, she was not able to maintain her stance. Therefore, we see that the raw data can be very useful in further differentiating a patient's performance. For Case 3, the inconsistent performance on Condition 4 is explained by this patient's 50–60% reduction in the limits of sway, as tested in the manner described above. Effectively, the *Fall* line for the Equilibrium Score graph can be thought of as positioned at approximately the position of the result from the limit of sway test (equilibrium score of 50–60%). If this is done in Case 3, it is apparent that the patient's performance on Condition 4 is very close to his perceived limits of sway, and therefore the three trials do not actually represent any significant difference. He has the ability to perform under Condition 4, yet his fear of falling and his problems with peripheral neuropathy have established a limit as to how far he will let his center of mass move prior to taking a step, as he did in the first and third trials of

Condition 4. This illustrates the use of the limits of sway information in helping to explain what would otherwise be a very inconsistent performance. This situation was easily corrected with a vestibular rehabilitation program, returning Condition 4 to a normal range with increases in the patient's limits of sway. Conditions 5 and 6 for this patient remain as shown, because there is a sensory system (peripheral vestibular system) missing. This implies that the suggested normal sensitivity of the vestibular system at frequencies at or greater than 1 Hz are not functionally of significance in maintaining quiet stance. This would be consistent with the data showing that this task falls in the frequency range dominated below 1 Hz (see Chapters 1 and 2). Of great interest is the question of why we are unable to use the residual frequency information above 1 Hz to reduce the oscillopsia that patients have when there is bilateral paresis, even with attempts at reduction with vestibular rehabilitation programs (Acierno, Trobe, Shepard, & Toglia, 1996; Bhansali & Bojrab, 1993).

Another aspect of postural control revealed in the sensory organization test is that of average position of the center of mass during the 20-second trial. If the patients have a tendency to maintain their center of mass positioned over the heel of the foot as opposed to the normal positioning, just anterior to the ankle joint, they reduce their backward range of motion for sway. Consequently, this also may be an explanation for an apparent inconsistent result on particular conditions of the testing, if their fall reactions resulted from backward movements. Review of raw data is necessary to identify this situation.

The use of dynamic posturography has been proposed for identification of patients that may be malingering, or for whatever the reason, exaggerating their condition. Recent work by several investigators (not all with EquiTest) has attempted to quantify the use of this tool to identify these patients (Allum, Huwiler, & Honegger, 1994; Cevette, Puetz, Marion, Wertz, & Muenter, 1995; Hamid, Huges, & Kinney, 1991). Even qualitatively, suspicion should be raised if any of the following conditions are met:

1. Performance on Condition 1 is abnormal, yet the patient is able to ambulate to the platform and mount the platform with no apparent difficulty.
2. Performance on Conditions 1, 2, and 3 are poorer than on Conditions 4, 5, and 6.
3. The raw data demonstrate that observed abnormalities in sway are consistent, repeatable, large amplitude sine wave movements of the center of mass.
4. When repeating the test within 1 hour and randomizing the conditions, and trials within the conditions, the pattern of abnormality changes significantly. For normal subjects and patients with documented pathologic conditions, randomizing the order of presentation does not alter the performance pattern.

Further discussion of interpreting of the sensory organization test will proceed as the interpretation of other components of dynamic posturography are introduced below.

Motor Control Test

This study is used less as a functional evaluation than the sensory organization test, and more to evaluate the long-loop pathway introduced in Chapters 1 and 2. This pathway begins with inputs from the ankle region (tendon and muscle stretch receptors), then projects to the motor cortex and back to the various muscles of postural control, including upper and lower body. When an abnormal latency to onset of active recovery from induced sway is noted, then problems in the long-loop pathway should be considered. The explanation may be as simple as ongoing joint or back pain, a congenital condition of the back or lower limbs, or an acquired lesion involving the neural pathways of the tracts on either the afferent or efferent side. Therefore, abnormalities of the motor control test related to latency are nonspecific indicators of potential problems in the long-tracts or the musculo-skeletal system needed to coordinate recovery from unexpectedly induced sway in the sagittal plane. Other abnormalities from this portion of the testing include inappropriate

weight bearing or an inability to properly scale the strength of the response to the increasing size of the perturbations. Such findings may provide information that helps explain the patient's complaints of disequilibrium. These abnormalities are unlikely to directly implicate neurological involvement if the latency findings are normal. In many cases, the weight shift or scaling problems may be maladaptive behaviors developed in response to the initial symptoms of the vestibular disorder. Case 1 is an example of this situation. Figure 7–5 A–D presents the sensory organization test results (A), the motor control test latency results (B), weight symmetry data (C, obtained prior to platform movement) and the amplitude scaling results (D), prior to a vestibular rehabilitation program. The patient's sensory organization test shows another example of a vestibular dysfunction pattern. This finding, along with other test data, suggests lack of both physiologic and functional compensation. His motor control test shows abnormalities only in persistent weight distribution onto his left lower extremity and the predominant use of the left side for recovery from translation of the platform. The use of the left leg for recovery was a direct reflection of his propensity for weight bearing on the left leg, not a result of a neurological or musculoskeletal problem. The patient had good range of motion, strength, and sensation in his lower extremities. When instructed, he could shift his weight solely onto his right leg. Therefore, it was hypothesized that the weight-bearing abnormality was a maladaptive behavior developed by the patient following the labyrinthectomy to somehow diminish his symptoms. Yet it seems that he did not aban-don this strategy as he underwent the compensation process. This was suspected to be the cause of the patient's left lower limb swelling and discomfort at the end of the day, presumably an overuse syndrome. In addition to his habituation exercises for reducing sensitivity to head movement, his vestibular rehabilitation program included balance and gait exercises focused on equal weight distribution. Figure 7–6 A–C presents this patient's test results after therapy, showing compensated functional abili-

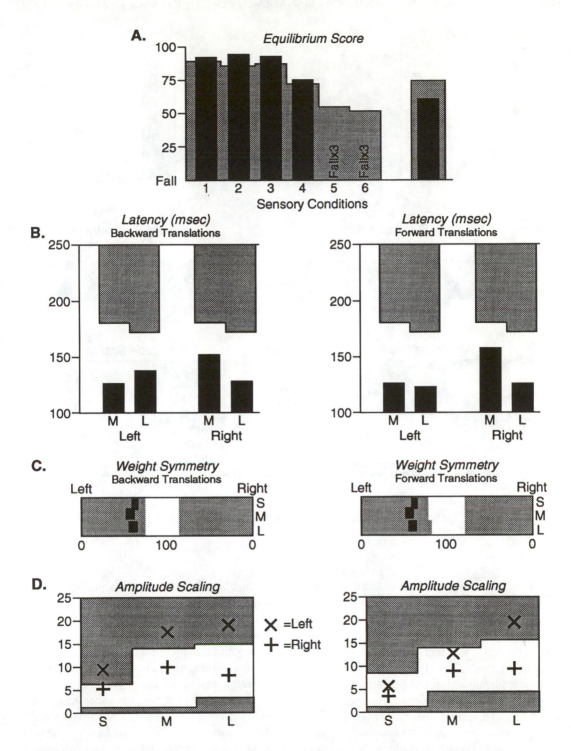

FIGURE 7–5. Pretherapy results for Case 1. **A.** Sensory organization test results. **B.** Latency results from motor control test. **C.** Weight bearing during the motor control test. **D.** Relative strength response for each lower limb in recovery from the translational perturbations from the motor control test.

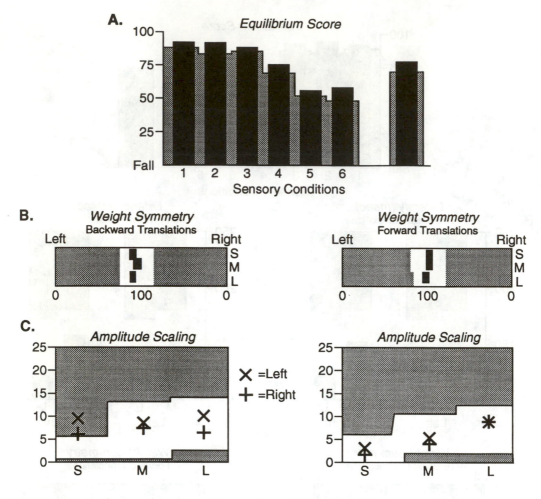

FIGURE 7–6. Posttherapy dynamic posturography results for Case 1. Latency results were not repeated, as they did not change.

ty on the sensory organization test and equal weight distribution. Subjectively, he was also virtually asymptomatic for head movements, and no longer experienced swelling or discomfort in the left lower leg.

In contrast, Case 19 (Figure 7–7) shows significant abnormalities of the latencies on the motor control test, with normal findings related to scaling and weight distribution. This patient also shows a severe pattern on sensory organization testing. The ENG, oculomotor tests, and rotary chair studies on this patient were noted to be well within normal limits. Yet, clearly, the greatest difficulty on the sensory organization test was experienced with Conditions 5 and 6.

From the discussion on interpretation of the sensory organization test, these results would indicate inadequate ability to use any combination of sensory inputs for maintaining quiet stance and complete inability to use vestibular system information alone. Does this finding reflect a lesion in the peripheral or central vestibular system? No, his other test results indicate completely normal functioning within their limits of sensitivity. In fact, he seems to acquire and use vestibular system information to discern his position in space and to activate muscle responses for repositioning the center of mass. This is seen from the motor control test latency results. This patient has no sensations

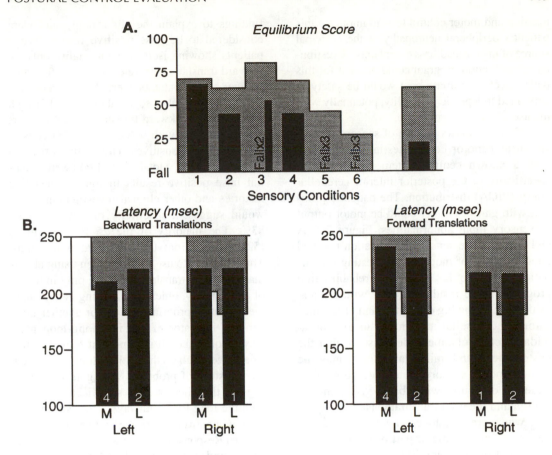

FIGURE 7–7. A. Sensory organization test results. **B.** Latency results from motor control test for Case 19. In B the number in the bar on the latency plots indicates the number of algorithms that agreed (out of a total of 4) on the latency shown. When the number is 1, the most conservative (shortest) value is given.

below his knees, due to his documented peripheral sensory neuropathy. Yet by the motor control test he is able to activate the appropriate musculature to recover from either forward or backward induced sway. Given the frequency response (above 1.5 Hz) needed for this task, he would have to be using his vestibular system to activate the response rather than vision. When the vestibular system is used to substitute in this manner, a minimum of 50–75 msec is added to the latency. This was discussed in Chapter 2 as an example of a way to modify behaviorally this automatic response. This would explain a portion of the delay in his latency findings. Therefore, his repeated falls on Conditions 5 and 6 were speculated to be accounted for by his in-

ability to feel his foot placement on a moving surface, even though he could probably detect his movement and send the correct signals to the lower limbs. His performance was hindered by the lack of any feedback from the plantar (underneath) surface of the foot relative to the force of his foot against the surface. So as he attempted corrections, a progressively accumulating error in the response developed, resulting ultimately in a fall. This is discussed here to emphasize the point that sensory organization testing is a only a test of functional ability to use the inputs available and does not imply a lesion in any given system when appropriate use of a particular input is not demonstrated. This also illustrates the combined use of the sensory organization and motor control tests to implicate this patient's peripheral neuropathy as the principal source of his unsteadiness complaints. A vestibular rehabilitation program could be used for this patient, yet its primary goal would be safety in continued independent mobility, potentially with the use of an assistive device.

Case 17 shows the use of sensory organization and motor control testing in a patient with a known central system lesion, related specifically to the posterior inferior cerebellar artery (PICA) distribution. The patient's problem with gait instability could be motor output or sensory input abnormalities. Figure 7–8 A and B shows the sensory organization test and latency results of motor control testing for this patient prior to his vestibular rehabilitation program. These results, together with clinical evaluations showing dysmetria and other indicators of cerebellar, pyramidal, or extrapyramidal tract involvement, demonstrate that the unsteadiness and mild gait ataxia may be related only to sensory input integration. This patient's difficulty with absent visual in-formation and the use of accurate visual information when present, together with gait activities, constituted a major part of his vestibular rehabilitation program. The results after therapy are given in Figure 7–8 C and D. Although he reported mild symptoms remaining, he had major subjective improvement.

As the motor control test has developed over the years and the algorithms for detection of the latency have changed, a significant increase in sensitivity to backward translations, producing forward sway, has been noted. This was investigated (in our facility) using a group of 150 randomly selected patients, with 25 of these patients showing abnormal latencies only on backward translation. Out of this group of 25, 12 patients had a history of possible biomechanical, musculoskeletal, or central nervous system problems which may have explained the abnormal findings. A major recurring theme in these clinical histories was complaints of pain involving the back, hip, or knee joints severe enough to cause the patient to report or demonstrate limitation of movement. The other 13 patients did not have positive histories or other findings to explain the abnormality and were considered to be false positive results. When patients showing isolated abnormality only on forward translations were evaluated in the same manner, three patients were felt to represent false positives out of seven abnormals. For both forward and backward translations, 28 patients were abnormal, with 9 (out of the 28) considered to be false positives. Therefore, of the 150 patients sampled, a total of 25 (17%) were potential false positive results in light of negative histories and other clinical investigations. This would suggest a specificity of approximately 83%. The majority of the 25 false positives (52%) came from the backward translations. Thus it is best to use caution when using abnormal backward translations as the only indicator of abnormality, unless this finding is accompanied by an appropriate history or another independent indicator of possible long-loop pathway involvement. It is important to realize that a negative result on the testing along with a negative history of problems with gait and stance suggest that there are no significant problems with the long-loop pathways. This became evident when investigating the use of Postural Evoked Responses to determine estimates of sensitivity and specificity of the EMG study reported above. Of the 25 patients with well-defined neurological disorders that affect this pathway, 68% had EMG abnormalities but only 9 (36%) had abnormal movement coordination test results. On the other side of the problem, 19 had histories of back or joint pain, all of whom had an abnormal motor control test results. However, only seven (37%) had abnormalities on Postural Evoked Response testing (Shepard, Lawson, Boismier, Oviatt, & Wang, 1994). The point to this discussion is that identifying abnormalities in a complex sensorimotor mechanism such as the long-loop pathway requires multiple indicators. It is perfectly consistent to have delayed mechanical latencies in the coordinated movement across the joints of the body, yet have normal latency to onset of isolated muscle groups in the distal lower limbs. The reverse can be equally true, with abnormal latencies or amplitudes of contraction of isolated muscle groups, yet normal coordinated movement

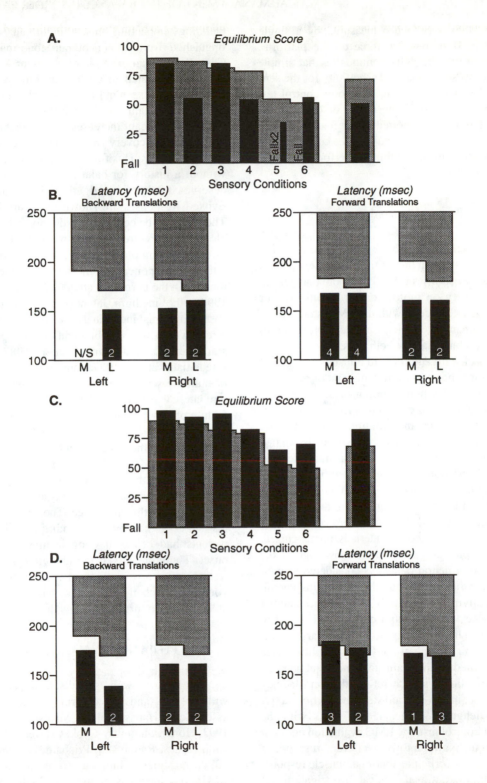

FIGURE 7–8. A and **B.** Sensory organization test and latency results pretherapy, respectively. **C** and **D.** Sensory organization test and latency results posttherapy for Case 17, respectively.

across the joints, when measured by a single point of floor reaction force on the platform. Recognizing this issue reminds us that simple studies of sensitivity and specificity for the sensory organization test or the motor control test cannot fully reflect the utility of this clinical tool. The studies reported here reflect the results for isolated patient groups and should not be interpreted as the definitive performance figures for the test.

Postural Evoked Responses

In light of the above discussion, it should be apparent that the decision to use Postural Evoked Responses is based on more than just an abnormality on motor control testing. In our facility, we proceed with the EMG study: (a) if the mechanical latencies of the motor control test are abnormal for both lower limbs and on both backward and forward translations or (b) if the patient has a primary complaint of persistent unsteadiness when standing or walking. The EMG patterns for contraction from the gastrocnemius and the anterior tibialis muscles are compared to those that have been associated with specific pathologies, such as multiple sclerosis, Parkinson's disease, or specific neurologic lesions. Patterns have been described for lesions in the anterior cerebellum and the basal ganglia, as well as for spinal cord compression. When the contraction pattern is unrecognized, the interpretation is based on knowledge of the underlying neural pathways considered responsible for the specific muscle activity. In general, these involve mediation of the short latency response via the spinal cord (H-reflex). The medium latency response is primarily controlled via the spinal cord, with amplitude size determined by the brain stem and basal ganglia. The functional stretch reflex, the long latency response, involves brain stem and cortical activity (Dichgans & Diener, 1987). As with the motor control test, the EMG evaluation does not distinguish afferent from efferent disruptions that may underlie the abnormal muscle responses. With additional clinical investigations of sensitivity in the lower limbs, and/or the use of lower limb somatosensory evoked responses,

pathology impacting sensory input can be distinguished from motor output abnormalities. Case 48 gives an example of a patient with no complaints related to unsteadiness or balance difficulties. As seen in Figure 7–9, although her ability to maintain upright stance was excellent, she had significant increases in her mechanical latencies for recovery from induced forward or backward sway. This finding in a young person without a history for balance or gait problems deserves further investigation. Her Postural Evoked Responses are shown in Figure 7–10. These should be compared to the normal example given in Figure 7–2. The most striking feature is the complete absence of the medium latency component from the gastrocnemius muscle. In the normative studies (Lawson et al., 1994), the medium latency component was absent in normal individuals 6% of the time, but rarely would they be bilateral. In the profile studies by Dichgans and Diener (1987) and Friedemann et al. (1987), approximately 30% of multiple sclerosis patients had absent medium latency responses. The second abnormal feature of this patient's test was a delayed onset of the long latency response (LL1 in Figure 7–10) for both the left and right anterior tibialis, with values of 149 and 147 msec, respectively. These are well beyond the value of 142 msec, which is two standard deviations above normal for females in this age range. The profile studies suggest that 69% of multiple sclerosis patients had delays in long latency response onset. Therefore, given the abnormal postural testing, a strong suspicion of involvement beyond the peripheral vestibular system is justifiable and led to further investigation.

PEDIATRIC EVALUATION

Children, as well as adults, have problems with postural and gait control, and also need assessment (Harris, Reidel, Matesi, & Smith, 1993; Horak, Shumway-Cook, Crowe, & Black, 1988; Jones, Radomskij, Prichard, & Snashall, 1990; Nashner, Shumway-Cook, & Marin, 1983; Woollacott & Shumway-Cook, 1989). The subject weights that are allowed while still permitting accurate EquiTest output is deter-

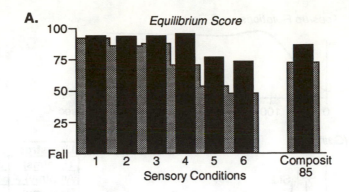

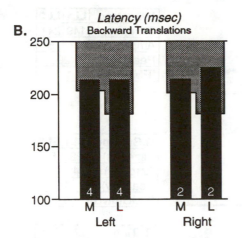

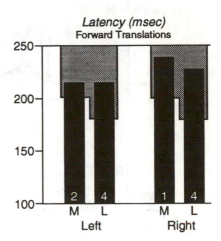

FIGURE 7–9. Sensory organization test (A) and latency results from motor control test (B), respectively for Case 48.

mined by the calibration of the equipment. This is typically set for a range of 40–300 lb. Therefore, most older children can be tested using the equipment. The younger child is typically too light to be tested, unless a change in the operating range of the equipment is made. Because of the cooperation needed from the subject, we find it easier to use a modified version of the Clinical Test of Sensory Interaction and Balance (CTSIB) to grossly approximate the ability of the child under 5 years of age to use vision, foot support cues, and vestibular information for maintaining stance. This is done with a qualitative assessment of stance on a flat firm surface in a lighted and then darkened room. The same visual conditions are repeated while the child is standing on a compressible surface. Having the examiner touch the fingers of the child during testing in darkness is adequate to tell if a fall reaction is to occur, and reassures the child. It should be noted that this touch does significantly expand the base of support of the child, and may obviate mild difficulty that otherwise would be detected. Most children in the 14–30-month age range are referred for complaints of difficulty learning to walk, or difficulty walking after meningitis. For these children, the use of rotational chair and simple postural control assessment can be very powerful for ruling out or defining the extent of bilat-

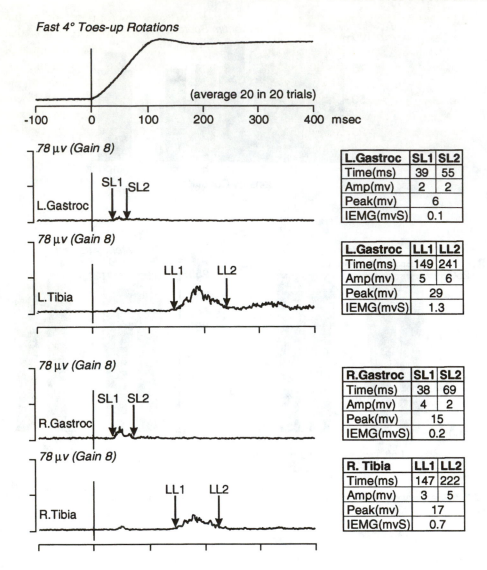

FIGURE 7–10. Postural Evoked Response results for Case 48; see legend of Figure 7–2 for explanation of figure. Note the absence of the medium latency response bilaterally.

eral peripheral involvement. The examiner must be aware that the child under the age of 5–7 years uses the three input systems differently than the older child and the adult (Forssberg & Nashner, 1982). This relates primarily to the use of visual cues and the ability to suppress the conflicting visual information that develops later in life.

NORMATIVE DATA

A large and reliable database for normal performance has been developed by the manufacturer, in conjunction with EquiTest users, for the age range of 16–79 years. This is appropriately divided by age groups to account for the effects of aging. For patients above or below this range, the testing facility must develop its own normal ranges. Unlike the normative data discussed for rotational chair and ocular-motor work, data from postural control testing (except EMG data) tend to be highly skewed toward good performance and thus are not normally distributed. Therefore, although two standard deviations have been taken to represent a normal range for the other investigations, this is not statistically appropriate for posturography. Therefore, the 5th percentile values are usually taken as the cutoff for normal performance. As with ocular-motor testing, age is a critical factor in the assessment of postural control performance, and age-related normative data are required for accurate clinical evaluations, independent of which method of testing is utilized.

8

INTEGRATED MANAGEMENT AND INTERPRETATION OF VESTIBULAR TEST RESULTS

RATIONALE

Discussion to this point has focused on laboratory tools for vestibular assessment, the clinical history, and physical examination. Cases introduced or completed in Chapter 7 demonstrate the benefit of integrating information from multiple tests with the patient's presenting history to develop a working diagnosis that allows the clinician to begin a treatment program. While the goal of establishing a working diagnosis and beginning management is a common theme, the tools used and the complexity of the treatment plan are different for the acute versus the chronic balance disorder patient. When evaluating a patient with the acute onset of vertigo for the first time, establishing a preliminary diagnosis, ruling out life-threatening causes of a neurological or cardiovascular nature, is of primary importance. This is typically accomplished with the use of the history, clinical examinations, perhaps an emergency CT scan, and screening cardiovascular testing. It is unlikely that vestibular testing

would be needed in this process. If auditory symptoms were reported, the patient should get a thorough audiometric evaluation and radiographic studies to rule out a cerebellopontine angle lesion, for which balance testing would not be required. In certain cases where eye movement abnormalities on the clinical examination suggest central involvement, use of ENG with extensive ocular-motor evaluation would be a reasonable follow-up study. When managing the acute onset of vertigo, after significant neurological and cardiovascular causes have been ruled out, the judicious use of medications to control symptoms is appropriate, as will be discussed in Chapter 9. The clinician should recommend that the patient return to normal activities as soon as possible. Counseling the patient not to avoid activities that provoke mild symptoms may help facilitate the natural compensation process. The patient should then be scheduled for follow up within 3 weeks for a progress check. If the patient continues to have symptoms, episodic or continuously, for longer than 6–8 weeks, one can assume that there is either incomplete compensation or an ongoing pathologic process in the vestibular system.

The chronic balance disorder patient is managed somewhat differently, assuming the above acute evaluation has been performed. Reassessment of the preliminary diagnosis and determination of the factors preventing recovery now must be addressed. As introduced in Chapter 3, this lack of improvement could involve a progressive or unstable peripheral or central system lesion, or a stable lesion with poor central system compensation. Determining which of these situations exists requires detailed historical information, assisted by results from the various laboratory studies. Perhaps more important than the actual diagnosis is the determination of which of these situations is responsible for the continued symptoms, as this strongly influences the formulation of the diagnostic and treatment plan. This plan may involve a medical or surgical intervention, or possibly a vestibular rehabilitation program. With many of the chronic patients, a combination of treatments is required. Chapters 10, 11, and 12 provide the reader with a brief discussion of these treatment options and their indications. Chapter 12 extensively reviews the decision process (philosophy) used by the authors to map out a treatment plan with a particular emphasis on avoiding the injudicious use of surgical procedures. By far, the use of a vestibular rehabilitation program is the most common form of treatment for the chronic balance disorder patients served in our facility. In the survey of 2266 patients introduced in previous chapters, 74% had recommendations for a vestibular rehabilitation program as part of their treatment plan. In general, less than 10% of chronic balance disorder patients are candidates for surgical procedures, unless the physician has a referral pattern that specifically selects only surgical candidates from the chronic balance disorder patients for inclusion in his or her practice.

When considering studies for a chronic balance disorder patient, is it appropriate to simply perform all of the tests discussed so far on all patients? This question will be addressed in two parts. First, which tests of balance system function discussed in Chapters 4–7 are appropriate for which patients? This will be considered in the next section of this chapter. Second, which audiometric tests, neuroradiographic or laboratory studies are needed? These issues, together with guidelines for subspecialist referrals, will be taken up in Chapter 9.

PROTOCOL FOR USE OF BALANCE FUNCTION STUDIES

To simplify decision making, it would be easiest to perform ENG, ocular-motor, rotary chair, and postural control assessment on all patients. This can be defended if the patients have had symptoms for an extended interval, usually greater than 1 year. If multiple inconclusive evaluations have been performed by other specialists, with no conclusive opinion as to the nature of the problem and no resolution of symptoms, a comprehensive series of studies is especially appropriate. However, even with this type of patient, an ENG with extended ocular-motor evaluation alone will often identify the structures of the balance system that are involved. It can also provide insight into the compensation status. The functional status of a chronic patient can be addressed using posturography, but it may well be clear after reviewing the presenting history and performing a few brief clinical screening tests. Being selective with test utilization becomes increasingly important with recently symptomatic patients undergoing their first formal laboratory study of the balance system. Additionally, in the current environment of strict medical cost containment programs and increasing managed care programs, routinely performing all tests for all patients may not be practical. Second, not all facilities will be willing to expend the amount of money needed to provide ENG, rotary chair, and posturography studies, yet need to provide initial services to many chronic balance disorder patients. Given these considerations, considerable effort has been put forth in our facility to develop a core of balance function tests that allows a thorough preliminary review of the chronic patient. Guidelines for additional testing by rotational chair and/or dynamic posturography have also been established. The protocol discussed below is based on the clinical utility information from the patient survey discussed earlier, together with formal research comparison of clinical screening tests such as Clinical Test of Sensory Interaction and Balance (CTSIB) with dynamic posturography (see Chapters 3 and 7).

Each patient referred for evaluation of a chronic balance disorder receives an evaluation including at least:

1. ENG, as described in Chapter 4
2. Ocular-motor evaluation as described in Chapter 5
3. A complete neuro-otologic history as described in Chapter 3
4. A modified CTSIB (no visual conflict conditions) as described in Chapter 3.

Based on the results from the core studies and history, the following guidelines are used for determining whether to include rotary chair and/or dynamic posturography:

Rotary Chair would be used

■ if the ENG is normal, and ocular-motor results are either normal or observed abnormalities would not invalidate rotational chair results (for example, Case 17 in Chapter 5 and 6). Chair testing is used here to expand the investigation of peripheral system involvement and compensation status.

■ if the ENG suggests a well-compensated status (no spontaneous or positional nystagmus), despite the presence of a clinically significant unilateral caloric weakness and ongoing symptoms complaints. Chair testing is used here to expand the investigation of compensation in a patient with a known lesion site and complaints suggesting poor compensation.

■ if the caloric irrigations are below 10°/sec bilaterally, when caloric irrigations cannot be performed, or when results in the two ears may not be compared reliably due to anatomic variability. Chair testing is used in these cases to verify and define the extent of a bilateral weakness, or to further investigate the relative responsiveness of the peripheral

vestibular apparatus in each ear when calorics studies are unreliable or unavailable (see Case 47, Chapter 7; Case 45, Chapter 6).

■ if a baseline is needed to follow the natural history of the patient's disorder (such as possible early endolymphatic hydrops) or for assessing the effectiveness of a particular treatment, like that of chemical ablation of one or both peripheral vestibular systems (see Chapter 11 and 12).

Dynamic Posturography would be used

■ if the CTSIB was abnormal with a fall reaction, significantly increased sway, or a sudden change of strategy for maintaining stance during a trial. Based on the comparison between CTSIB and dynamic posturography, we know that the patient who can perform CTSIB in the normal range is very unlikely to fail the sensory organization portion of dynamic posturography. On the other hand, dynamic posturography is needed to further delineate postural control difficulties when abnormal performance is noted on the CTSIB.

■ if the patient has a major complaint involving unsteadiness when standing or walking, independent of the CTSIB results. Dynamic posturography, especially movement coordination testing, is used in this case to further investigate postural control. This patient would also be a candidate for Postural Evoked Response testing.

■ if the patient had a history of known pathology involving the postural control pathways that may influence the patient's overall performance, even though unsteadiness is not a major complaint (see Case 35, Chapter 7).

When these criteria were applied to over 4000 patients tested in our facility, 30% would have completed only the core testing. The remaining 70% would have gone on for combinations of rotary chair and dynamic posturography. The reader is advised that this estimate is dependent on the demographics of patients referred for testing in our facility. These can serve as general guidelines, but they may need to be altered for the specific setting in other institutions.

INTEGRATED TEST REPORTING

When multiple tests are used on a patient, it is best to report the results in a way that integrates the findings in the following areas:

1. Presence or absence of peripheral system involvement, the side of the lesion, and compensation status.
2. Presence or absence of central vestibulo-ocular or ocular-motor pathway involvement and, if possible, lesion localization within the central system.
3. Status of postural control ability for maintenance of upright stance and status of coordinated response to recovery from unexpected sway.

Recommendations based on these impressions and the patient's presenting clinical history will depend on the organizational nature of the testing facility. In the authors' institution, patients may be referred for evaluation by any discipline, in an open service model not unlike a radiology department. If this model is followed, the recommendations returned with the test results should cover the following issues:

1. The need for additional specialty referral for diagnostic evaluation and treatment, such as otology, neurology, physical medicine, and rehabilitation, and so on.
2. The potential benefit of a vestibular rehabilitation program.

If the patients evaluated in a balance function laboratory were all primarily managed by an otologist or neurologist knowledgeable in balance disorders, the recommendations might be less specific or unnecessary. On the other hand, the testing facility should not allow an inexperienced clinician to assume that a mass lesion or degenerative condition has been ruled out by balance testing. When unexplained findings are detected, the report should be prepared in a way that prompts the clinician to pursue additional studies, if necessary. This continues to be the responsibility of the physician.

In order to give integrated impressions as suggested above, certain test results should influence the interpretation of others. Case 17, presented throughout Chapters 5–7, illustrates the common situation where ocular-motor results influence the interpretation of other test results that could represent either peripheral or central involvement. In this case, the increased phase lead on rotary chair and the positional nystagmus from the ENG were felt to be secondary to a central system lesion based on the ocular-motor results. Case 18, from Chapter 7, demonstrates the integration of limited chair results with dynamic posturography and the caloric findings to give the impression of a mild bilateral peripheral system paresis. It was this unexplained bilateral paresis, along with the patient's asymmetric loss of hearing, that stimulated the recommendation for MRI investigation. This led to the discovery of bilateral cerebellopontine angle mass lesions. Impressions for Case 20 (Chapter 6) were also an integrated effort. The presence of clinically significant positional nystagmus could have been from peripheral or central involvement, and given the patient's history of symptoms starting after a motor vehicle accident, central involvement was a strong possibility. Yet the normal ocular-motor findings and the strongly positive chair results collectively suggested peripheral system involvement exclusively. The other features of his presenting symptoms, including spontaneous events of vertigo and motion-provoked symptoms, assisted in implicating the peripheral vestibular system.

The patient's presenting history may be as influential in shaping the impressions as the test results themselves. Case 19 (Chapter 7) provided no test findings suggestive of peripheral or central system involvement. However, it is known that patients with classic Ménière's disease frequently have completely normal findings, so this finding in itself does not rule out peripheral labyrinthine pathology. This patient's history together with the dynamic posturography findings collectively provide the impression that the symptoms were secondary to severe peripheral sensory neuropathy.

In summary, the various case examples given throughout the text emphasize the relationship between the test results and the importance of the patient's presenting complaints. Interpreting findings in isolation from other aspects of the test battery and the patient's history may produce significant diagnostic confusion and ultimately lead to delays in diagnosis and appropriate treatment.

9

▪ DIAGNOSTIC TEST SELECTION IN THE EVALUATION OF THE BALANCE DISORDER PATIENT

*T*he methods of vestibular diagnosis using the patient's clinical history, physical examination, and various vestibular testing protocols have been comprehensively reviewed in Chapters 3 through 7 of this textbook. Chapter 8 integrated this information into a format useful for guiding vestibular test selection and interpretation of the resulting diagnostic information in the clinical setting. This chapter is designed to review the role of other diagnostic procedures that may play an important role in the assessment of individuals with dizziness or other disturbances of balance function.

AUDIOMETRIC TESTING

It is not unusual to be confronted with a patient whose balance test results suggest dysfunction of the peripheral vestibular system. Unfortunately, these tests cannot distinguish a lesion in the labyrinth itself from those involving the VIIIth nerve or even the vestibular nucleus. On the other hand, audiometric test results frequently can determine the specific anatomic location of a peripheral lesion that impairs auditory function and may be associated with vertigo. The diagnostic utility of audiometric testing is briefly reviewed here, and the interested reader is referred to standard works for a more complete discussion (Jacobson & Northern, 1991; Katz, 1994).

Conventional diagnostic audiometry evaluates auditory sensitivity to identify either conductive or sensorineural hearing loss. A complete audiometric evaluation includes a pure tone audiogram, speech audiometry, tympanometry, and acoustic reflex testing.

Pure Tone Audiometry

The patient's threshold for detecting pure tones is obtained by both air and bone conduction, with the proper use of clinical masking when indicated. Conductive hearing loss is evident when sensitivity to air-conducted signals is impaired relative to the bone-conduction threshold, resulting in an air-bone gap. The diagnostic interpretation of a conductive hearing loss hinges on the history and the otoscopic examination. If the external ear, tympanic membrane, and middle ear appear to be normal, otosclerosis is suspected. If the hearing loss began after trauma, an ossicular disruption is suspected. The otologic exam may reveal evidence for acute or chronic otitis media. Either of these conditions may be associated with dizziness, as discussed in Chapter 3. Sensorineural hearing loss results in equal impairment of air and bone conduction thresholds. This finding on the audiogram localizes the lesion either to the cochlea or to the VIIIth cranial nerve but cannot distinguish between the two.

Speech Audiometry

The speech reception threshold may be useful whenever the pure tone audiogram is abnormal. This value should be similar to the average of the thresholds obtained in the low to mid frequency range during pure tone testing. This test primarily serves to verify the reliability of the behavioral audiogram. Speech discrimination ability is assessed by presenting phonetically balanced monosyllabic words to one ear at a comfortable suprathreshold intensity. The test is scored as a percentage of correct responses. Cochlear lesions are usually associated with an impairment of speech discrimination that is proportional to the configuration and degree of the pure tone hearing loss. Unexpectedly poor speech discrimination scores suggest a retrocochlear process, such as acoustic neuroma or multiple sclerosis. VIIIth cranial nerve lesions can result in severely impaired speech discrimination despite normal or near normal pure tone thresholds. As the intensity of test presentation is increased, the patient with a cochlear lesion will show improved performance, whereas an VIIIth nerve lesion may cause performance to deteriorate, a phenomenon known as *rollover*. In the early 1980s, the wide availability of sophisticated neurodiagnostic testing and the introduction of noninvasive radiographic studies dramatically reduced the clinical utility of performing tests for rollover

and other indicators of possible retrocochlear pathology.

Tympanometry and Acoustic Reflex Testing

The tympanogram provides a rapid means of assessing tympanic membrane integrity and middle ear compliance. The *acoustic reflex* refers to the reflex contraction of the stapedius muscle in response to a loud sound. The stapedius muscle contracts bilaterally when either ear is stimulated, causing a decrease in the compliance of the middle ear system as measured by a change in acoustic immittance. By systematically recording the acoustic reflex findings in each ear stimulated ipsilaterally and contralaterally, the integrity of the middle ear system, the VIIth and VIIIth cranial nerves, and related brainstem pathways can be evaluated. Reflexes generally are absent when a significant conductive hearing loss is present. On the other hand, the acoustic reflex is particularly useful when evaluating a sensorineural hearing loss. Hearing loss due to a purely cochlear lesion must be severe before the acoustic reflex is lost. Unexpectedly elevated or absent acoustic reflex thresholds, or rapid decay of the acoustic reflex response, suggests retrocochlear pathology.

The presence of an asymmetrical sensorineural hearing loss is a strong lateralizing sign for labyrinthine pathology. In the absence of a conflicting clinical history or vestibular test results, the symptomatic vestibular system is almost invariably associated with the ear demonstrating a sensorineural hearing loss (Shone et al., 1991). Serial audiograms may show progression or fluctuation of sensorineural hearing loss, documenting inner ear dysfunction in some puzzling cases. If there is great difficulty lateralizing the ear that is causing a peripheral vestibular disturbance, it may be helpful to have the patient's hearing tested during an acute episode of vertigo to see if fluctuating hearing loss can be detected. If no hearing loss is ever detected in a patient with recurring severe spontaneous spells of vertigo without associated auditory symptoms, the likelihood of endolymphatic hydrops decreases. This patient is more likely to be suffering from a migraine variant than a pure labyrinthine disorder.

Auditory Brain Stem Response Testing

The auditory brain stem response (ABR) is a far field potential that reflects the function of the external, middle, and inner ear together with the VIIIth cranial nerve and brainstem auditory pathways. The response is generated by presenting a series of clicks (and sometimes tone bursts, Telian & Kileny, 1989) by earphone or an insert transducer sequentially to each ear. The ABR is recorded by scalp electrodes, amplified and filtered, and the signals that result are averaged by computer after multiple repetitions. The resulting waveform represents the specific neural responses that are time-locked to the auditory stimulus, and is generally divided into waves I–V for analysis. Wave I results from activation of the VIIIth cranial nerve terminals near the cochlea. Wave II is generated by the medial portion of the cochlear nerve, prior to entry into the cochlear nucleus. Wave III is felt to be generated by the cochlear nuclei. The exact neuroanatomic generators of waves IV and V, along with two late waves sometimes detected (waves VI and VII) are uncertain, but involve other brain stem structures involved in central auditory processing, such as the superior olivary complex, the lateral lemniscus, and the inferior colliculus. A lesion along the auditory pathway may result in decreased amplitude, increased latency, or absence of subsequent waves. In general, waves I, III, and V are the most robust and reliable for determining response abnormalities and measuring conduction through the auditory system. Auditory brain stem response tests are very effective in screening for cerebellopontine angle tumors. Absent wave III and/or wave V in the presence of a replicable wave I suggests a retrocochlear lesion. The ABR is relatively insensitive to metabolic abnormalities and is useful in distinguishing metabolic from structural causes of brain stem dysfunction. The ABR also may be used to confirm the true hearing sensitivity when behavioral audiometric results are suspect.

The ABR is not performed routinely in the evaluation of the vestibular disorder patient. In the past, ABR has been used as an excellent non-invasive screening test for vestibular schwannoma (acoustic neuroma). The introduction of magnetic resonance imaging (MRI), a safe and highly sensitive imaging modality, has largely displaced the use of ABR when a mass lesion is strongly suspected. The utility of ABR as a screening tool also diminishes as the cost differential between this study and MRI decreases. Because a small tumor (< 0.8 cm) may not produce ABR abnormalities, one should be cautious about using ABR alone to rule out this diagnosis (Telian, Kileny, Kemink, Niparko, & Graham, 1989). However, when clinical suspicion is low or when MRI is not readily available, an abnormal ABR may serve as an impetus to pursue a definitive imaging study. ABR testing is sometimes pursued when the MRI is negative but other clinical information suggests VIIIth nerve dysfunction. An increased I–III interpeak latency might increase the suspicion of demyelinating disease or a vascular loop compression syndrome in this setting.

Electrocochleography

Electrical potentials generated within the cochlea and in the proximal auditory nerve fibers can be evaluated by electrocochleography (ECoG). This is accomplished by the delivery of an auditory stimulus similar to that used in ABR testing, but requires the placement of a recording electrode near the tympanic membrane or transtympanically onto the promontory of the cochlea. The transtympanic placement is preferred due to improved detection and repeatability of responses, but introduces the risk of infection and tympanic membrane perforation. The responses that are clinically important are the summating potential (SP) and the N1 action potential (AP). The AP corresponds to wave I of the ABR and can be used to help identify wave I if the ABR morphology is poor. As the amplitude of these potentials is variable, the SP/AP ratio has been the most widely used measurement clinically. This ratio is generally below .35 in normal ears when click stimuli are employed. Elevations of the SP/AP ratio have been thought to reflect altered hydrodynamic pressure relationships within the inner ear, as might be encountered in endolymphatic hydrops or perilymphatic fistula. However, the significant variability of the SP/AP ratio in disease states and in normal ears results in considerable overlap, dramatically reducing the test sensitivity and specificity. Thus, the clinician generally must make diagnostic and treatment decisions based on the patient's history and other test data regardless of the ECoG results. For this reason, the authors rarely use electrocochleography to guide clinical decisions. One exception might be a very puzzling case where atypical Ménière's disease was suspected. An ECoG might be performed if the clinician had insufficient grounds to proceed with definitive treatment, especially if no hearing loss was present. If the ECoG results document a dramatically elevated SP/AP ratio in one ear, the finding could be extremely helpful in identifying the offending ear and increasing the suspicion of endolymphatic hydrops.

RADIOGRAPHIC STUDIES

Radiologic evaluation of the temporal bone and posterior cranial fossa is indicated in the presence of asymmetrical sensorineural hearing loss or significant unilateral abnormalities on vestibular testing. A variety of temporal bone lesions may present initially with vertigo. These include congenital and acquired cholesteatoma, glomus tumors, and giant cholesterol cysts of the temporal bone. Some of these abnormalities, especially cholesteatoma, will be suspected from the clinical history and physical examination. If so, imaging studies are only performed if they are required to confirm the diagnosis or plan treatment. On the other hand, most posterior fossa lesions cannot be diagnosed with confidence until confirmed by a suitable imaging study. The vast majority of these lesions are acoustic neuromas and, less commonly, meningiomas of the cerebellopon-

tine angle. Other benign tumors, metastatic tumors, and brain stem lesions are exceedingly rare. High resolution computed tomography (CT) is preferred for the assessment of intrinsic lesions of the temporal bone and for preoperative evaluation of bony anatomy. Magnetic resonance imaging, expecially with gadolinium enhancement, is exquisitely sensitive in the detection of mass lesions of the internal auditory canal and cerebellopontine angle. In addition, the MRI will sometimes identify ischemic or demyelinating disease of the brainstem that cannot be detected by CT.

OTHER LABORATORY STUDIES

Dizziness is a nonspecific symptom that may be associated with a variety of metabolic disturbances or other medical problems unrelated to the ear or central nervous system. Laboratory studies ordered for a patient with dizziness or vertigo should be guided by information obtained from the history and physical examination. Routine hematologic and chemical tests to be considered include a complete blood count, serum electrolytes, glucose, thyroid function tests, blood urea nitrogen, and creatinine. Special studies that should be considered when evaluating vestibular dysfunction associated with fluctuating or rapidly progressive sensorineural hearing loss include the fluorescent treponemal antibody test for possible otosyphilis and tests that may indicate possible autoimmune disease, such as an erythrocyte sedimentation rate, antinuclear antibody, and rheumatoid factor. Although these tests are rarely abnormal, they occasionally recognize an important systemic condition that could negatively impact both hearing and general health if unrecognized. In addition, abnormalities in these tests may indicate that specific unique treatment measures should be considered. When otosyphilis is suspected, treatment with antibiotics and corticosteroids may eliminate or reduce the severity of symptoms. Unfortunately, a reliable and specific serologic test for autoimmune inner ear disease has not yet been developed. However, patients who have clinical symptoms and test results that suggest this diagnosis may benefit from treatment with corticosteroids or immunosuppression with cytotoxic agents. Urinalysis is sometimes performed for a toxicology screen if substance abuse is suspected.

When no vestibular cause for dizziness can be identified after careful evaluation, it is reasonable to refer the patient back to the primary care physician or an internist for a complete medical evaluation. General health measures such as weight reduction and a suitable exercise program may eliminate some nonspecific symptoms. Arterial blood gases, pulse oximetry, chest X-ray, EKG, or noninvasive carotid artery studies may be appropriate if cardiovascular insufficiency is suspected. Patients who have severe nonspecific dizziness only when standing, especially if associated with fainting or near-syncope, should undergo a tilt table evaluation to evaluate the regulatory function of the autonomic nervous system in blood pressure control.

GUIDELINES FOR SPECIALTY REFERRAL

The average patient with a self-limited vertigo syndrome (typical stable peripheral lesion) can be managed successfully by the primary care physician who is familiar with common vestibular disorders. The otolaryngologist frequently is consulted when there is a hearing loss, when the primary care physician is uncertain about the diagnosis, or when symptoms persist. Together, these physicians should be able to properly evaluate and manage the vast majority of patients with dizziness. The otolaryngologist can prevent unnecessary and costly testing by carefully selecting the appropriate diagnostic evaluation. An otolaryngologist with special training or experience in neurotology can provide help with the differential diagnosis in difficult cases and provide surgical management when indicated. The number of regional centers that provide comprehensive vestibular testing capabilities are increasing. These facilities play an important role in the evaluation of puzzling cases or those that present special treatment challenges.

Routine neurological consultation is not necessary when dizziness results from vestibular pathology. However, a neurologic evaluation should be considered when the screening neurological exam is abnormal, when there are positive findings on the MRI, or when abnormalities are noted in the oculomotor test battery that cannot be explained by small ischemic lesions in the brain stem on the MRI. Otherwise, it is unlikely that a significant neurologic condition that would influence the patient's clinical course will be detected. Sometimes a physical medicine and rehabilitation consultation is helpful in disability assessment or in assisting the impaired patient who is properly motivated to return to the workplace.

Psychiatric disorders will sometimes cause subjective complaints of dizziness or complicate the management of a patient with a primary vestibular disorder. Patients with panic disorder, agoraphobia, and generalized anxiety disorder frequently complain of dizziness or disorientation (Jacob 1988). Reactive depression may complicate any chronic illness and is particularly likely to develop in the setting of chronic vestibular dysfunction (see Chapter 11). Although these patients generally appear to be well, they cannot function in society in a way that is satisfactory to their family, friends, coworkers, and employers. If they are frustrated with the medical community's inability to successfully diagnose and treat their condition, this may add to their sense of hopelessness. Sometimes, a trusted primary care physician can successfully manage the anxiety disorder or depression that is negatively impacting the vestibular patient's functional capacity. If not, a psychiatric consultation should be pursued. Unfortunately, referral for psychiatric consultation carries a negative stigma with much of the population that must be overcome. In addition, one must recognize that many of these patients have been dismissed as simply "crazy" by the family or other physicians. If psychiatric referral is suggested, patients may feel that the current physician also disregards the importance of their physical symptoms. The treating physician must affirm the authenticity of the symptoms that are reported, and supportively place the psychiatric referral into proper context. Panic disorder and depression in particular have underlying neurochemical substrates that can almost always be successfully manipulated by psychoactive medications. The patient should be helped to understand that psychiatrists are simply the specialists who best understand these disorders and their treatment. The selection of the proper antidepressant or anti-anxiety medication, as well as necessary dosage adjustments, can be a complex task. This is especially true in panic disorder patients, many of whom consider themselves to be "highly sensitive" to all medications. They may tend to abandon recommended treatment at the first hint of side effects. For this reason, it is often helpful to have an expert assist in the treatment decisions. Many of these individuals also may benefit from additional services that the mental health community can provide, such as behavioral therapy or counseling. It is important to emphasize to the patient that accepting the reality of a psychological component to their illness is not an admission of weakness. Rather, it opens the door to move toward effective treatment and recovery.

10

■ VESTIBULAR REHABILITATION PROGRAMS

Vertigo or disequilibrium may persist due to poor central nervous system compensation after any acute injury to the vestibular system, even if there is no ongoing labyrinthine dysfunction (see Case 5 in Chapter 7). In addition, some patients will develop maladaptive postural control strategies that are destabilizing or bothersome in certain settings (see Case 1 in Chapter 7). These patients often benefit from a program of vestibular rehabilitation like those given as examples in Chapters 4–7. Such programs are most effective when customized to the needs of the individual patient and supervised by an appropriately trained physical therapist (Shepard & Telian, 1995; Shepard, Telian, Smith-Wheelock, & Raj, 1993; Shumway-Cook & Horak, 1990).

PHYSIOLOGIC BASIS AND THERAPEUTIC IMPLICATIONS

Current knowledge about the process of central compensation (see Chapter 3) for vestibular lesions suggests that avoidance of movements and body positions that provoke vertigo, as well as the traditional practice of prescribing vestibular suppressants for these patients, may be counterproductive. The stimulus for recovery from an acute vestibular lesion seems to be repeated exposure to the sensory conflicts produced by movement (habituation). Therefore, once the severe symptoms are resolved, the patient's medications should be discontinued and an informal program of increased activities that help toward recovery should be encouraged. For most individuals, recovery will be rapid and nearly complete. For some, the symptoms of vestibular dysfunction may persist. These chronic balance disorder patients are candidates for formal programs of vestibular rehabilitation. Four features of the nervous system underlie the physiologic basis behind vestibular rehabilitation. These qualities collectively enhance the therapeutic effect of specific, customized exercise programs. These areas are:

1. Adaptive plasticity of the central nervous system for balance system control. Examples of this were given in Chapters 2 and 3 illustrating modifications of postural control, the vestibulo-ocular reflex, and the ocular control mechanisms for saccades. These activities take advantage of short-term central nervous system adaptation to produce a change in the automatic mapped response to a familiar stimulus (Zee, 1994). To accom-

plish this, repeated exposure to particular environmental conditions or specific stimuli is needed. This factor is exploited primarily for treating disorders of postural control and gait difficulties.

2. Central sensory substitution involves the nervous system's limited ability to substitute one of the sensory inputs (vision, vestibular, or somatosensory/proprioception) for another one that is virtually absent. For example, vision may substitute for loss of cutaneous proprioceptive inputs in the plantar surface of the foot, or it may help control eye movements in patients with bilateral peripheral vestibular system paresis (see Chapter 2). While many patients naturally use substitution, some may require specific targeted activities from a vestibular rehabilitation program to optimize this effect.

3. Tonic rebalancing of neural activity at the level of the vestibular nuclei, in response to a persistent asymmetry of input from the two sides of the peripheral vestibular system. This usually results from an acute peripheral system insult or an ablative surgical procedure. The acute *(static compensation)* phase of recovery should take place without active head movement exercises. However, some patients (see, for example, Case 43, Chapter 3) fail to progress through the chronic *(dynamic compensation)* phase and require a formalized program of head movement exercises to promote this process.

4. Habituation is the long-term reduction in a neurologic response to a particular noxious stimulus that is facilitated by repeated exposure to the stimulus. In the vestibular system, the unpleasant response is usually a vertiginous sensation, often associated with nausea, in response to certain head movements. Even with the mechanisms described in numbers 1–3 firmly in place and functioning properly, deficiencies in the overall compensation process may persist. If so, certain specific head movements, position changes, or motion in the visual environment may predictably provoke brief spells of vertigo or disequilibrium. To reduce or eliminate these undesirable responses to daily activity, habituation exercises are prescribed that repeatedly expose the patient to the stimuli that provoke the abnormal responses. When this process is complete, the changes appear to be long lasting (Smith-Wheelock, Shepard, & Telian, 1991b).

The general principles of designing vestibular rehabilitation programs involve exposing the patient to the stimuli that provoke vertigo and challenging areas of deficiency in postural control. First, the therapist must identify those activities or environmental situations that provoke symptoms. Habituation exercises present repeated, brief, and controlled exposure to these stimuli to reduce the response. Second, the patient's functional deficits regarding balance and gait must be identified. These may be caused by the vestibular symptoms or by maladaptive behavior that has developed in response to the symptoms. Balance and gait retraining exercises may be prescribed that will alter the stimulus-coded response mapping and eliminate or reduce the deficits. Lastly, it is desirable to challenge the sedentary life-style that vestibular disorder patients often adopt. An active life-style including regular exercise that accounts for age and other health constraints will serve as a maintenance program once active therapy is completed. Therefore, in the development of any customized therapy exercise program, three areas should always be given consideration:

1. Habituation exercises
2. Balance and gait exercises
3. General conditioning exercises.

The specific details of the physical therapy evaluation needed to arrive a customized plan for treatment varies depending on the therapist. Detailed literature exists describing this evaluation process and will not be repeated here, except in a general manner. The reader requiring greater detail is referred to other sources (Borello-France, Whitney, & Herdman, 1994; Herdman, 1994b; Shumway-Cook & Horak, 1990; Smith-Wheelock, Shepard, & Telian, 1991a)

COMMON TECHNIQUES

Although minor details may vary among patient groups, the general approach to the physical therapy evaluation in our vestibular rehabilitation program is the same. First, a complete systems evaluation is performed. This evaluates the individual systems that make up the balance system, as discussed in Chapters 1 and 2. The physical therapist may not personally perform all the assessments used in this review, as many of these are evaluated by the test batteries discussed in Chapters 4–7. Nevertheless, the therapist must be familiar with the test results and their interpretation in light of the presenting history. The systems reviewed are:

Visual system

Vestibular system, peripheral and central

Ocular-motor control

Neurological, limb coordination, and sensation in the distal lower limbs

Musculoskeletal, including range of motion and strength

Cognition, the ability to remember and follow instructions.

The evaluation of these systems *does not* provide sufficient information to establish the treatment plan. These evaluations, in the context of the patient's presenting history, determine the limits on the therapy program because of severe, permanent dysfunction in one or more of these systems. Cases 19 and 3 from Chapters 6 and 7 are examples of situations where the prognosis was limited due to severe peripheral sensory neuropathy in the first case, and severe bilateral peripheral vestibular system paresis in the other. The actual treatment program is developed from the patient's presenting history and the systems integration evaluation. This evaluation examines the entire system as a whole for activities that provoke difficulties with dizziness or balance disturbance, as well as the functional deficits that may result. The areas we review during this phase of the evaluation are:

1. Static and dynamic postural control, including sensory organization and movement coordination (performed in clinical tests or with equipment like that discussed in Chapter 7)
2. Gait evaluation, to include gait at different speeds, with reciprocal horizontal and vertical head rotations, tandem gait, and eyes-closed gait
3. Sensitivity to rapid changes in head position. We utilize 16 rapid positional head movements. Each response is characterized by asking the patient to rate symptom intensity on a scale from 0 to 5, also accounting for the length of time the symptoms last, and the total number of position changes that produce symptoms. These three characterizing features are combined to produce a single number called the Motion Sensitivity Quotient (MSQ), ranging from 0 to 100%. If any of these three features change, this change will be reflected in the motion sensitivity quotient. Details of the movements and the formula used for the motion sensitivity quotient are given in a paper by Smith-Wheelock et al. (1991a) and the formula is repeated in Table 10–1.

The systems integration evaluation is used to develop the specific exercise activities that will comprise the vestibular rehabilitation program. A variety of clinical evaluations have been used to assess the sensorimotor systems that facilitate postural control and gait. In the same way that the MSQ score can quantify motion sensitivity, a quantifiable approach for scoring each of the clinical tests of systems integration has been developed. A group of normal subjects between age 20 and 79 years, with a minimum of 10 subjects per decade, were used to evaluate the effects of age and gender on the clinical tests used in our assessment protocol, as well as to establish normative data for use in the clinic. The goal is to use simple measures of postural control and gait with a high degree of test-retest reliability, so that experienced therapists repeating the exam on the same patient will obtain virtually the same scores. Table 10–1 gives the cutoff values for normal performance, as a function of age. Details of the study are

TABLE 10–1. Normative Data: Clinical Tests for Physical Therapy Evaluation

Variable\Age	20-49 Years	50-59 Years	60-69 Years	70-79 Years
*Dyn. Post. Comp.	725 (704)	620 (704)	660 (676)	630 (638)
Bal. Mast. St. Swy.	998	996	995	997
Bal. Mast. St. Pos.	767	653	703	860
*Bal. Mast. Dyn.	519	247 (318)	318	281
Clinic Static	750	633 (679)	679	663
Clinic Dynamic	969	850 (888)	844 (888)	888
CTSIB	177 (180)	180	178	151
*SOLEO RT.	18	5	9	3
*SOLEO LT.	19	6	8	4
*SOLEC RT.	3	3	2	1
*SOLEC LT.	3	2	2	1
TREO RT.	24 (30)	30	12 (30)	30
TREO LT.	30	6 (30)	30	30
*TREC RT.	6	3	4	5
*TREC LT.	7	4	2	6
*STAND TOTAL	120	64 (86)	86	84
*STEP	16	8	9	8
GAIT NML	20	20	20	20
GAIT FAST	20	20	20	20
GAIT SLOW	20	20	20	20
*GAIT TANDEM	20	13	15	15
*GAIT EYES CL.	16	13	15	15
GAIT ROTATION	18 (20)	20	20	19
GAIT FLEXION	20	20	20	20
*GAIT TOTAL	136	126 (135)	135	132
MOTION SENSITIVITY QUOTIENT	1.7 (1.6)	5.1 (1.6)	1.6	2.1 (1.6)

NOTES: Each cell shows the calculated 5th percentile clinical limit of normal. If a number is in () in a cell, that is the figure to be used in clinical evaluations. For all variables, except **Motion Sensitivity Quotient**, values less than the 5th percentile limit are considered outside the normal range.

* Indicates variables for which age had a statistically significant impact ($p < .05$).

Dyn. Post. Comp.—Dynamic posturography composite score from sensory organization of EquiTest. Normative data from NeuroCom given in () for each cell.

Bal. Mast. St. Sway.—The cumulative area of sway from Balance Master static test on EO, EC Romberg, and EO Romberg with a visual target was subtracted from 300 and the result divided by 0.3 to give the score, with maximum performance 999.

(continued)

TABLE 10–1. (*continued*)

Bal. Mast. St. Pos.—The cumulative percentage of time that mean center of gravity (from Balance Master static test) was away from the target on the three conditions EO, EC Romberg, and EO Romberg with a visual target subtracted from 300 and divided by 0.3 to give the score, with maximum performance 999.

Bal. Mast. Dyn.—The maximum limits of sway area able to be achieved (on three trials) multiplied by 10, with the maximum score of 1000.

Clinic Static—Combined measure of clinical measures of static balance. Represents the combined performance on CTSIB + STAND TOTAL, adjusted for maximum performance of 1000. Clinic Static = ((CTSIB ÷ 180) + (Stand total ÷ 240)) × 500.

Clinic Dynamic—Combined measure of clinical measures of dynamic balance.

Represents the sum of the performance on STEP + GAIT TOTAL, adjusted for maximum performance of 1000. Clinic Dynamic = (Step + Gait total) ÷ 0.16

CTSIB—*Clinical Test of Sensory Interaction and Balance.* 30-second maximum for each condition, with up to three trials (using the average of the three): one trial for Condition 1, two for Condition 2, and three for Conditions 3–6. Time was stopped when the patient underwent a fall reaction type of behavior with a step or sudden, significant sway movement with reaching. Maximum score was 180.

SOLEO—Standing on one leg eyes open, right leg. 30 second maximum with the average of three trials, unless the 30 seconds achieved on two of the three trials, then score taken as 30. Subsequent conditions involve standing, eyes open, on the left leg; eyes closed, on the right then left leg.

TREO—Tandem standing, eyes open, with the right leg in the rear. Scoring is the same as for SOLEO. Subsequent conditions involve tandem standing, eyes open, with the left leg in the rear; tandem standing, eyes closed, right then left leg in the rear.

STAND TOTAL—The sum of each of the SOLEO/EC and TREO/EC conditions for right and left legs combined. Maximum score of 240.

STEP—Stepping up and down from a 10″ stool as many times as possible within a 10-second interval. Three intervals performed, with the first practice and scores for the last two added for the final score..

GAIT NML—Gait at the patient's normal pace without head movement. Twenty-foot walk with turn and return. Walk within an 18″ set of parallel lines. The score is the number of steps within the lines for a total of twenty steps. Each step on or outside the line subtracts one from the maximum. Subsequent conditions involve gait at a fast pace (116 steps per minute, timed by a metronome); gait at a slow pace (66 steps per minute); tandem gait on a 5-cm-wide line, scoring is as with the gait between the lines, each step off is subtracted from the maximum of twenty; gait with eyes closed following the start (scored as above between the 18″ separated lines; gait with horizontal head rotation at the rate of the normal walk; gait with head flexion and extension at the rate of the normal pace.

GAIT TOTAL—The sum of the scores of all of the gait conditions. Maximum score was 140.

MOTION SENSITIVITY QUOTIENT—A composite score from 16 rapid positioning maneuvers. Motion Sensitivity Quotient = ((# of positions × Total score) ÷ 2048) × 100%). The specific positional movements are given in Smith-Wheelock et al. (1991b).

given by El-Kashlan et al. (1996; see Chapter 3). Note that the normative data for the CTSIB (Clinical Test of Sensory Interaction and Balance) test was obtained using the technique originally described by Shumway-Cook and Horak (1986), although the type of foam pad utilized was different. This technique was compared to the sensory organization test of EquiTest.

Another important concern in vestibular rehabilitation programs is the ability to measure treatment outcome. Although the clinic tests used for evaluation (Table 10–1) provide a numerical baseline against which to compare over time, some of these are specifically practiced during therapy, which could bias the outcome measures. Assessment tools that are not specifically practiced during the therapy exercises are important in helping to verify the effectiveness of the treatment. The one exception is the use of the motion sensitivity quotient to determine the effects of habituation exercises. This practice is defensible since the habituation effect is thought to be a physiological change in activity at the synaptic level in the vestibular system, as opposed to learned or modified behavior as is the case with gait and postural control (Shumway-Cook &

Horak, 1990). Activities such as the four graded mobility tests discussed in the opening of Chapter 7 (Gavie et al., 1994) could be one tool for evaluation before and after therapy. Other types of outcome measures are more global, involving scales of performance. Two that the authors have used for years, and validated against the Dizziness Handicap Inventory (see Chapter 7), involve independently assessing degree of disability and intensity of residual symptoms at the end of the active therapy program. Distinguishing between symptom control and disability is important, as the primary goal of any vestibular rehabilitation program is to reduce the patient's level of disability. It has become clear that the level of disability may be reduced even if symptoms are not significantly reduced. For some patients, reducing anxiety about their symptoms, and showing that they can remain in control even while symptoms occur, may significantly improve disability and allow for a more active life-style. The two scales used for these measures are given in Tables 10–2 (disability) and 10–3 (symptom control). As indicated in Chapter 7, the DHI is also a reasonable outcome measure for changes during therapy.

The following section will review the features of a vestibular rehabilitation program in slightly more detail and discuss the role of the therapist and the physician in the rehabilitation process.

Habituation of Pathologic Responses

For most patients with positional or motion-provoked symptoms, the primary goal is to extinguish the pathologic responses that remain due to incomplete or disordered compensation. The therapist identifies the typical movements that produce the most intense symptoms and provides the patient with a list of exercises that reproduce these movements. These are performed twice daily, unless limited by severe nausea or dizziness. In the experience of the authors, for greater than 85% of the patients this can be handled with a home program, without the need for direct supervision other than infrequent visits with the therapist for modifications. The patients are counseled that symptoms typically are aggravated by the exercises at first, but that gradual improvement will follow. Patients are often encouraged by experiencing short-term adaptation at the end of an exercise session. If they can persevere with their program, most patients will begin to note improvement of positional vertigo within 4 to 6 weeks.

It is not uncommon for patients with motion-provoked symptoms to note that motion in the visual environment reproduces similar symptoms, even without movement of the head. In a smaller group of patients, visual sensitivity is the primary or only complaint. These symptoms must be addressed by exercises other than movement of the head. Head movement activities with the eyes open provide some of the visual-vestibular interaction work desired, but this does not seem to be sufficient for those with specific visual motion sensitivity (Herdman, Borello-France, & Whitney, 1994b). Specific visual motion activities such as visual-vestibular interaction exercises are needed. These are similar to those discussed below for patients

TABLE 10–2. Disability Scale

Score	Description
0	No disability; negligible symptoms
1	No disability; bothersome symptoms
2	Mild disability; performs usual work duties, but symptoms interfere with outside activities
3	Moderate disability; symptoms disrupt performance of both usual work duties and outside activities
4	Recent severe disability; on medical leave or had to change job because of symptoms
5	Long-term severe disability; unable to work for over 1 year or established permanent disability with compensation payments

TABLE 10–3. Post-therapy Symptoms Scoring

Score	Description
0	No symptoms remaining at the end of therapy
1	Marked improvement in symptoms, mild symptoms remaining
2	Mild improvement, definite persistent symptoms remaining
3	No change in symptoms relative to pretherapy period
4	Symptoms worsened with therapy activities on a persistent basis relative to pretherapy period

with bilateral vestibular system paresis and oscillopsia.

Postural Control and Gait Exercises

When abnormalities of postural control or difficulty with gait are detected in the assessment, they may be specifically addressed in the prescribed exercise program. Programs can be designed to correct weight-bearing asymmetries, limited mobility about the center of gravity, and sensory input selection problems. For example, if the patient is found to depend on somatosensory input despite the availability of accurate visual cues, the program may involve exercises that require balancing on thick foam. This would be performed initially with eyes open and eventually with eyes closed. Difficulty with gait, if not noticed during routine walking, may often be exposed if head movements are added during ambulation. It should not be assumed that improvements in static or even dynamic postural control will result in improved gait. Although there are shared functional activities involved in both tasks, such as weight shifting, the overall mechanisms for postural control and gait are different. Therefore, specific evaluation of gait and exercise activities to address gait problems may be needed. This is especially true in the bilateral peripheral vestibular paresis patient. For these individuals, gait is highly dependent on the proprioceptive and visual information available in the environment. Specific walking programs are used for all bilateral paresis patients. Each begins with a program that has them walking independently (contingent on other health factors) on a flat

firm surface in good lighting. They then work on the flat firm surface in poorer lighting until reasonable control of gait is achieved. Next, they focus on attempting to traverse irregular or compressible surfaces in good lighting. When this can be accomplished, the patient attempts to work on the disruptive surface in poor lighting, with assistance from another person or an assistive devise. Depending on the extent of the bilateral loss (as assessed by rotational chair testing), this last condition may never be negotiated without assistance. Such was the situation for the patient presented in Chapter 7 as Case 3. The extent of his loss prohibited gait control in a dark environment with an irregular support surface. Yet with practice, he was able to accomplish this task using a cane lightly touching the ground, giving a much expanded base of support. This patient's active therapy also was focused on increasing his volitional limits of sway in the sagittal plane, as evidenced functionally with his performance on Condition 4 of sensory organization (see Figure 7–4, Chapter 7). In the bilateral peripheral paresis patients, the extent and site-of-lesion studies (caloric irrigations and rotational chair) directly impact on the design and prognosis of the therapy program. In Case 3, with reduced vestibulo-ocular reflex (VOR) gain for all frequencies below .32 Hz, one should never expect return of function under Conditions 5 and 6 of sensory organization testing. Therefore, although practice in situations with altered vision and proprioception were part of his program, this was done primarily to increase his functional capacity by teaching him to use his assistive device and to recognize the difficulties he could expect in these environmental conditions. In contrast, a bilateral weakness patient with return of normal peripheral sensitivity on rotational chair by 0.16 Hz might be expected to improve performance on Conditions 5 and 6 of the sensory organization test, and may have a more ambitious therapy program prescribed.

Visual-Vestibular Interaction

For patients with bilateral vestibular paresis or disorders of visual-vestibular interaction, exercises may be required that optimize the use of the visual system inputs for maintaining equilibrium and gaze stability (Telian, Shepard, Smith-Wheelock, & Hoberg, 1991). These may be incorporated with hand-eye coordination exercises when needed (Herdman, 1994b). An example would be to have a visual target in an outstretched hand, maintaining gaze as the head is reciprocally moved in the horizontal or vertical plane with the hand moving in the opposite direction.

Conditioning Activities

Most patients with vertigo and balance disorders have adopted a sedentary life-style to avoid their symptoms. While this is an understandable behavior, it unfortunately contributes to their ongoing perceived and actual disability, while helping to prevent their recovery. All patients who receive customized vestibular rehabilitation programs are also provided with suggestions for a general exercise program that is suited to their age, health, and interests. For most individuals, this would involve at least a graduated walking program. These activities are done once a day, 5 days per week. For some, a more strenuous program is suggested that may include jogging, treadmill, aerobics, or bicycling. Activities that involve coordinated eye, head, and body movements such as golf or racquet sports may be appropriate. Swimming is approached cautiously because of the disorientation experienced by many vestibular patients in the relative weightlessness of the aquatic environment. These activities will form the cornerstone of the maintenance program that the patient will be advised to follow after the active therapy phase of the program. It is important

that the patient realize the conditioning activities must include head movements to be effective for purposes related to maintaining compensation status. These head movements should exceed those required for the patient's routine activities. Habituation of a response in one plane of motion does not seem to generalize to other planes of motion. In fact, there is significant anecdotal evidence to conclude the opposite. Therefore, no matter how physically active the patient is during the daily routine, the initial program and the maintenance program both should include active head movements in different planes.

Maintenance of Initial Results

Once the patient has completed the initial period of treatment (typically 2–6 weeks), progress is assessed and adjustments are made in the program. Exercises that no longer produce symptoms are eliminated and replaced by others that were not originally included because of lower priority. This process is continued until the improvements begin to plateau. When this point is reached (8–10 weeks is the average for the home program patients), it is important to provide the patient with counseling and a program of maintenance exercises to ensure stability of the initial improvements. The maintenance program typically includes continuing the prescribed conditioning exercises, as well as any unique postural control activities that were required. The patient is instructed to resume the habituation exercises if a relapse of positional symptoms should occur. Although relapses may be anticipated during periods of illness or fatigue, experienced patients will reinstitute their exercise program and regain a well-compensated state. If this is not successful, the patient should be re-evaluated by the physician and therapist.

In an effort to determine the long-term effects of therapy and our success in changing the life-style of the patients, a 20% random sample of 152 patients who had completed a customized program 12 to 30 months earlier were questioned. The 152 patients were the subjects of a prospective observational study and were well characterized as to post-therapy disability and symptoms (Shepard, Telian, Smith-Wheelock, & Raj, 1993). Each patient within the 20% sample was personally interviewed by phone to obtain his or her current status (Smith-Wheelock et al., 1991b). Eighty-seven percent of the sampled patients described their post-therapy disability and symptoms scores as being equal to or improved from what it was at the completion of therapy. Additionally, 47% were continuing to perform their maintenance program at least three times per week. Twenty-seven percent of the patients had experienced an interval of increased symptoms since they had completed their therapy, but reinstituted their therapy program and regained their compensated state. In summary, this review suggested that the effects of therapy can be long lasting and that a reasonable percentage of patients did change their life-style.

Role of Therapist in Patient Education

A key role of the therapist in the management of balance disorder patients is to educate patients about their illness. Often, considerable misinformation must be addressed. This supportive function of the therapist is particularly essential for the management of patients with a less favorable prognosis. Patients who are well educated regarding the nature of vestibular dysfunction will understand the rationale for vestibular rehabilitation. They will recognize that these measures are primarily a management technique instead of a cure. The patient takes significant responsibility for his or her therapy outcome. This focus takes the patient from a passive to an active role in recovery from dizziness and disequilibrium. The patients with significant bilateral peripheral vestibular system paresis are major benefactors of this education process. In a recent study, 13 such patients underwent complete re-evaluation at least 6 months after completion of active therapy. No changes in the extent of the lesion were noted, nor were there any changes in oscillopsia or the functional impact on postural control (as measured by EquiTest). In spite of the lack of measurable physiologic improvement, all patients reported improved postural control and reduced symptoms of oscillopsia following their therapy program. Although some of the perceptual changes probably resulted from practicing activities that had been avoided previously, the extensive survey that was taken in this study indicated that the education process was of great importance (Acierno et al., 1996).

Role of the Physician

Otologists increasingly recognize the need to develop a successful program of vestibular rehabilitation to serve their patients with balance complaints. This is best pursued by assembling a qualified team of professionals including the otologist, vestibular testing personnel, and a physical therapist specifically trained in vestibular assessment and treatment. A working relationship with insightful neurologic and psychiatric consultants also is very helpful. Optimally, the physical therapist will understand something of the diagnostic aspects of neurotology, as well as the strengths and limitations of conventional medical and surgical modalities. The otologist likewise must appreciate the role that the therapist can hope to play in the treatment of this challenging patient population. A mutually supportive and interactive environment is ideal for responding to the diverse needs encountered in a busy vestibular treatment program. The otologist will find that the time investment required for education and team development will pay considerable dividends in terms of treatment outcome and patient satisfaction.

TREATMENT EFFICACY

The utility and success of vestibular rehabilitation programs appear to be population-specific. Generally patients with uncompensated or decompensated unilateral peripheral lesions have the best overall prognosis. The percentage of patients who dramatically or completely improve increases from 30% among those having a history of head injury at onset of symptoms to better than 90% for those without head injury, provided they have good postural control and if their symptoms only occur with rapid head movement.

When patients have substantial loss of function in one or more systems responsible for balance function (vestibular, visual, somatosensory), prognosis for therapy success would necessarily be limited. However, this does not imply that treatment should be withheld in these groups. The impact of oscillopsia and deficits due to bilateral vestibular paresis may be reduced primarily from the repeated practice activities and to the extensive educational benefit of the therapy program.

Controlled Studies of Efficacy

Norré (1987) has demonstrated that patients with benign paroxysmal positional vertigo (BPPV) seem to benefit from habituation exercises in a controlled study. The active treatment group demonstrated a dramatically superior result when compared with a sham exercise group and a nontreated control group. He also studied the use of traditional vestibular suppressant therapy during habituation training, and noted that those on medications were approximately half as likely to achieve complete resolution of symptoms.

Horak and colleagues (Horak, Jones-Rycewicz, Black, & Shumway-Cook, 1992) performed a controlled study comparing the benefits of a customized program of vestibular rehabilitation to two control groups. One group received medical therapy with meclizine or diazepam, and the other group performed a program of sham exercises, involving aerobic exercise and strength training. All three groups reported some subjective decreases in dizziness, with a dramatic benefit in the vestibular rehabilitation group. Posturography and other measures of balance ability documented a beneficial effect only in the vestibular exercise group.

Shepard and Telian (1995) completed a randomized trial comparing the efficacy of a customized vestibular rehabilitation program with a generic program of vestibular exercises. The customized therapy group showed statistically significant resolution of spontaneous nystagmus and rotational chair asymmetries by the end of therapy, as well as significant reduction in motion sensitivity. They also had improved performance on clinical measures of static and dynamic balance ability. The only statistically significant change in the performance measures for the generic program was in static balance ability, probably reflecting the fact that one of the generic exercises was identical to one of the performance measures in this category. This study suggests that the level of vestibular compensation achieved in a customized program is far superior to the level that can be anticipated from a generic program, and justifies the expense required to involve a trained physical therapist in the treatment of patients with chronic vestibular symptoms.

Three other special applications of vestibular rehabilitation now each have controlled studies showing statistically significant improvement over a control group. The first is loosely referred to as a vestibular rehabilitation program because it is actually a single office treatment procedure for benign positional vertigo, the particle repositioning maneuver. This procedure has become popular in the 1990s and will be discussed in more detail below. Lynn and colleagues (Lynn, Pool, Rose, & Suman,1995) randomized 36 patients with confirmed, unilateral BPPV, into a treatment group that went through a modified Epley procedure (Epley, 1992) or to a control group that underwent a sham procedure. Patients and the evaluating audiologist were blinded to the group assignments. At the 1 month follow-up, 89% of the treatment group and only 27% of the control group had negative Hallpike maneuvers, a highly significant difference. A controlled study of another particle repositioning maneuver compared a treatment group to no treatment and reported no significant difference in outcome (Blakley, 1994). This latter study cautioned that the natural history of BPPV is spontaneous resolution in many patients within the first 4–8 weeks.

Another area of study with a randomized control group involved therapy for gait in patients with significant bilateral peripheral vestibular system paresis (Krebs, Gill-Body, Riley, & Parker, 1993). This study, despite a small group of subjects, was able to demonstrate a statistically significant improvement in measures of gait performance in the treatment group compared to the control group.

One area where the authors have found a generic exercise program to be useful is in the postoperative care of patients after any surgical procedure that produces unilateral vestibular loss, such as vestibular nerve section, labyrinthectomy, or vestibular schwannoma resection (Shepard, Telian, Smith-Wheelock, Kemink, & Boismier, 1993). The generic program is initiated as soon as the patient is out of intensive care. If the patient does not demonstrate significantly improved postural control and resolution of motion-provoked symptoms after 4 weeks, a customized program is instituted. Use of this generic program (detailed in Shepard, Telian, Smith-Wheelock, Kemink, & Boismier, 1993) over 3 years and ongoing suggests that less than 5% of the postoperative patients will require a customized program. A randomized study (Herdman, Clendaniel, Mattox, Holliday, & Niparko, 1995) was performed in patients following acoustic neuroma resection, with postoperative activities beginning on postoperative day 3 for both groups. The control group performed eye movement exercises and walking, while the experimental group performed a series of activities designed to increase vestibulo-ocular reflex gain, including head and eye movements, plus a walking program (a generic program). The authors were able to demonstrate a significantly superior improvement in postural control, as assessed by EquiTest, in the experimental group. There was also significantly less subjective disequilibrium reported by postoperative days 5 and 6 in the experimental group.

While the above review is not meant to be exhaustive, it does present an impressive and growing body of literature clearly demonstrating the statistically verifiable efficacy of this management technique in a wide variety of balance disorder patients.

PATIENT SELECTION CRITERIA

This section will discuss specific patient populations that may benefit from vestibular rehabilitation therapy and the expected results for each group.

Uncompensated Unilateral Peripheral Lesions

Vestibular rehabilitation therapy is appropriate in any condition characterized by a stable unilateral vestibular deficit when the patient's natural compensation process appears to be incomplete. If the medical evaluation reveals no evidence of a progressive process, it is likely that a vestibular rehabilitation program will produce a satisfactory resolution of symptoms. This intervention is certainly preferable to long-term use of vestibular suppressants, and may contribute meaningfully to the patient's future well-being and productivity. Regarding the patient's suitability for vestibular rehabilitation, the nature of the described condition is *more important* than the underlying diagnosis. Even chronic lightheadedness or disequilibrium may be treatable, provided that there is evidence for underlying poor vestibular compensation. If any intense vertigo is experienced, it should be produced primarily by head or visual motion. There should be no evidence for progressive or fluctuating labyrinthine dysfunction, leading to spontaneous vertigo spells such as those resulting from endolymphatic hydrops.

Although therapy activities are customized to the needs of the individual patient, an illustrative example of a patient with an uncompensated peripheral lesion is now presented.

CASE 50

History: A 41-year-old male with the diagnosis of uncompensated vestibular neuritis complained of a sudden onset of motion-provoked vertigo without a particularly severe peripheral vestibular crisis at onset. Symptoms improved over 6 months but then suddenly returned, with vertigo spells lasting for less than a minute experienced several times each day. Multiple head movements could cause the symptoms, as well as visual scanning tasks such as shopping in store aisles. Aural fullness was noted in the left ear, without hearing loss. Balance testing showed persistent low-amplitude left-beating nystagmus throughout the study. All other test results were normal. Initial therapy work-up showed a Motion Sensitivity Quotient of 21% and moderate to severe disability. There were no balance or gait difficulties unless his head was moving while he was walking.

Treatment: Based on the therapist's findings, the following customized program of exercises was suggested for twice daily use:

1. Sit upright with your legs in front of you. Rapidly lay straight down on your back with eyes open, wait 10 seconds or until symptoms return to baseline, and rapidly roll to the right side. Again wait 10 seconds or until symptoms return to baseline, and roll to your back. Wait 10 seconds or until symptoms return to baseline and quickly sit back upright. Repeat 3 times.
2. From a sitting position, rapidly bend down with nose to right knee, wait 10 seconds or until symptoms return to baseline, and rapidly sit back upright. Repeat 3 times.
3. While sitting, turn your head to the right and then to the left, leading your head with your eyes as if you are watching a tennis match. Go back and forth 5 times, then wait for 10 seconds or until symptoms return to baseline, and repeat the entire process 3 times.
4. While sitting, bend your head down, looking at the floor, then look up at the ceiling, moving both your head and eyes. Repeat this 5 times. Then wait 10 seconds or until symptoms return to baseline and repeat the entire process 3 times.
5. While standing, make a rapid left "about face" pivot with eyes open, wait until symptoms return to baseline, and repeat. Then wait 20 seconds or until symptoms return to baseline and repeat the entire process to the right. Repeat this entire activity 3 times.
6. Begin a walking program, with up to a 30-minute walk at a comfortable pace, using head movements as if your are "window shopping." Perform this walk once a day for 5 days per week.

Outcome: Patient was 100% compliant with the program for 6 weeks. At his follow-up visit, the motion sensitivity quotient was reduced to 7% and he reported significant subjective improvement, with occasional symptoms. There was no residual disability. He was advised to continue the exercise program for several weeks and then change to a maintenance program.

Central Lesions

Patients with stable central nervous system lesions or mixed central and peripheral lesions need not be excluded from treatment, although their prognosis may be more limited than the average patient with a stable peripheral injury. This was clearly demonstrated in Case 17, discussed in Chapters 6 and 7. In the observational study by Shepard, Telian, Smith-Wheelock, and Raj (1993b), the only difference in outcome between stable central lesions and stable peripheral lesions was that the central group took longer to achieve the final result. Limited anecdotal experience with progressive central nervous system disorders, such as olivopontocerebellar atrophy and multisystem atrophy, has suggested that, although gait or postural control deficits cannot be improved, it may be possible to reduce the sensitivity to head movements with habituation exercises. This same result was seen in a formal trial of therapy with patients who had stable or progressive cerebellar lesions (Suarez, Caffa, & Macadar, 1992). Combined peripheral and central vestibular system lesions are most often seen in the head injured population and will be discussed separately below.

Positional Vertigo

One important subset of vestibular patients that has been treated with exercises are those with benign paroxysmal positional vertigo. In the studies cited above, the authors included patients with BPPV who were treated with conventional rehabilitation protocols. This approach was universally effective and is recommended as an appropriate treatment modality for patients with this diagnosis. The use of noncustomized generic programs such as Cawthorne exercises has a long and fairly successful history for the management of this problem (Cawthorne, 1944). For many patients, the Cawthorne program is too intensive and provokes disturbing vestibular symptoms, often associated with nausea or vomiting, that may discourage the patient from continuing. A preferred noncustomized program for BPPV that addresses the needs of most patients with BPPV is provided in Table 10–4. When this program fails to bring relief, it is appropriate to refer the patient for a customized program.

Specific treatment programs have been proposed that attempt to reposition particulate material, perhaps displaced otoconia, pathologically located in the ampulla or floating freely in the endolymphatic compartment of the posterior semicircular canal. Brandt and Daroff (1980) advocated that the patient repeatedly lie down quickly from the sitting position onto the side that provoked the vertigo. After waiting for the vertigo to abate, the patient is to sit up quickly, wait again for symptoms to clear, and then lie quickly onto the other ear. The patient was instructed to perform the maneuver repeatedly at each session until no vertigo was noted, and to repeat the exercises every three hours until he or she could no longer induce vertigo. Most of those who benefited from this approach were probably habituating centrally, although sudden cures did result occa-

sionally, possibly from repositioning of the offending particles. The *liberatory maneuver* of Semont, Freyss, and Vitte, (1988) utilizes similar planes of motion yet attempts to dislodge and reposition the otoconia in a single session. Usually a physician or therapist has the patient quickly assume the offending position, wait for 2 to 3 minutes, then rapidly turns the patient through the original sitting position and onto the other ear. The patient is returned to the sitting position and advised to remain upright for the next 48 hours. Semont et al. report over a 90% rate of complete symptomatic relief after one or two treatments with this technique in over 700 patients. Epley (1992) and Parnes and Price-Jones (1993) have reported similarly high rates of success using techniques that feature deliberately slow passive manipulation of the head through planes of rotation that are designed to allow the particles in the posterior canal to filter back into the vestibule. For a more thorough review of the different procedures and results to date the reader is referred to Herdman (1994b); Brandt, Steddin, Erg, and Daroff (1994); and Beynon (1996).

TABLE 10–4. Generic Exercises for Benign Paroxysmal Positional Vertigo

INSTRUCTIONS

Perform the following exercises TWICE DAILY, once in the morning and again in the evening. Perform them in an OPEN AREA, where you cannot injure yourself in the event of a fall. If any of the exercises cause PAIN, then stop and notify your physician or therapist so the program can be modified. It is expected that you will become dizzy while performing these exercises. This dizziness may become worse over the first week. If the dizziness continues to worsen after 7 days, then discontinue the program and contact your physician or therapist. Perform these exercises faithfully until they no longer cause dizziness. From that point, continue to perform them twice daily for at least two more weeks to ensure complete relief of symptoms. You may wish to continue them on a once-daily basis indefinitely. If your dizziness should return in the future, you should reinstate this program. If you do not notice an improvement in your symptoms within 6 weeks, then you may require an exercise program customized to your particular needs. In this event, contact your physician or therapist for more information.

EXERCISES

1. Sit upright on the edge of the bed with your feet flat on the floor or dangling straight down. Quickly lie down onto your LEFT/RIGHT side, swinging your feet up onto the bed. Remain in this position for 30 seconds, (even if dizziness occurs) or until symptoms subside. Then swing your feet back over the edge of the bed and sit up quickly into the original position. Wait 30 seconds, or until symptoms subside, and then repeat this exercise three more times.
2. Sit upright in a comfortable chair and bend your head quickly up and down (as if nodding your head "yes") looking alternately at the floor and the ceiling five times. Stop, wait 10 seconds or longer until the dizziness passes, and repeat the whole exercise three more times.
3. Still sitting in the chair, tilt your head up and to the LEFT/RIGHT looking up at the ceiling. Hold the position for 30 seconds, then return your head to the original neutral position. Wait 30 seconds again, or until symptoms subside. Then repeat the exercise three times.

The physician should attempt to distinguish between pure BPPV and positional vertigo resulting from poor compensation after a labyrinthine injury. The key distinguishing feature is the lack of a significant vestibular crisis at the onset of symptoms in BPPV and the lack of any other positive findings on clinical or laboratory testing. Although the first attack of BPPV is usually memorable because of its novelty to the patient, it is rarely any more intense than the subsequent attacks. This distinction is now especially significant since the development of the particle repositioning techniques. In cases of positional vertigo due to poor compensation after a vestibular crisis, even when positive Hallpike maneuvers are observed, such specific treatments are much less likely to successfully remove all symptoms. This point is illustrated by the authors' experience in a recent prospective observational study with 51 patients having classical Hallpike responses. Using the particle repositioning maneuver (PRM) as described by Parnes and Price-Jones (1993), 28% of patients felt to have pure BPPV required further habituation programs for residual symptoms following the PRM, whereas 70% of those felt to have positional vertigo (secondary BPPV) from uncompensated vestibular lesions required additional rehabilitation programs. The residual symptoms included continued positive Hallpike responses or symptoms in other planes of motion. The PRM was successful in eliminating the Hallpike response in over 85% of the 51 patients, and the additional customized programs were typically used for other symptoms. Interestingly, 63% of patients in the secondary positional vertigo group did report significant reduction of symptoms after the PRM.

Disequilibrium of Aging

Another indication for the use of a vestibular rehabilitation program is multifactorial balance difficulties in the elderly (Smith-Wheelock, Shepard, Telian, & Boismier, 1992). This becomes especially important when other treatment options are unavailable or have been exhausted. These individuals may benefit greatly from balance retraining exercises and individualized conditioning programs. Frequently, the relationship with the therapist assumes a strong counseling function, and the use of assistive devices for safety in ambulation can be introduced as needed. Given the potential public health impact of complications from falls in the elderly, any therapeutic program that can decrease the functional impact of disequilibrium, balance, and/or gait problems is highly desirable. The authors are not aware of any controlled studies investigating a customized vestibular rehabilitation program in this population. However, our prospective observational results suggest that both objective and subjective therapy outcome measures were not significantly poorer for those over 65 years relative to younger subjects. The only significant difference noted for the older population was the length of time required to maximize the benefit from therapy (Shepard, Telian, Smith-Wheelock, & Raj, 1993). We also find that a higher percentage of elderly patients need repeated contact with a therapist instead of an independent home-based program. A representative customized program for an elderly individual with balance and dizziness complaints is presented below.

CASE 51

History: An 84-year-old female complains of a gradual onset of unsteadiness while standing and walking, without a history of falls. She denies any vertigo and reports unsteadiness as provoked whenever she is up moving, and she is free of symptoms if sitting or lying down. She has arthritis, osteoporosis, and medically controlled hypertension. Mild bilateral hearing loss requires hearing aids. Balance testing showed evidence for an abnormally low time constant on rotational chair testing, suggesting peripheral involvement, normal findings on all oculomotor tests, and sporadic left-beating positional nystagmus. Caloric irrigations produced normal responses. Posturography showed abnormal results on Condition 6 only, suggesting sensitivity to visual motion stimuli when foot support surface cues are not accurate. Initial therapy evaluation showed no motion sensitivity. The patient could not stand on thin or thick foam with eyes closed without a fall or step within 10 seconds. While walking she drifted to the right, and this problem was increased with head movements. She could perform an unsteady tandem walk, stepping off the line 3 times out of 20 steps. She was able to rise from a chair without use of hands. The functional problems appeared to result from possible peripheral vestibular involvement and significant fear of falling.

Treatment: The patient was treated in a supervised outpatient setting twice per week for 3 weeks with the following supplementary customized home program: Find a straight path in your house. Place a chair at each end of the path. Now set a timer for 5–10 minutes and perform the following activities:

1. Walk from one chair to the other, turning your head slowly from side to side.
2. When you get to the other chair (the back of the chair will be facing you) practice standing on one leg while you lightly touch the chair.
   Shift weight onto the right. Slowly lift and lower the left leg 5 times.
   Shift weight onto the left. Slowly lift and lower the right leg 5 times.
3. Now turn and walk back to the other chair, slowly tilting your head up and down.
4. When you get to the chair practice standing on one leg again.

Outcome: At the final therapy visit, the patient could stand with eyes open or closed on a firm surface and thin foam without falls, and on thick foam with minimal fall reactions, even with eyes closed. Walking with head movements still caused some drift, but she was able to correct this without stumbling or fall reactions. She was now able to step up and down a 6–8 inch curb without assistance for the first time in several years. She remains fearful of falling but notes significant subjective improvements in her balance. She was placed on a maintenance program (15–20-minute walks, 3–5 times per week with "window shopping" head movements) to be continued indefinitely. Significant effort was provided in explaining her problem with balance, and means for continued, safe mobility.

Use After Vestibular Surgery

As introduced above, when a patient with an unstable vestibular condition undergoes a labyrinthectomy or vestibular nerve section, a stable unilateral vestibular lesion is created. It is possible that many of the unsatisfactory outcomes following such surgery can be attributed to incomplete or delayed postoperative compensation (Monsell, Brackman, & Linthicum, 1988). All operative patients should be instructed regarding the importance of central compensation for the success of vestibular surgery, and routine use of a vestibular rehabilitation program (generic or customized) can be helpful in optimizing the outcome achieved. It is appropriate for the therapist to offer counseling and general instructions to any patient who undergoes a procedure that results in a unilateral loss of vestibular function. Those who demonstrate a particularly slow recovery should be referred for a customized vestibular rehabilitation program. Those individuals who are at particular risk for poor recovery because of complicating CNS conditions, sedating medications, or poor motivation for recovery should be encouraged to pursue a customized program early in their postoperative course.

Head Injury

Vestibular rehabilitation may play a role in other conditions that include a component of balance complaints. Frequently, patients who have suffered head injuries have significant disability from vestibular symptoms. As their conditions often include cognitive and central vestibular involvement along with the peripheral component, vestibular rehabilitation program techniques are best used as a supplement to a comprehensive, multidisciplinary traumatic brain injury program, rather than as the primary rehabilitative measure. A review of therapy with this specific group is provided by Shumway-Cook (1994). An important subgroup within this population involves those suspicious for perilymphatic fistula. Vestibular rehabilitation may seem counterintuitive for these patients, as rapid head movements should make the symptoms worse. However, a diagnostic trial of therapy has been used for individuals in whom hearing is stable. Symptom improvement, ranging from mild improvement to complete resolution of dizziness, was noted in 63% of patients suspect for fistula. There was no change in symptoms in 25%, and worsening of symptoms in 12%. Surgical exploration is recommended to those who become worse during the course of therapy, as the therapy failure provides stronger evidence for an unstable labyrinth (Shepard et al., 1992).

Malingering

When faced with the patient who is thought to be malingering or embellishing the degree of disability associated with vestibular complaints, it may be helpful to refer for vestibular testing and a vestibular therapy evaluation. Dynamic posturography can often identify malingerers, as they typically demonstrate inconsistent or nonphysiologic results (see Chapter 7 for discussion). They may perform poorly on the easier tasks despite being able to perform the Romberg test without difficulty in the clinic. Often, their performance is within the normal range on the more difficult trials, despite poor performance on the simpler trials. Experience suggests that both those who are seeking or receiving disability compensation and those involved with pending litigation are unlikely to experience significant functional gains in vestibular rehabilitation therapy. Nevertheless, the therapist who is experienced in treating vestibular disorder patients can be very helpful in discriminating true physiologic disability from the psychological or socioeconomic issues. This information may be helpful to the physician called upon to provide written documentation or verbal testimony in such cases. If the patient seems to have legitimate dysfunction and demonstrates a good faith effort to cooperate with the therapy program, the physician is much more likely to feel comfortable in supporting a disability claim or testifying favorably on the patient's behalf.

Panic Disorder and Other Anxiety Disorders

Patients with panic disorder and other anxiety disorders often present seeking management of ill-defined vestibular symptoms. After a suitable evaluation is performed, a vestibular rehabilitation program may be recommended as an adjunctive measure for their condition as many do have head or visual motion provoked symptoms. If the anxiety is mild, the vestibular rehabilitation program functions as a behavioral intervention similar to exposure therapy for treatment of phobias. As with other habituation exercise groupings, this is a progressive program increasing the exposures to various movements over time. These programs for the mild cases are well handled by the physical therapist. If the anxiety component is significant, and particularly if panic attacks are frequent, psychiatric intervention will be required as well.

Ménière's Disease

Occasionally, patients with Ménière's disease will complain of positional vertigo or other chronic vestibular complaints between their definitive attacks. Although such patients are candidates for a vestibular rehabilitation program, they must proceed with the understanding that the prognosis for lasting relief of chronic symptoms is reduced if the severe spontaneous attacks of Ménière's disease occur more than monthly. If the attacks are rare, or the Ménière's disease is inactive, the prognosis is considerably improved.

Diagnostic Trial

It is not always possible for the physician to determine whether the patient's complaints are due to stable vestibular disease with inadequate central compensation or to unstable labyrinthine function. In this setting of diagnostic uncertainty, a trial of vestibular rehabilitation is appropriate. This measure may help clarify this important distinction and prevents premature surgery when a course of therapy will suffice. On the other hand, failure to improve in a vestibular rehabilitation program lends further credibility to the diagnostic impression that the lesion is unstable or progressive. It is then suitable to proceed with appropriate surgical management.

Inappropriate Candidates

These whose symptoms occur only in spontaneous episodes, such as is seen with Ménière's patients who have no residual symptoms between spontaneous events, will not benefit from a vestibular rehabilitation program. If there are no provocative movements or body positions that reliably produce spells, and no postural control abnormalities are noted during the evaluation, the patient is best managed with alternative medical or surgical strategies. Nonetheless, such patients should be encouraged to remain active and optimize their general health through physical activities performed at a level that is appropriate for their age and general health.

In conclusion, the use of vestibular rehabilitation programs for a wide range of patients with complaints of balance and dizziness is not only appropriate but quite efficacious. The use of therapy measures, like those discussed, have significantly expanded our ability to care for the chronic balance disorder patient.

PEDIATRIC PATIENTS

In general, the selection criteria, and overall program assessment and treatment plan development, are as described for the adults. In many cases encouraging normal childhood play, or when applicable, use of sports such as soccer serve well as the therapy program. In cases of bilateral paresis, considerable counseling for parents is necessary to help encourage normal childhood activities and to present basic safety issues regarding bicycle and water sports. The counseling helps physical education instructors to understand what may appear as inconsistent performance in various activities. No population studies using these techniques with children have been reported. Yet, our experience with a small number of children has been equally as positive as with adults.

11

■ MEDICAL THERAPY FOR THE BALANCE DISORDER PATIENT

*F*or most chronic vestibular disorders, no disease-specific pharmacological treatment is available. Stimulant medications such as caffeine and amphetamines have not generally been employed in the clinical setting, despite animal research suggesting that they may enhance vestibular compensation. The use of medications in the treatment of balance disorder patients falls into three major categories: (a) general suppression of vestibular symptoms; (b) pharmacological treatment of specific conditions that cause vestibular symptoms, such as Ménière's disease or migraine variants; and (c) treatment of the patient who has developed a reactive clinical depression in response to troubling vestibular symptoms.

VESTIBULAR SUPPRESSION

The agents typically prescribed for symptomatic relief of dizziness include benzodiazepines, antihistamines, and anticholinergic agents (Zee, 1985). In general, these medications are ineffective in preventing acute vertiginous spells, yet they may be quite effective in reducing the inten-

sity of a spell and controlling the associated nausea and vomiting. However, the physician must remember that all of these agents are centrally sedating. Active head and eye movements produce sensory error signals that trigger compensation mechanisms in the central nervous system after injuries to the peripheral vestibular system. It is almost certain that vestibular suppressants for dizziness inhibit the brain's ability to properly apprehend the sensory conflicts in the balance system, inhibiting central compensation (Peppard, 1986). Thus, although vestibular suppressants are appropriate for the short-term control of acute symptoms, they may be counterproductive with respect to the eventual desired outcome. This is particularly true in the setting of a fixed unilateral lesion, such as is seen after an episode of acute labyrinthitis or vestibular neuritis. Some patients with long-standing vestibular complaints after a peripheral injury may improve simply by weaning them from their vestibular suppressants.

Benzodiazepines

Although the individual's response to any medication is unpredictable, diazepam (Valium®) is generally the single most effective drug for the suppression of severe vertigo. For acute episodes requiring emergency room visits, intravenous diazepam is often effective in controlling symptoms, even in low doses of 1 to 2 mg. Once the symptoms are reduced, additional oral diazepam can be administered and continued as needed until the symptoms subside. The research data regarding the use of diazepam after vestibular insults is reviewed in Chapter 2. There appears to be a strong scientific basis for the use of this medication in the setting of an acute vestibular injury. It appears to assist in the early phases of compensation, perhaps by allowing for earlier ambulation as well as the head movements that are required to initiate the dynamic aspects of vestibular compensation. It would seem logical to wean the patient from this medication once the acute symptoms are resolved to prevent physiological addiction and to facilitate central compensation. The use of diazepam is also recommended for the symptomatic relief of severe recurring attacks of Ménière's disease. Other benzodiazepines such as clonazepam (Klonopin®) and alprazolam (Xanax®) have also been used for treatment of dizziness. Alprazolam is particularly effective in controlling dizziness associated with panic disorder, although other medications less likely to result in psychological or physiologic dependence are generally preferred.

Antihistamines

Milder medications used as vestibular suppressants include the antihistamines, especially meclizine (Antivert®) and dimenhydrinate (Dramamine®). Their efficacy is probably due in part to their significant anticholinergic side effects. Any antihistamine that crosses the blood-brain barrier would be expected to provide some benefit. Meclizine has considerable popularity among primary care physicians for the treatment of dizziness. Although there is no strong physiologic rationale for prophylactic use of this medication to prevent the spells of Ménière's disease, many patients have come to use it on a daily basis. Some patients cannot be dissuaded from regular use, convinced that their disease will relapse. Most clinicians advise patients to use the medication at the first sign of a Ménière's attack, especially if there is a predictable interval between the onset of hearing symptoms and the actual episode of vertigo. This safe and well-tolerated medication is sometimes completely adequate for symptomatic management of Ménière's spells, but is unlikely to be effective if no benefit is seen from a 25-mg dose. The prescribed dose may range from 12.5 to 50 mg three times daily, and can be titrated based on sedative side effects. Some patients who have Ménière's disease or nonspecific dizziness syndromes associated with allergic symptoms note considerable benefit from the regular use of oral antihistamines.

Anticholinergics

Oral propantheline (ProBanthine®) or transdermal scopolamine (Transderm Scop®) may be helpful in the management of dizziness, particularly for patients with chronic continuous symptoms. This may be partially explained because of the cholinergic transmitter influence in the peripheral and possibly, central vestibular system. Their use is often limited by the side effects of dry mouth and blurred vision. These preparations should be used cautiously in elderly individuals who may develop confusion or other more disturbing mental status changes. Dermatologic sensitivity to the transdermal patch may occur. Some patients believe that the patch must be worn in the postauricular region, so that it is near the inner ear. Although this belief may provide an additional placebo effect, there is no rational basis for this pattern of application because the medication is absorbed transcutaneously into the circulation. Therefore, at the first indication of dermatitis developing at the site of patch application, the patient should be encouraged to rotate the application to other thin hairless skin surfaces. Those who develop a dramatic dermatologic sensitivity must discontinue use of this product, and may occasionally require topical or systemic corticosteroids to control the skin reaction.

TREATMENT OF THE ACUTE VESTIBULAR CRISIS

When treating the patient with a new onset of severe vertigo due to presumed labyrinthitis or vestibular neuritis, it is appropriate to select a vestibular suppressant, as discussed above. In addition, it may be desirable to prescribe a burst of oral corticosteroid therapy, as this has been demonstrated to reduce symptom intensity and abbreviate the time required to resolve the disabling vertigo symptoms (Ariyasu, Byl, Sprague, & Adour, 1990).

TREATMENT OF MÉNIÈRE'S DISEASE

The diagnosis of Ménière's disease is based on the clinical history and confirmed by appropriate diagnostic testing. This diagnostic classification must be accurate, as the management of Ménière's disease involves several unique dietary, medical, and operative treatments that are not appropriate for other vestibular disorders. Control of vertigo is frequently accompanied by stabilization of hearing and a decreased sensation of tinnitus and aural fullness.

Restriction of salt intake together with a high volume of fresh water intake (48–64 oz per day) is the cornerstone of any dietary program for Ménière's disease. The typical American diet contains between 8 and 14 grams of sodium per day. Although most physicians simply instruct their patients to prepare meals without additional salt, strict low-salt diets between 1.5 and 2 grams of sodium per day are preferred when the Ménière's attacks are frequent and severe. Most patients who believe they are observing a salt-restricted diet are actually taking in amounts significantly higher than this ideal level, usually because of eating outside the home or using prepared foods that are high in sodium. It is best when the low-salt diet can be established and strictly monitored with the help of an experienced dietician. While such low sodium diets are very restrictive, many patients testify that this stringent reduction of salt is sufficient to control their symptoms. Some patients note that caffeine ingestion, nicotine use, or certain specific foods may exacerbate their symptoms.

Medications used to control the symptoms of Ménière's disease may simply provide symptomatic relief by suppressing vestibular activity during acute spells (discussed above), or may attempt to reduce the underlying problem of endolymphatic hydrops. If a low-sodium diet is insufficient, the use of thiazide diuretics with or without triamterene may help minimize the endolymphatic hydrops associated with Ménière's disease. The occasional patient will note a strong association between activity of Ménière's disease and allergic symptoms. These patients may be treated with regular use of an antihistamine preparation during the peak seasons of allergy sensitivity. Some will benefit from allergic desensitization therapy.

Intramuscular injections of streptomycin sulfate have been used for treatment of bilateral Ménière's disease or when the involved ear is the only ear with residual hearing. Medical ablation of peripheral vestibular function by intramuscular streptomycin was first reported by Schuknecht (1956). Streptomycin, an aminoglycoside antibiotic widely used at that time for the treatment of tuberculosis, was found to have ototoxic side effects. This property was initially exploited to produce complete vestibular ablation. This approach was complicated almost universally by oscillopsia, although most patients reported improved functional capacity compared to their pretreatment level. In an attempt to avoid the permanent and potentially disabling symptom of oscillopsia, methods to produce a reduction in symptoms by subtotally ablating vestibular function were advocated in later years. Graham and Kemink (1984) reported the use of titration streptomycin therapy (1 g intramuscularly twice daily for 5 days per week), with careful monitoring of inner ear function by audiometric and electronystagmographic testing. Total streptomycin dosages required usually ranged from 10 to 25 g, with some patients requiring up to 50 g to control symptoms. Response to therapy is best monitored by serial measurements of vestibulo-ocular reflex gain using the computerized rotational chair. Therapy is discontinued when low-frequency gain measurements begin to decrease or when 20 g have been administered. The patient is then observed for a clinical remission of the Ménière's symptoms. If symptoms persist, additional doses of streptomycin can be provided, as the therapeutic effects appear to be cumulative despite intervals between times of administration.

In recent years, interest has developed in the topical application of ototoxic aminoglycoside antibiotics into the middle ear cleft to produce selective ototoxicity in the ear with active Ménière's disease. Theoretically, the drug is absorbed into the inner ear fluids through the round window membrane. Gentamicin has been the preferred agent for this indication because of its wide clinical availability, and a variety of treatment protocols have been studied (Monsell, Cass, & Rybak, 1993; Nedzelski, Schessel, Bryce, & Pfleiderer, 1992). Although gentamicin is less toxic to the cochlea than the vestibular tissues, no ideal protocol has yet been established that will predictably produce a complete "chemical labyrinthectomy" with a satisfactorily low incidence of hearing loss. Nevertheless, this promising modality has the potential to replace the use of ablative surgical procedures for the control of vertigo due to Ménière's disease.

TREATMENT OF VERTIGO DUE TO MIGRAINE

Some patients with classic migraine headaches may experience vertigo as an aura prior to the onset of headache. These individuals, and others without a clear personal history of migraine headaches, may experience episodic spells of vertigo as a migraine variant without an associated headache (Cutrer & Baloh, 1992; Harker, 1994; Harker & Rassekh, 1988). The diagnosis in this latter group is obviously more elusive, due to the absence of associated headache. The spells typically last from 20 minutes up to several hours. They resemble in character the spells of vertigo seen with Ménière's disease, except for the absence of associated auditory symptoms. There are typically no clinically significant abnormalities on auditory or vestibular testing, although this is also frequently true in early cases of Ménière's disease. The key to the diagnosis of migrainous vertigo without headache is the consistent absence of auditory symptoms or aural fullness with the attacks. The hypothesis in this setting is that vasospasm in the brain stem, or possibly in the vessels supplying the peripheral vestibular structures, is the initiating event. Thus, it is rational to institute a trial of prophylactic vasodilator therapy. A calcium channel blocker, such as nifedipine (Procardia®) or nicardipine (Cardene SR®) can be prescribed. Use of a long acting beta-blocker, such as propranolol (Inderal LA®) or atenolol (Tenormin®) is a suitable alternative that will frequently prevent migraine events. Therapy may need to be continued for several weeks, with gradual increases in dosage to achieve a therapeutic effect. If the spells abate with any of these medications, there is strong evidence that the symptoms were due to the central vasomotor instability characteristic of migraine sufferers. More sophisticated management of the suspected migraine patient is best deferred to a neurological consultant.

TREATMENT OF REACTIVE DEPRESSION

Any patient with a chronic illness can develop a reactive clinical depression, especially when the symptoms are severe and unpredictable as seen in some vestibular disorders. A poor understanding of the nature of vestibular disorders by the patients' family, employer, and treating physician may contribute to their sense of discouragement and hopelessness. The presence of a significant depression is often overlooked as a contributing factor in the overall disability produced by the illness, and the physician does well to explore this possibility. Depression should be suspected whenever the patient admits to sleep disturbances, unexplained weight loss or gain, significant disruption of close relationships, loss of sexual desire, or suicidal thoughts.

Major advances have been made in understanding the biochemical basis for depression and its treatment in recent years (Goldberg, 1995). The physician should emphasize this fact to the patient and attempt to remove the negative stigma that the patient may associate with mental illness. It should also be stressed that referral for treatment of reactive depression does not mean that the physician does not take seriously the vestibular impairment that the patient is experiencing.

Many patients report a dramatic improvement in functional capacity after treatment for reactive depression, even if the vestibular symptoms persist. The tricyclic antidepressants have a long history of relative effectiveness in the control of depression, but are plagued with a fairly high incidence of troublesome side effects, some of which may compound the problems experienced by the balance disorder patient. Newer compounds such as sertraline hydrochloride (Zoloft®) and fluoxetine hydrochloride (Prozac®) are usually better tolerated and quite effective for the relief of serious depression. Often the patient's primary care provider will be experienced in the medical management of depression, but the otolaryngologist should not hesitate to seek expert psychiatric consultation on behalf of the vestibular disorder patient when needed.

CONCLUSION

Managing the complex vestibular disorder patient can be a challenging, even daunting task. The authors contend that an essential part of the care of this patient population is a careful and thorough evaluation followed by comprehensive counseling about the nature of vestibular dysfunction. This will allay many of the patients' fears and produce an understanding of their disease that will allow them to participate meaningfully in management decisions. An informed patient, along with the judicious selection of medical, surgical, and/or rehabilitative measures, will result in a positive outcome in most any case of vestibular dysfunction, even if the symptoms cannot be entirely eliminated.

CONCLUSION

12

SURGICAL MANAGEMENT OF THE BALANCE DISORDER PATIENT

*I*t is not unusual to encounter patients with intense episodes of vertigo who have already seen several physicians and tried multiple medical treatments without success. Those who are disabled by their symptoms are often desperate for relief. While it is proper to consider surgical treatment in this setting, the physician must recognize that unsuccessful surgery may greatly aggravate the patient's discouragement with his or her disease and the medical profession. The astute clinician recognizes the vulnerability of this patient population and seeks to guide them toward rational and effective surgical options when available, while sheltering them from unvalidated treatment practices. It is beyond the scope of this text to discuss the technical aspects of the surgical procedures that are available for the treatment of vertigo. These are available in standard reference materials. Rather, the authors intend to provide principles that will allow the clinician to understand the benefits and limitations of surgical treatments for vertigo, with the expectation that these will assist in proper patient selection and successful outcomes when surgery is undertaken.

THE RATIONALE FOR SURGICAL TREATMENT OF VESTIBULAR DISORDERS

In most cases, the process of central vestibular compensation reliably relieves dizziness resulting from insults to the peripheral vestibular system, provided that the lesion is either stable (e.g., viral labyrinthitis) or produces only an insidious progressive deterioration (e.g., vestibular schwannoma). On the other hand, if the lesion is unstable or rapidly progressive, compensation is not possible unless the lesion can be stabilized by medical or surgical treatment. Ménière's disease is the prototypical disorder in this latter category, wherein the ear may fluctuate between normal labyrinthine function and dramatic cochleovestibular symptoms. Vestibular system surgery seeks to stabilize inner ear function in the setting of an unstable system, whether by correcting a defect that underlies the disorder or by ablating function in the pathologic ear.

Certain surgical procedures are applicable only to a particular diagnosis. Some of these are widely accepted as both rational and effective, such as posterior semicircular canal occlusion and singular neurectomy procedures for intractable benign paroxysmal positional vertigo (Gacek & Gacek, 1994; Parnes & McClure, 1991). Other disease-specific operations, such as endolymphatic sac surgery for Ménière's disease, repair of perilymph fistula, and microvascular decompression of the VIIIth nerve, continue to generate controversy. These operations are enthusiastically embraced by some practitioners, while others have abandoned their use. All of the operations in this group have as their unifying feature the desirable goal of correcting a pathologic process that is unique to the particular diagnosis, while preserving any portion of inner ear function that is unaffected by the disease process. Success in this setting obviously hinges on making an exact diagnosis and selecting operations with proven efficacy.

On the other hand, procedures designed to ablate unilateral vestibular function, such as labyrinthectomy and vestibular nerve section, may be applied to any peripheral vestibular disorder. In this setting, an exact etiologic diagnosis is less critical. Instead, the physician must be certain that the problem is attributable to peripheral system dysfunction and that the pathologic ear has been correctly identified. In addition, it should be clear that the peripheral labyrinthine disorder is fluctuating or rapidly progressive in nature, rather than simply a failure of central compensation for a stable lesion. On the other hand, if the ongoing vertigo represents poor initial central vestibular compensation or recent decompensation following a stable vestibular lesion, ablative surgery is not likely to be necessary or particularly effective.

SURGICAL PATIENT SELECTION: THE PRIORITY OF DISTINGUISHING POOR COMPENSATION FROM UNSTABLE LABYRINTHINE DISEASE

Although the specific etiology of dizziness may at times be elusive, it is usually possible to distinguish individuals whose symptoms are caused by a stable but uncompensated lesion from those with unstable or progressive disease in the vestibular system. This categorical distinction has important treatment implications, especially as our understanding of vestibular compensation and the application of rehabilitative techniques have evolved. It is generally believed that an operation designed to ablate unilateral vestibular function can effectively relieve vertigo due to labyrinthine dysfunction of any cause. However, failure to recognize that the patient's symptoms result from poor vestibular compensation for a stable lesion may lead to inappropriate and fruitless surgical intervention. Prior to the availability of vestibular rehabilitation programs, surgery to ablate vestibular function was offered to any patient whose vestibular injuries were clearly peripheral in nature. However, it has subsequently been demonstrated that the results of vestibular rehabilitation are markedly superior to vestibular nerve section for the control of symptoms caused by uncompensated vestibular neuritis (Table 12–1). Thus, surgery is rarely recommended for this indication today. If surgery is undertaken as a last resort for the patient with an uncompensated lesion, both the surgeon and the patient should be aware that the prognosis

TABLE 12–1. University of Michigan Treatment Results in Uncompensated Vestibular Neuritis: Vestibular Nerve Section vs. Vestibular Rehabilitation

	Vestibular Nerve Section $n = 16$	Vestibular Rehabilitation $n = 59$
Complete Improvement	0%	25%
Dramatic Improvement	25%	47%
Mild Improvement	45%	13%
No Improvement	25%	15%
Worse	5%	0%

for success is dramatically lower than for disorders causing fluctuations in labyrinthine function. Perhaps in the future, more effective treatments such as better vestibular rehabilitation methods or specific neuropharmaceuticals geared toward enhancing compensation will replace surgery altogether for the treatment of incomplete vestibular compensation. This topic was introduced in Chapter 3 but will be expanded here, because the methods available to help the physician differentiate the uncompensated patient from those with unstable labyrinthine pathology are important in surgical patient selection. These methods include recognition of key features in the clinical history, the use of vestibular testing, and the possible use of a therapeutic trial of vestibular rehabilitation.

Distinctions in the Clinical History

It has been stated that a complete neuro-otologic history is the most important single component in the diagnostic evaluation of the balance disorder patient. This is also true in the assessment of the patient's compensation status. Certain clues in the history suggest the patient suffers from incomplete compensation despite the fact that the vestibular lesion is stable. If the patient describes a severe vestibular crisis at onset without equally intense symptoms on any occasion since that time, an uncompensated lesion is more likely. This is particularly true if the current symptoms are characterized as a continuous unsteadiness following recovery from the severe crisis. Although there still may be intermittent vertigo, it would be exclusively provoked by rapid head motions or certain head positions. On the other hand, if the intensity and duration of the current spells are equal to or greater than the initial insult, an unstable or progressive vestibular lesion is suggested.

As discussed in Chapter 3, the documentation of fluctuating or progressive sensorineural hearing loss also provides a strong indication of unstable inner ear function. Sometimes the patient is uncertain about the nature of an associated hearing loss. A review of serial audiograms may be helpful in this setting. Occasionally, it is desirable to obtain an audiogram during an episode of vertigo to determine if subtle changes in auditory function are occurring that may be imperceptible to the patient.

Role of Vestibular Testing in the Assessment of Compensation

The purpose of balance function testing encompasses three major goals. The most traditional is site-of-lesion localization. Second, if posturography is available, an assessment of the patient's ability to use available sensory input systems in an integrated fashion may be completed. A third goal is to evaluate the level of physiologic and functional vestibular compensation.

Clinically significant spontaneous nystagmus, positional nystagmus, or a directional preponderance on the ENG provide evidence for failure of physiologic compensation in the vestibulo-ocular reflex. Rotational chair testing provides additional information about the vestibulo-ocular reflex that cannot be obtained from the ENG. In general, although abnormalities in the timing (phase) or amplitude (gain) of the eye movements produced by the vestibulo-ocular reflex in response to head acceleration provide evidence for peripheral vestibular dysfunction, they do not address the issue of compensation within the central system. On the other hand, persistent asymmetry (bias) in the slow-component eye velocity responses produced by rightward versus leftward rotation strongly suggests that the peripheral lesion is physiologically uncompensated. For rotation toward the paretic side, the maximum slow-component velocity is reduced from normal, resulting in asymmetry of the gain observed for rotations toward or away from the lesion. As the compensation process proceeds, the asymmetry often resolves. However this is not always the case (Shepard et al., 1992). Therefore, given the lack of strong functional implications from the extent and site-of-lesion studies (see Chapter 7), and the possibility of an asymptomatic state with ongoing nystagmus or abnormal chair asymmetries, routine use of ENG or chair testing as outcome measures for a vestibular rehabilitation program would not be recommended. The studies can be useful if a change in compensation status is suspected, by worsening of symptoms. The nature of rotational stimuli also allows for testing of visual-vestibular interactions, such as enhancement or suppression of the vestibulo-ocular reflex, that assist in the evaluation of the status of the central vestibulo-ocular pathways. Abnormalities in these measures may help to explain an observed lack of central compensation.

Dynamic posturography provides adjunctive functional information about the balance system. Sometimes a patient with significant complaints related to the vestibular system will have normal findings on ENG and rotational chair testing. Posturography may help to demonstrate that there continues to be functional impairment despite relatively normal physiologic responsiveness (as measured by the other studies) in both inner ears (see Case 19, Chapter 7, as an example). By measuring the degree of postural sway under several test conditions, this test may document that the patient is unable to make proper use of sensory inputs from the visual, vestibular, and somatosensory systems for maintaining stable stance, suggesting incomplete or maladaptive compensation for the prior vestibular lesion. It may also demonstrate sensory preference abnormalities, in which the incorrect conflicting sensory cues are selected inappropriately. Such information is helpful in patient counseling and the design of

rehabilitation programs. Dynamic posturography is justifiably used for an outcome measure of a vestibular rehabilitation program given the strong relationship between the test results of sensory organization testing and patients' functional abilities and perceptions of their problems (see Chapter 7).

In summary, a complete battery of vestibular testing may be quite helpful in assessing compensation status or explaining poor compensation by identifying pathology in the central nervous system. The selection of the tests to start a laboratory evaluation and criteria for expansion to studies such as rotary chair and dynamic posturography are given in Chapter 8. The specific vestibular test results that may be helpful in these distinctions are summarized in Table 12–2.

Therapeutic Trial of Vestibular Rehabilitation

Ultimately, even with the best clinical history and vestibular test capabilities, the clinician often is faced with diagnostic uncertainty when treating patients with dizziness. For an extreme example, consider the head injury patient who may have a mix of spontaneous and motion-provoked symptoms, as well as evidence of both central and peripheral vestibular

---

TABLE 12–2. Clinical Utility of Vestibular Test Results

■ Evidence for peripheral labyrinthine dysfunction:
  Unilateral caloric weakness
  Spontaneous/positional nystagmus with normal oculomotor findings
  Classic nystagmus after Hallpike maneuver
  Rotational chair phase or asymmetry abnormalities with normal oculomotor findings
■ Evidence for uncompensated status:
  Clinically significant spontaneous or positional nystagmus
  Rotational chair asymmetry
  Abnormalities on sensory organization posturography test
■ Explanations for poor compensation due to CNS pathology:
  Vertical or perverted nystagmus*
  Oculomotor test abnormalities on ENG battery
  Failure of visual suppression of nystagmus*
  Failure of visual enhancement of nystagmus*
  Abnormalities on motor coordination posturography test with musculoskeletal issues resolved

*These are used independently if a noncomputerized screening ocular-motor evaluation is used as opposed to the extensive work-up given in Chapter 5.

dysfunction. There also may be impairment of cognitive function and reactive depression. In situations such as this, it may be difficult or impossible to identify the primary cause of ongoing disability. In settings of diagnostic uncertainty, a program of supervised vestibular rehabilitation may be very helpful from a diagnostic standpoint. The patient may make outstanding progress, suggesting that the primary problem was poor compensation for a stable lesion in the vestibular system. There may be continued spontaneous spells with improvement of the functional baseline between spells. If the patient fails to improve at all or seems to be worse after 4–6 weeks of therapy, an unstable lesion of the labyrinth is considerably more likely. Such an outcome may provide additional credibility to a clinical diagnosis of perilymph fistula.

MÉNIÈRE'S DISEASE

There are many issues that the otologic surgeon must address in selecting a surgical approach to patients with Ménière's disease. The first is a diagnostic question. Does the patient really have Ménière's disease? Physicians, in their eagerness to assign a diagnosis, may inaccurately label a patient when proper diagnostic criteria have not been fulfilled. If the diagnosis is uncertain, the physician should be less inclined to suggest operations designed to address the specific disorder of endolymphatic hydrops. Then there are issues of when to intervene surgically. The general teaching is that surgery is reserved for patients with "intractable vertigo who have failed medical therapy." Experience suggests that otologists differ significantly in their standards for determining medical failure. Some require 6 to 12 months of frequent and severe spells of vertigo before undertaking surgery. Others are willing to proceed much more quickly. These differences are important to remember in evaluating uncontrolled clinical studies of surgical efficacy, especially in light of the spontaneous remissions that characterize this disorder.

When the decision is made to proceed with surgery, questions arise regarding the choice of operation. Although vestibular nerve section or labyrinthectomy reliably relieves vertigo from Ménière's disease, they require ablation of function in the affected inner ear. The ideal procedure would restore function, or at least preserve residual function, while stabilizing the ear. The cochlear endolymphatic shunt (cochleosacculotomy procedure) is one operation that has been proposed as a method to create a permanent communication between the perilymphatic space and the hydropic endolymphatic compartment (Schuknecht, & Bartley, 1985). The goal is to equalize endolymphatic and perilymphatic pressure by creating a small fistula in the osseous spiral lamina of the cochlea. As might be expected, the operation has been associated with a significant incidence of high-frequency sensorineural hearing loss. Despite reports of fair success in controlling vertigo, the operation has had only limited application, perhaps due to general unfamiliarity with the surgical anatomy of the cochlea. A variety of surgical procedures on the endolymphatic sac have also been advocated in an attempt to relieve vertigo while retaining inner ear function. The efficacy of these procedures has been widely questioned and debated. Advocates of sac surgery argue that a 50–70% success rate improves upon the anticipated natural history in this patient population, making an initial endolymphatic sac procedure preferable to ablative procedures (Telischi & Luxford, 1993). Detractors argue that this success rate, even if accurate, is unsatisfactory and may even reflect the natural history of the disorder rather than a therapeutic benefit (Silverstein, Smouha, & Jones 1989; Snow & Kimmelman, 1979). In the absence of properly controlled clinical trials, the physician must answer several questions in choosing whether to recommend or perform endolymphatic sac procedures: Is endolymphatic sac surgery efficacious, and if so, do the results deteriorate as the disease progresses? Is the efficacy of sac surgery reported in uncontrolled observational studies inflated, given the retrospective nature of the studies? Are the reports reliable given the lack of standardized, validated outcome measures? Is the observed benefit attributable to the placebo effect or another nonspecific effect of mastoid surgery, as suggested by the Danish sham surgery study (Bretlau,Thomsen, Tos, & Johnsen, 1989)? If so, is it ethical to perform this surgery? Is there evidence that any specific manipulation of the sac or duct improves the outcome, or are all approaches equally successful (Jackson et al., 1988)? Is it reasonable to perform revision surgery after initial failure of an endolymphatic sac procedure? These unresolved issues significantly complicate the management of this important patient population. Continued uncertainty about these questions after 30 years of wide clinical experience suggests the need for properly designed multi-institutional clinical trials to address the role of endolymphatic sac surgery in Ménière's disease.

If sac surgery is rejected or unsuccessful, questions arise regarding the next surgical option. What is the procedure of choice to provide definitive control of vertigo? What is the likelihood of the patient developing Ménière's disease in the contralateral ear and how should this influence the choice of surgery? These questions bring us to the subject of procedures designed to ablate unilateral peripheral vestibular function.

UNILATERAL ABLATION OF VESTIBULAR FUNCTION

The patient with recurrent vertigo refractory to medical or conservative surgical management is a candidate to undergo a procedure that will ablate the residual vestibular function in the involved ear. The authors consider the transmastoid labyrinthectomy to be the gold standard for surgical relief of vertigo from inner ear pathology. However, because complete loss of residual hearing is inevitable after this operation, it is reserved for those patients who have extremely poor hearing in the affected ear. When hearing must be preserved, a selective vestibular nerve section procedure may be undertaken. Although more risky (due to the intracranial nature of the procedure) and slightly less reliable, vestibular neurectomy also has a proven track record in the surgical relief of vertigo in properly selected patients. Both of these procedures are designed to produce a total loss of afferent input from the offending vestibular periphery. Although these procedures

are most often applied in Ménière's disease, they may be effective in any peripheral vestibular disorder (Benecke, 1994; Kemink, Telian, El-Kashlan, & Langman, 1991). To optimize chances of a successful outcome, several factors must be considered in patient selection, as detailed below.

Unstable Function Versus Poor Compensation

The vestibular symptoms experienced by the patient should be a result of an unstable labyrinth, rather than an uncompensated stable lesion. This issue has already been discussed at length in this chapter. The patient with fluctuating or rapidly progressive unilateral dysfunction is the ideal surgical patient. On occasion, if appropriate rehabilitative measures fail to relieve symptoms in a patient who is uncompensated after a stable lesion, surgery on the offending side may be considered as a last hope of cure. In this case, the patient should be counseled regarding a less favorable prognosis for relief of symptoms.

Identification of the Offending Labyrinth

If there is uncertainty regarding the ear that is causing vertigo, ablative surgery should not be considered. Reliable lateralizing features include fluctuating or progressive unilateral sensorineural hearing loss and a consistently reproducible unilateral reduction of responsiveness to caloric irrigations. The asymmetric hearing loss in one ear is by far the best indicator of the pathologic side. An extended duration of pre-existing hearing loss need not dissuade the physician from incriminating the involved ear as the cause of vertigo (see Delayed Onset Vertigo Syndrome, Chapter 3). Less reliable features include tinnitus, aural fullness, direction of observed spontaneous or positional nystagmus, and rotary chair asymmetries. The latter findings are best used only as confirmatory evidence when the more convincing features are present. Although audiologic and vestibular test results usually are reliable in determining the involved ear, they must always be interpreted in light of the entire clinical presentation to avoid a serious error in diagnosis. For example, if there is a significant unilateral sensorineural hearing loss and the ENG shows a unilateral vestibular weakness on the same side, the clinician can be confident that the suspect labyrinth is indeed pathological. However, if the patient reports that roaring tinnitus or fluctuations of hearing in the better ear are associated with the spells of vertigo, it is likely that the second ear has now become involved. In this case, surgery is ill-advised.

Identification of Intracranial Pathology

Acoustic neuroma and other lesions of the posterior fossa may present with clinical features indistinguishable from classical vertigo syndromes. It is appropriate to perform a definitive radiographic imaging study before undertaking vestibular surgery of any type (see Case 18 from Chapter 7). Magnetic resonance imaging (MRI) of the posterior fossa with gadolinium enhancement provides a reliable means of detecting tumors even of small size, early stages of demyelinating disease, and subtle ischemic lesions of the brainstem. Even when the MRI is normal, vestibular test findings that suggest central pathology should be recognized and evaluated prior to considering vestibular surgery. Worrisome findings on the ENG include vertical or perverted nystagmus (nystagmus where direction of the fast component is opposite the direction expected during caloric irrigations) and oculomotor test abnormalities, as discussed in Chapter 5. When a noncomputerized approach to ocular-motor evaluation is used, other potential central findings also include failure of visual suppression or visual enhancement of nystagmus in the rotary chair battery. As illustrated in Case 48 from Chapter 7, dramatic abnormalities on the motor coordination test during dynamic posturography raise important suspicions that must be addressed.

Consideration of Other Potential Treatments

Although labyrinthectomy and vestibular nerve section may be applied in any peripheral vestibular disorder, certain patients may be effectively treated by simpler procedures. As mentioned above, classical benign paroxysmal positional vertigo is best addressed surgically by specific procedures designed to disrupt posterior semicircular canal function. These include surgical section of the nerve to the posterior canal ampulla (singular neurectomy), or procedures that occlude the lumen of this canal. In cases where the history strongly suggests a perilymph fistula, it is desirable to perform an exploratory tympanotomy prior to undertaking a definitive procedure. One exception to this rule may be the patient with long-standing symptoms who already has a profound sensorineural hearing loss on the suspect side. In such cases, it may be preferable to proceed directly to labyrinthectomy.

There has been a great deal of discussion in the medical literature regarding the best approach to unilateral ablation of vestibular function. Recently, the use of ototoxic aminoglycoside antibiotics has been advocated to produce a chemical labyrinthectomy, usually by topical instillation into the middle ear (Monsell et al., 1993; Nedzelski et al., 1992). The dosage of the drug that is absorbed into the inner ear is somewhat uncontrolled when administered transtympanically. Nevertheless, the procedure holds some promise for future therapy once reliable clinical protocols and the preferred agent have been identified in experimental settings.

Determination of the Utility of Residual Hearing

Generally, labyrinthectomy operations are reserved for patients with extremely poor residual hearing in the involved ear. Rather than setting a specific hearing threshold and/or speech discrimination score as the criteria for suggesting a vestibular nerve section instead of a labyrinthectomy, the authors prefer to consider each case on an individual basis. Ultimately, in order to desire hearing preservation, the patient must appreciate that the residual hearing in the diseased ear has some potential future value. The patient's perception of the usefulness of the current residual hearing is the most important factor. Some patients swear that they receive benefit from hearing aid use in ears that the medical community would deem useless compared to the better ear. Others fail to recognize any functional utility to an ear that should provide some benefit. Clearly, such perceptions should influence the choice of surgical procedure. Other factors that influence this equation are the patient's age, health status, and the likelihood that the hearing loss will progress to profound deafness in the near future, even if hearing is initially preserved. Some authors argue that labyrinthectomy should never be performed if there is any residual hearing. This is because they fear the unlikely scenario that the better ear would develop a hearing loss in the future that is greater than the loss in the diseased ear. This approach is too dogmatic to be practical, especially when one considers the additional risks of vestibular nerve section. If this rare outcome should occur, a cochlear implant in the most recently deafened ear would almost certainly rehabilitate the patient successfully.

Selection of the Surgical Procedure

Surgery for vertigo is virtually always elective. A well-informed patient can and should participate meaningfully in surgical decision making, both regarding timing of surgery and the operation to be performed. Patients must decide when their vertigo has produced sufficient disability in their life-style to outweigh the consequences and risks of surgery. Certainly a patient who has come to this juncture without coercion by family or the physician is most prepared to face the surgery and recovery phase with a positive outlook. It is appropriate to perform a labyrinthectomy instead of a selective vestibular nerve section if the better ear is stable, if the patient is convinced that the involved ear is functionally useless, and if he or she is unwilling to accept the incremental risks of intracranial surgery. A vestibular neurectomy is appropriate when the ear is deemed useful by both the clinician and the patient, especially when the hearing in the involved ear is unlikely to deteriorate in the near future.

The transcanal oval window labyrinthectomy provides fairly reliable results, especially if performed by surgeons experienced with this technique. The additional administration of ototoxic aminoglycosides into the vestibule further enhances the likelihood of success (Schuknecht, 1991).

The transmastoid labyrinthectomy is the most reliable method for ablating the labyrinth, as all neuroepithelial elements can be directly visualized and removed (Kemink, Telian, Graham, & Joynt, 1989). Although the facial nerve is at risk, physicians experienced in neurotologic surgery of the temporal bone can accomplish this procedure quickly and safely. As the surgery does not violate the dura of the posterior cranial fossa or the internal auditory canal, there should not be any significant risks of meningitis or cerebrospinal fluid leak.

Some have argued that the addition of a translabyrinthine vestibular nerve section to a labyrinthectomy provides incremental benefits sufficient to justify the additional risks. It is difficult to understand the rationale for such an argument in light of the excellent results experienced with the labyrinthectomy alone (Langman & Lindeman, 1993). Other authorities have advocated opening the internal auditory canal to section the cochlear nerve, arguing that this may eliminate or decrease the incidence of tinnitus after the procedure (Jones, Silverstein, & Smouha, 1989). This approach currently has few adherents, as most reports of cochlear nerve section for tinnitus have shown a dismal success rate.

The best surgical approach for vestibular nerve section also remains a controversial issue. The middle fossa approach is technically the most demanding of the conventional approaches (Garcia-Ibanez & Garcia-Ibanez, 1980). It allows for a definitive identification of the vestibular fibers within the internal auditory canal, but carries significant danger to hearing and facial nerve function when performed by surgeons unfamiliar with the fine points of this approach. The retrolabyrinthine approach is technically simpler for most neurotologic surgeons, but provides a view of the VIIIth cranial nerve in a location where it may be difficult to distinguish the cochlear from vestibular fibers of the nerve. This approach is satisfactory if the observed hearing results are equivalent to other methods (Kemink & Hoff, 1986). The retrosigmoid and the combined retrolabyrinthine-retrosigmoid approaches allow for the ability to drill away bone behind the internal auditory canal, if needed, to better distinguish the cochlear and vestibular fibers (Silverstein, Norrell, & Smouha, 1987). The infralabyrinthine approach for vestibular nerve section is rarely used (Vernick, 1990). As the name implies, the surgeon approaches the internal auditory canal by outlining the posterior semicircular canal and drilling inferior to the bony labyrinth. Although there are some theoretical advantages to this approach, it is possible only in temporal bones with an extensively pneumatized mastoid air cell system.

POSTOPERATIVE VESTIBULAR REHABILITATION

The compensation process is particularly critical for recovery from ablative vestibular surgery. When counseling preoperative patients, it is important to remember that the process of vestibular compensation is variable. Not all patients will compensate fully for the loss of unilateral vestibular function, and some may be left with considerable chronic disequilibrium or motion-provoked vertigo. The phenomenon of incomplete or delayed postoperative compensation may explain many of the unsatisfactory outcomes from vestibular surgery. Those who are at particular risk for poor recovery include patients with additional sensory deficits, complicating neurological conditions, centrally sedating medications, or poor psychological motivation for recovery. Such patients should be encouraged to pursue a customized program early in their postoperative course. The routine use of vestibular rehabilitation exercises has been shown to help optimize balance function after labyrinthectomy, vestibular neurectomy, or any operation that results in unilateral loss of labyrinthine function (see Chapter 10 for a complete discussion). It is appropriate for the therapist to offer counseling and instruction in a generic exercise program to all postoperative patients, and any who demonstrate a poor early recovery should be referred for a customized program of vestibular rehabilitation.

Beyond the acute phase of recovery, it may be difficult to determine if a postoperative relapse of vestibular symptoms represents disease progression or merely central nervous system decompensation. The phenomenon of decompensation may be observed following initially complete recovery from any peripheral lesion, including vestibular surgery (see the Case 1 example in Chapter 7). Early failures after labyrinthectomy are best attributed to incorrect diagnosis, incomplete surgical removal of the neuroepithelium, or inadequate initial vestibular compensation. Late failures might be due to central decompensation, which should respond briskly to vestibular rehabilitation (Katsarkas & Segal, 1988). Failures after vestibular nerve section may be due to an incomplete division of the vestibular fibers, and occasionally a labyrinthectomy or a revision procedure to complete the neurectomy is required. However, a therapeutic trial of vestibular rehabilitation is appropriate prior to considering additional surgery whenever the possibility of incomplete compensation or decompensation remains.

■ REFERENCES

Acierno MD, Trobe JD, Shepard NT, Taglia DM, (1996). Long-term disability related oscillopsia and imbalance caused by aminoglycoside treatment. Manuscript submitted for publication.

Alexander NB, (1994). Postural control in older adults. *J Am Gerontol Soc, 2,* 93–108.

Alexander NB, Shepard N, Gu MJ, Schultz A, (1992). Postural control in young and elderly adults when stance is perturbed: Kinematics. *J of Gerontology: Medical Sciences, 47,* 79–87.

Allum JH, (1983). Organization of stabilizing reflex responses in tibialis anterior muscles following ankle flexion pertubations of standing man. *Brain Res, 264,* 297–301.

Allum JH, Pfaltz CR, (1985). Visual and vestibular contributions to pitch sway stabilization in the ankle muscles of normals and patients with bilateral peripheral vestibular deficits. *Exp Brain Res, 58,* 82–94.

Allum JHJ, (1990). Posturography Systems: Current measurement concepts and possible improvements. In Brandt T, Paulus W, Bles W, Dieterich M, Krafczyk S, Straube A, (eds.), *Disorder of Posture and Gait (pp 16–28).* New York: Georg Thiem Verlag.

Allum JHJ, Honegger F, Schicks H, (1993). Vestibular and proprioceptive modulation of postural synergies in normal subjects. *J Vest Res, 3,* 59–85.

Allum JHJ, Huwiler M, Honegger F, (1994a). Objective measures of non–organic vertigo using dynamic posturography. In Taguchi K, Igarashi M, Mori S, (eds). *Vestibular and neural front: Proceedings of the 12th International Symposium on Posture and Gait (pp 51–55).* Amsterdam: Elsevier.

Allum JHJ, Schicks H, Honegger F, (1994b). The influence of a bilateral peripheral vestibular deficit on prostural synergies. *J Vest Res, 4,* 49–70.

Arenberg IK, (ed), (1993). *Dizziness and Balance Disorders.* Amsterdam/New York: Kugler Publications.

Ariyasu L, Byl FM, Sprague MS, Adour KK, (1990). The beneficial effect of methylprednisolone in acute vestibular vertigo. *Arch Otolaryngol Head Neck Surg, 116,* 700–703.

Baloh R, Honrubia V, (1990). *Clinical Neurophysiology of the Vestibular System, (2nd ed.).* Philadelphia: F. A. Davis.

Baloh RW, Harker LA, (1993). Meniere's disease and other peripheral vestibular disorders. In Cummings CW (ed.), *Otolaryngology–Head and Neck Surgery, (2nd ed., pp. 3177–3198).* St. Louis: Mosby Year Book.

Baloh RW, Honrubia V, Jacobson K, (1987), Benign positional vertigo: Clinical and oculographic features in 240 cases. *Neurology, 37,* 371–378.

Baloh RW, Jacobson KM, Socotch TM, (1993). The effect of aging on visual–vestibuloocular responses. *Exp Brain Res, 95,* 509–516.

Barany R, (1906). Untersuchungen uber den vom Vestibularapparat des Ohres reflectorisch ausgelosten rhytmischen Nystagmus und seine begleiterscheinungen. *Monatschr Ohrenheilk, 40*, 193–297.

Barany R, (1907). *Physiologie and Pathologie des Bogengangsapparates beim Menschen.* Vienna: Deuticke.

Barany R, Witmaack K, (1911). Funktionelle prufung des vestibularapparates verhandl. *Dtsch Otolog Gesllsch, 20*, 37–184.

Barber HO, Sharpe JA, (1988). *Vestibular disorders.* Chicago: Year Book Medical Publishers, Inc.

Barber HO, Stockwell CW, (1980). *Manual of Electronystagmography,* (2nd. ed.). St. Louis, MO: C.V. Mosby.

Barin K, (1987). Human postural sway responses to translational movements of the support surface. *Proceedings of the Ninth Annual Conference of the IEEE Engineering in Medicine and Biology Society, Boston.* 745–747.

Barin K, Seitz CM, Welling DB, (1992). Effect of head orientation on the diagnostic sensitivity of posturography in patients with compensated unilateral lesions. *Otolaryngol Head Neck Surg, 106*, 355–362.

Ben–David J, Podoshin Left, Fradis M, Faraggi D, (1993). Is the vestibular system affected by middle ear effusion? *Otolaryngol Head Neck Surg, 109*, 421–426.

Benecke JE, (1994). Surgery for non–Meniere's vertigo. *Acta Otolaryngol Suppl (Stockh), 513*, 37–39.

Bernstein P, McCabe BF, Ryu JM, (1974). The effect of diazepam on vestibular compensation. *Laryngoscope, 84*, 267–272.

Berthoz A, Lacour M, Soechting JF, Vidal PP, (1979). The role of vision in the control of posture during linear motion. In Granit, Pompeiano O, (eds), *Progress in Brain Research. Reflex Control of Posture and Movement, 50.* Amsterdam: Elsevier Science Publishers B.V.

Berthoz A, Pozzo T, (1988). Intermittent head stabilization during postural and locomotory tasks in humans. In Amblard B, Berthoz A, Clarac F, (eds.), *Posture and Gait: Development, adaptation and Modulation (pp 189–198).* Amsterdam–NewYork–Oxford: Excerpta Medica.

Beynon G, (1996). A review of management of benign paroxysmal positional vertigo by exercise therapy and repositioning manoeuvers. *British Journal of Audiology,* in press.

Beynon G, Shepard NT, (1996). Dizziness handicap inventory: Clinical utility in assessment and rehabilitation of the balance disorder patient. In preparation.

Bhansali SA, Bojrab DI, (1993). Oscillopsia. In Arenberg IK, (ed), *Dizziness and Balance Dis-*

orders, *(pp 587–590).* Amsterdam/New York: Kugler Publications.

Bienhold H, Abeln W, Flohr H, (1981). Drug effects on vestibular compensation. In Flohr H, Precht W. (Eds.) *Lesion–Induced Neuronal Plasticity in Sensorinotor Systems (pp 265–273).* New York, Springer–Verlag

Black FO, Pabski WH, Reschke MF, Calkins DS, Shupert CL, (1993). Vestibular ataxia following shuttle flights: effects of microgravity on otolith–mediated sensorimotor control of posture. *Amer J Otol, 14*, 9–17.

Blake AJ, Morgan K, Bendall MJ, et al, (1988). Falls by elderly people at home: Prevalence and associated factors. *Age and Aging, 17*, 365–372.

Blakely B, (1994). A randomized, controlled assessment of the canalith repositioning maneuver. *Otolaryngol Head Neck Surg, 110*, 391–396.

Boismier TE, Shepard NT, (1991). Test retest variability of dynamic posturography in a patient population. *Abstracts for Association for Research in Otolaryngology, Fourteenth Midwinter meeting, (p 91).* St. Petersburg Beach, FL.

Borello-France DF, Whitney SL, Herdman SJ, (1994). Rehabilitation assessment and management. In Herdman SJ, (ed), *Vestibular Rehabilitation, (pp 287–315).* Philadelphia: F.A. Davis.

Brandt T, Daroff RB, (1980). Physical therapy for benign paroxysmal positional vertigo. *Arch Otol Rhinol Laryngol, 106*, 484–485.

Brandt T, Steddin S, (1993). Current view of the mechanism of benign paroxysmal positioning vertigo: cupulolithiasis or canalolithiasis? *J Vestib Res, 3*, 373–382.

Brandt Th, Steddin S, Eng D, Daroff RB, (1994). Therapy for benign parozysmal positioning vertigo, revisited. *Neurology, 44*, 796–800.

Bretlau P, Thomsen J, Tos M, Johnsen NJ, (1989). Placebo effect in surgery for Meniere's disease: Nine–year follow–up. *Am J Otol, 10*, 259–261.

Bronstein AM, (1992). Plastic changes in the human cervicoocular reflex. *Annal of the NY Acad of Sciences, 656*, 708–715.

Brookler KH, (1976). The simultaneous binaural bithermal: A caloric test utilizing electronystagmography. *Laryngoscope, 86*, 1241–1250.

Brookler KH, (1990). Electronystagmography. *Neurologic Clinics, 8(2)*, 235–259.

Brown JJ, Baloh RW, (1987), Persistent Mal de Debarquement syndrome: A motion–induced subjective disorder of balance. *Am J Otolaryngol, 8*, 219–222.

Campbell, AJ, Reinken J, Allan BC, Martinez GS, (1981). Falls in old age: A study of frequency and related clinical factors. *Age and Aging, 10*, 264–270.

Cass SP, Furman JMR, (1993). Medications and their effects on vestibular function testing. *ENG Report, November.* ICS Medical Corporation.

Casselbrant ML, Furman JM, Rubenstein E, Mandel EM, (1995). Effect of otits media on the vestibular system in children. *Ann Otol Rhinol Laryngol, 104,* 620–624.

Cawthorne T, (1944). The physiological basis for head exercises. *J Chart Soc Physiother, 106–107.*

Cevette MJ, Puetz B, Marion MS, Wertz ML, Muenter MD, (1995). Aphysiologic performance on dynamic posturography. *Otolaryngol Head Neck Surg, 112,* 676–688.

Chandra NS, Shepard NT, (1996). Clinical utility of lateral head tilt posturography. *Am J of Otology,* in press.

Cohen B, Buttner–Ennever JA, (1984). Projections from the superior colliculus to a region of the central mesencephalic reticular formation (cMRF) associated with horizontal saccadic eye movements. *Exp Brain Res, 57,* 167–176.

Cohen B, Henn V, Raphan T, Dennett D, (1981). Velocity storage, nystagmus, and visual–vestibular interactions in humans. *Ann NY Acad Sci, 374,* 421–433.

Cohen B, Matsuo V, Fradin J, Raphan T, (1985). Horizontal saccades induced by stimulation of the central mesencephalic reticular formation. *Exp Brain Res, 57,* 605–616.

Cohen B, Uemure T, Takemore S, (1973). Effects of labyrinthectomy on optokinetic nystagmus (OKN) and optokinetic after–nystagmus (OKAN). *Equilibrium Research, 3,* 88–93.

Courjon JH, Jeannerod M, (1979). Visual substitution of labyrinthine defects. In Granit Right, Pompeiano O, (eds), *Progress in Brain Research. Reflex control of Posture and Movement, 50.* Amsterdam: Elsevier Science Publishers B.V.

Cramer RL, Dowd PJ, Helms DB, (1963). Vestibular responses to oscillations about the yaw axis. *Aerospace Med, 34,* 1031.

Curthoys IS, Halmagyi GM, (1995). Vestibular compensation: A review of the oculomotor, neural, and clinical consequences of unilateral vestibular loss. *J Vestib Res, 5,* 67–107.

Cutrer FM, Baloh RW, (1992). Migraine–associated dizziness. *Headache, 31,* 300–304.

Cyr DG, (1983). The vestibular system: Pediatric considerations. *Seminars in Hearing, 4(1),* 33–45.

Daroff RB, Troost BT, Dell–Osso LF, (1978). Nystagmus and related ocular oscillations. In Glaser JS, (ed), *Neuro–ophthalmology (pp 220–240).* Hagerstown, MD: Harper & Row.

Deiterich M, Brandt Th, (1994). Vestibular syndromes in the roll plane: Topographic diagnosis from brainstem to cortex. In Taguchi K, Igarashi M, Mori S, (eds). *Vestibular and Neural Front: Proceedings of the 12th International Symposium on Posture and Gait (pp 423–436).* Amsterdam: Elsevier.

Dener JL, (1994). Effects of aging on verticle visual tracking and visual–vestibular interactions. *J Vest Res, 4,* 355–370.

Dichgans J, Diener HC, (1987). The use of short– and long–latency reflex testing in leg muscles of neurological patients. In Struppler A, Weindl A, (eds), *Clinical Aspects of Sensory–motor Integration: Implications for Neurological Patients, (pp 165–175).* New York: Springer–Verlag.

Diener HC, Dichgans J, Guschlbauer B, Bacher M, (1986). Role of visual and static vestibular influences on dynamic posture control. *Hum Neurobiol,5,* 105–113.

Diener HC, Dichgans J, Hülser P–J, Buettner U–W, Bacher M, Guschlbauer B, (1984). The significance of delayed long–loop responses to ankle displacement for the diagnosis of multiple sclerosis. *Electroencephalogr Clin Neurophysiol, 57,* 336–342.

Eklund G, Hagbarth KE, (1966). Normal variability of tonic vibration reflexes in man. *Exp Neurology, 16,* 80–92.

Elidan J, et al, (1991). Short and middle latency vestibular evoked responses to acceleration in man. *Electroenceph Clin Neurophysiol, 80(2),* 140–145.

Elidan J, Langhofer Left, Honrubia V, (1987). Recording of short–latency vestibular evoked potentials induced by acceleration impulses in experimental animals: Current status of the method and its applications. *Elctoenceph Clin Neurophysiol, 68,* 58–69.

El–Kashlan H, Shepard NT,, Asher A, Smith–Wheelock M Telian SA, (1996). Evaluation of clinical measures of equilibrium: Vestibular rehabilitation program evaluation tools. Manuscript submitted for publication

Epley JM, (1992). The canalith repositioning procedure for treatment of benign paroxysmal positional vertigo. *Otolaryngol Head Neck Surg, 107,* 399–404.

Ewald R, (1892). *Physiologishc Untersuch hber das Endorgan des Nervous Octavus.* Wiesbaden: Bergmann.

Fitzgerald G, Hallpike CS, (1942). Studies in human vestibular function: I. Observations of the directional preponderance of caloric nystagmus resulting from cerebral lesions. *Brain, 65,* 115.

Fitzpatrick R, Burke D, Gandevia S, (1994). Task–dependent reflex responses and movement illusions evoked by galvanic vestibular stimulation in standing humans. *J Physiol London, 478,* 363–372.

Fletcher WA, Hain TC, Zee DS, (1990). Optokinetic nystagmus and afternystagmus in human beings: Relationship to nonlinear processing of information about retinal slip. *Exp Brain Res, 81,* 46–52.

Ford–Smith CD, Wyman JF, Elswick RK, Fernandez T, Newton RA, (1995). Test–retest reliability of the sensory organization test in noninstitutionalized older adults. *Arch Phys Med Rehabil, 76,* 77–81.

Forssberg H, Nashner LM, (1982). Ontogenetic development of postural control in man: Adaptation to altered support and visual conditions during stance. *The Journal of Neuroscience, 2(5),* 545–552.

Fortin M, Shepard NT, Diener HC, Lawson GD, (1996). Within and between laboratories reliability of the latency markings for the postural evoked response test. In preparation.

Francis DA, Bronstein AM, Rudge P, du Boulay EPGH, (1992). The site of brainstem lesions causing semicircular canal paresis: An MRI study. *J of Neurology Neurosurgery Psychiatry, 55,* 446–449.

Friedmann HH, Noth J, Diener HC, Bacher M, (1987). Long latency EMG responses in hand and leg muscles: Cerebellar disorder. *J Neurol Neurosurg Psychiatry, 50,* 71–77.

Fukuda T, (1959). The stepping test: Two phases of the labyrinthine reflex. *Acta Otolaryngol, 50,* 95.

Fukuda T, (1983). *Statokinetic Reflexes in Equilibrium and Movement*. Tokyo: University of Tokyo Press.

Furman JMR, (1993). Off–vertical axis rotational testing. In Sharpe JA, Barber HO, (eds), *The Vestibulo–Ocular Reflex and Vertigo, (pp 79–88).* New York: Raven Press, Ltd.

Furman JMR, Baloh RW, (1992). Otolith–ocular testing in human subjects. *Annals New York Academy of Sciences, 656,* 431–451.

Furman JMR, Schor RH, Kamerer DB, (1993). Off–vertical axis rotational responses in patients with unilateral peripheral vestibular lesions. *Ann Otol Rhinol Laryngol, 102,* 137–143.

Furman JMR, Wall C, Kamerer DB, (1988). Alternate and simultaneous binaural bithermal caloric testing a comparison. *Ann Otol Rhinol Laryngol, 97,* 359–364.

Furst EJ, Goldberg J, Jenkins HA, (1987). Voluntary modification of the rotatory induced vestibulo–ocular reflex by fixating imaginary targets. *Acta Otolaryngol (Stockh), 103,* 232–240.

Gacek RR, Gacek MR, (1994). Singular neurectomy in the management of paroxysmal positional vertigo. *Otolaryngol Clin North Am, 27,* 363–379.

Garcia–Ibanez E, Garcia–Ibanez JL, (1980). Middle fossa vestibular neurectomy: A report of 373 cases. *Otolaryngol Head Neck Surg, 88,* 486–490.

Gavie S, Shepard NT, Goldner N, Nihem C, (1994). Graded mobility tests: An assessment tool for balance disorders resulting from vestibular lesions. *Abstracts of the Seventeenth Midwinter Research Meeting.* St. Petersburg, FL: Association for Research in Otolaryngology.

Goebel JA, Hanson JM, Fishel DG, (1994). Age–related modulation of the vestibulo–ocular reflex using real and imaginary targets. *J Vest Res, 4,* 269–276.

Goebel JA, Hanson JM, Fishel DG, The Interlaboratory Rotational Chair Study Group, (1994). Interlaboratory variability of rotational chair test results. *Otolaryngol Head Neck Surg, 110,* 400–405.

Goebel JA, Hanson JM, Langhofer LR, Fishel DG, (1995). Head-shake vestibulo-ocular refex testing: Comparison of results with rotational chair testing. *Otolaryngol Head Neck Surg, 112,* 203–209.

Goldberg RJ, (1995). Diagnostic dilemmas presented by patients with anxiety and depression. *Am J Med, 98,* 278–284.

Gordon CR, Spitzer O, Doweck I, Melaned Y, Shupak A, (1995). Clinical features of Mal de Debarquement: Adaptation and habituation to sea conditions. *J Vest Res, 5(5),* 363–371.

Graham MD, Kemink JL, (1984). Titration streptomycin therapy for bilateral Meniere's disease. *Am J Otol, 5,* 534–535.

Gu MJ, Shepard NT, Schultz A, Fassois SD, (1992). Calculation of center of mass movements from center–of–reaction measurements. In Woollacott M, Horak F, (eds), *Posture and Gait: Control Mechanisms (pp 388–391)*. Portland, OR: University of Oregon Press.

Gurfinkel VS, Lipshits MI, Popv KY, (1974). Is the stretch reflex the main mechanism in the system of regulation of the vertical posture of man? *Biophysics, 19,* 744–748.

Hain T, (1993a). Background and technique of ocular motility testing. In Jacobson GP, Newman

CW, Kartush JM, (eds) *Handbook of Balance Function Testing (pp 83–100).* St. Louis MO: Mosby–Year Book, Inc.

Hain T, (1993b). Interpretation and usefulness of ocular motility testing. In Jacobson GP, Newman CW, Kartush JM, (eds), *Handbook of Balance Function Testing (pp 101–122).* St. Louis MO: Mosby–Year Book, Inc.

Hain TC, Fetter M, Zee DS, (1987). Head–shaking nystagmus in patients with unilateral peripheral vestibular lesions. *Am J Otolaryngol, 8,* 36–47.

Hain TC, Herdman SJ, Holliday M, Mattox D, Zee DS, Byskosh AT, (1994). Localizing value of optokinetic afternystagmus. *Ann Otol Rhinol Laryngol, 103,* 806–811.

Hain TC, Zee DS, (1991). Abolition of optokinetic afternystagmus by aminoglycoside ototoxicity. *Ann Otol Rhinol Laryngol, 100,* 580–583.

Halmagyi GM, Brandt Th, Dieterich M, Curthoys IS, Stark RJ, Hoyt WF, (1990). Tonic contraversive ocular tilt reaction due to unilateral meso–diencephalic lesion. *Neurology, 40,* 1503–1509.

Halmagyi GM, Curthoys IS, (1988). A clinical sign of canal paresis. *Arch Neurol, 45,* 737–739.

Halmagyi GM, Curthoys IS, Brandt Th, Dieterich M, (1991). Ocular tilt reaction: Clinical sign of vestibular lesion. *Acta Otolaryngol (Stockh), Suppl. 481,* 47–50.

Halmagyi GM, Curthoys IS, Dai MJ, (1993). The effects of unilateral vestibular deafferentation on human otolith function. In Sharpe JA, Barber HO, (eds), *The Vestibulo–Ocular Reflex and Vertigo, (pp 89–104).* New York: Raven Press, Ltd.

Halmagyi GM, Gresty MA, Gibson WPR, (1978). Ocular tilt reaction with peripheral vestibular lesion. *Ann Neurol, 6,* 80–83.

Hamid MA, Hughes GB, Kinney SE, (1991). Specificity and sensitivity of dynamic posturography—a retrospective analysis. *Acta Otolaryngol (Stockh), Suppl. 481,* 596–600.

Hamid MA, Hughes GB, O'Keefe M, (1985). Can the chair test determine the side of vestibular dysfunction? In Myers E (ed), *New Dimensions in Otolaryngology–Head and Neck Surgery, 2, (pp 285–286).* New York: Elsevier Science Publishers.

Harada Y, (1988). *The Vestibular Organs: S.E.M. Atlas of the Inner Ear.* Amsterdam/Berkeley/Milano: Kugler & Ghedini Publications.

Harker LA, Rassekh C, (1988). Migraine equivalent as a cause of episodic vertigo. *Laryngoscope, 98,* 160–164.

Harker LA, (1994). Migraine. In Jackler RK, Brackmann DE, (eds), *Neurotology (pp 463–470).* St. Louis: Mosby–Year Book, Inc.

Harris GF, Riedel SA, Matesi D, Smith P, (1993). Standing postural stability assessment and signal stationarity in children with cerebral palsy. *IEEE Trans Rehab Engineer, 1,* 35–42.

Herdman SJ, Clendaniel RA, Mattox DE, Holliday MJ, Niparko JK, (1995). Vestibular adaptation exercises and recovery: Acute stage after acoustic neuroma resection. *Otolaryngol Head Neck Surg, 113,* 77–87.

Herdman SJ, (1994a). Preface. In Herdman SJ, (ed), *Vestibular Rehabilitation (pp ix–x).* Philadelphia: F.A. Davis Co.

Herdman SJ, (ed), (1994b). *Vestibular Rehabilitation.* Philadelphia: F.A. Davis Company.

Herdman SJ, Borello–France DF, Whitney SL, (1994). Treatment of vestibular hypofunction. In Herdman SJ, (ed), *Vestibular Rehabilitation, (pp 287–315).* Philadelphia: F.A. Davis Co.

Hirsch C, (1940). A new labyrinthine reaction. The waltzing test. *Ann Otol,49,* 232.

Hoffman DL, O'Lear DP, Munjack DJ, (1994). Autorotation test abnormalities of the horizontal an vertical vestibulo–ocular reflexes in panic disorder. *Otolaryngol Head Neck Surg, 110,* 259–269.

Honrubia V, Baloh RW, Khalili R, (1989). Subjective and oculomotor responses during interaction of smooth pursuit with optokinetic and vestibular stimuli. *Abstracts of the Twelfth Midwinter Research Meeting.* St. Petersburg, FL: Association for Research in Otolaryngology.

Honrubia V, et al, (1968). Experimental studies on optokinetic nystagmus. II. Normal humans. *Acta Otolaryngol, 65,* 441.

Honrubia V, Jenkin HA, Baloh RW, Yee RD, Lau CGY, (1984). Vestibulo–ocular reflexes in peripheral labyrinthine lesions: I. Unilateral dysfunction. *Am J Otolaryngol, 5,* 15–26.

Horak F, Jones–Rycewicz C, Black FO, Shumway–Cook A, (1992). Effects of vestibular rehabilitation on dizziness and imbalance. *Otolaryngol Head Neck Surg, 106,* 175–180.

Horak FB, Diener HC, Nashner LM, (1989). Influence of central set on human postural responses. *J Neurophysiol, 62,* 841–853.

Horak FB, Nashner LM, (1986). Central programming of postural movements: Adaptation to altered support surface configurations. *J Neurophysiol, 55,* 1369–1381.

Horak FB, Nashner LM, Diener HC, (1990). Postural strategies associated with somatosensory and vestibular loss. *Exp Brain Res, 82,* 167–177.

Horak FB, Shumway–Cook A, Crowe TK, Black FO, (1988). Vestibular function and motor proficiency of children with impaired hearing, or with learning disability and motor impairment. *Dev Med Child Neurol, 30,* 64–79.

Igarashi M, (1984). Vestibular compensation: An overview. *Acta Otolaryngol (Stockh), Suppl 406,* 78–82.

Ishikawa K, Igarashi M, (1984). Effect of diazepam on vestibular compensation in squirrel monkeys. *Arch Otorhinolaryngol, 240,* 49–54.

Jackson CG, Dick JR, Glasscock ME, Fritsch MH, Graham SS, Dimitrov EA, (1988). Endolymphatic mastoid shunt surgery using the Denver inner ear shunt. *Otolaryngol Head Neck Surg, 99,* 282–285.

Jackson RT, Epstein CM, (1991). Effect of head extension on euilibrium in normal subjects. *Ann Otol Rhinol Laryngol, 100,* 63–67.

Jacob R, (1988). Panic disorder and the vestibular system. *Psychiatric Clinics of North America, 11,* 361–374

Jacobson GP, Calder JA, Shepherd VA, Rupp KA, Newman GW, (1995). Reappraisal of the monothermal warm caloric screening test. *Ann Otol Rhinol Laryngol, 104,* 942–945.

Jacobson GP, Newman CW, (1990). The development of the dizziness handicap inventory. *Arch Otolaryngol Head Nech Surg, 116,* 424–427.

Jacobson GP, Newman CW, Hunter Left, Balzer G, (1991). Balance function test correlates of the dizziness handicap inventory. *J Am Acad Audiol, 2,* 253–260.

Jacobson GP, Newman CW, Kartush JM, (eds), (1993). *Handbook of Balance Function Testing.* St. Louis MO: Mosby–Year Book, Inc.

Jacobson GP, Newman CW, Safadi I, (1990). Sensitivity and specificity of the head–shaking test for detecting vestibular system abnormalities. *Ann Otol Rhinolog Laryngolog, 99,* 539–542.

Jacobson JT, Northern JL, (eds.), (1991). *Diagnostic Audiology.* Austin, Texas: Pro–Ed.

Johansson R, Magnusson M, Ckesson M, (1988). Identification of human posutral dynamics. *IEEE Trans Biomedical Engineer, 35,* 858–869.

Johansson R, Magnusson M, Fransson PA, (1995). Galvanic vestibular stimulation for analysis of postural adaptation and stability. *IEEE Trans Biomedical Engineer, 42,* 282–292.

Jones NS, Radomskij P, Prichard AJN, Snashall SE, (1990). Imbalance and chronic secretory otitis media in children: Effect of myringotomy and insertion of ventilation tubes on body sway. *Ann Otol Rhinol Laryngol, 99,* 477–481.

Jones R, Silverstein H, Smouha E, (1989). Long–term results of transmeatal cochleo-

vestibular neurectomy: An analysis of 100 cases. *Otolaryngol Head Neck Surg, 100,* 22–29.

Karlberg M, Johansson R, Magnusson M, Fransson P, (1996). Dizziness of suspected cervical origin distinguished by posturographic assessment of human postural dynamics. *J Vest Res, 6,* 37–48.

Karlberg M, Persson L, Magnusson M, (1995). Reduced postural control in patients with chronic cervicobrachial pain syndrome. *Gair & Posture, 3,* 241–249.

Katsarkas A, Segal B, (1988). Unilateral loss of peripheral and vestibular function in patients: Degree of compensation and factors causing decompensation. *Otolaryngol Head Neck Surg, 98,* 45–47.

Katz J,(ed.), (1994). *Handbook of Clinical Audiology (4th edition).* Baltimore: Williams & Wilkins.

Kemink JL, Hoff JT, (1986). Retrolabyrinthine vestibular nerve section: Analysis of results. *Laryngoscope, 96,* 33–36.

Kemink JL, Telian SA, El–Kashlan H, Langman AW, (1991). Retrolabyrinthine vestibular nerve section: Efficacy in disorders other than Meniere's disease. *Laryngoscope, 101,* 523–528.

Kemink JL, Telian SA, Graham MD, Joynt L, (1989). Transmastoid labyrinthectomy: Reliable surgical management of vertigo. *Otolaryngol Head Neck Surg, 101,* 5–10.

Keshner EA, Woollacott MH, Debu B, (1988). Neck, trunk, and limb muscle responses during postural perturbations in humans. *Exp Brain Res, 71,* 455–466.

Kileny P, McCabe B, Ryu JH, (1989). Effects of attention–requiring tasks on vestibular nystagmus. *Ann Otol Rhinol Laryngol, 89,* 9–12.

Krebs DE, Gill–Body KM, Riley PO, Parker SW, (1993). Double–blind, placebo-controlled trial of rehabilitation for bilateral vestibular hypofunction: Preliminary report. *Otolaryngology Head Neck Surg, 109,* 735–741.

Kroenke K, Mangelsdorff AG, (1989). Common symptoms in ambulatory care: Incidence, evaluation, therapy and outcome. *Am J Med, 86,* 262–266.

Kubo N, Wall C, (1990). Serial data variation in the dynamic posturography. *Abstracts forAssociation for Research in Otolaryngology, thirteenth Midwinter meeting, (p 350).* St. Petersburg Beach, FL.

Kubo T, Igarashi M, Wright W, (1981). Eye–head coordination and lateral canal block in squirrel monkeys. *Ann Otol Rhinol Laryngol, 90,* 154–157.

Kumar A, (1981). Diagnostic advantages of the Torok monothermal differential caloric test. *Laryngoscope, 91*, 1679–1694.

Kumar A, Mafee M, Torok N, (1982). Anatomic specificity of central vestibular signs in posterior fossa lesions. *Ann Otol Rhinol Laryngol, 91*, 510–515.

Kveton JF, (1994). Symptoms of vestibular disease. In Jackler RK, Brackmann DE (eds.), *Neurotology (pp. 145–151)*. St. Louis: Mosby Year Book.

Lafortune SH, Ireland DJ, Jell RM, (1991). Suppression of OKN velocity storage in humans by statiotilt in roll. *J Vest Res, 1*, 347–355.

Lalwani AK, (1994). Vertigo, dysequilibrium, and imbalance with aging. In Jackler RK, Brackmann DE, (eds), *Neurotology (pp 527–534)*. St. Louis: Mosby–Year Book, Inc.

Langman AW, Lindeman RC, (1993). Surgery for vertigo in the nonserviceable hearing ear: Transmastoid labyrinthectomy or translabyrinthine vestibular nerve section. *Laryngoscope, 103*, 1321–1325.

Lawson GD, Shepard NT, Oviatt DL, Wang Y, (1994). Electromyographic responses of lower leg muscles to upward toe tilts as a function of age. *J Vest Res, 4*, 203–214.

Ledin T, Gupta A, Larsen LE, Ödkvist LM, (1993). Randomized perturbed posturography: Methodology and effects of midazolam sedation. *Acta Otolaryngol (Stockh), 113*, 245–248.

Ledin T, Loftås P, Öhman S, Ödkvist LM, (1993). Effects of alcohol in modified dynamic posturography and randomized perturbed posturography. *Acta Otolaryngol (Stockh), 113*, 252–255.

Ledin T, Ödkvist LM, (1993). Effects of increased inertial load in dynamic and randomized perturbed posturography. *Acta Otolaryngol (Stockh), 113*, 249–252.

Leigh RJ, Zee DS, (1982). The diagnostic value of abnormal eye movements: A pathophysiological approach. *The Johns Hopkins Medical Journal, 151*, 122–135.

Leigh RJ, Zee DS, (1991). *The Neurology of Eye Movements, (2nd ed.)*. Philadelphia: F.A. Davis Co.

Levens SL, (1988). Electronystagmography in normal children. *British J of Audiology, 22*, 51–56.

Lynn S, Pool A, Rose D, Brey R, Suman V, (1995). Randomized trial of the canalith repositioning procedure. *Otolaryngol Head Neck Surg, 113*, 712–720.

Magnusson M, Johansson R, (1993). Dynamic properties of feed back control of human posture in subjects with vestibular neuritis. *Acta Otolaryngol (Stockh), Suppl, 503*, 47–48.

Manusson M, Norrving B, (1993). Cerebellar infarctions and vestibular neuritis. *Acta Otolaryngol (Stockh), Suppl. 503*, 64–66.

Magnusson M, Petersen H, Harris S, Johansson R, (1995). Postural control and vestibulospinal function in patients selected for cochlear implantation. *British J Audiology, 29*, 231–236.

Maki BE, Holliday PJ, Fernie GR, (1987). A posture control model and balance test for the prediction of relative postural stability. *IEEE Trans Biomedical Engineer, 34*, 797–810.

Maki BE, Whitelaw RS, (1992). Influence of experience, expectation and arousal on posture control strategy and performance. In Woollacott M, Horak F, (eds), *Posture and Gait: Control Mechanisms (pp 123–126)*. Portland, OR: University of Oregon Press.

Manchester D, Woollacott M, Zederbauer–Hylton N, et al, (1989). Visual, vestibular and somatosensory contributions to balance control in the older adult. *J Gerontol, 44*, M118–127.

Mathog RH, (1972). Testing of the vestibular system by sinusoidal angular acceleration. *Acta Otolaryngol, 74*, 96–103.

Mathog RH, Peppard SB, (1982). Exercise and recovery from vestibular injury. *Am J Otolaryngol, 3*, 397–407.

Matthew NG, Davis LL, O'Leary DP, (1993). Autorotation test of the horizontal vestibulo–ocular reflex in Meniere's disease. *Otolaryngol Head Neck Surg, 109*, 339–412.

Mauritz KH, Dietz V, (1980). Characteristics of postural instability induced by ischemic blocking of leg afferents. *Exp Brain Res, 38*, 117–119.

Melvill JG, Berthoz A, Segal B, (1984). Adaptive modification of the vestibulo–ocular reflex by mental effort in darkness. *Exp Brain Res, 56*, 149–153.

Melvill JG, Guitton D, Berthoz A, (1988). Changing patterns of eye–head coordination during 6 hr of optically reversed vision. *Exp Brain Res, 69*, 531–544.

Melvill JG, Mandl G, (1981). Motion sickness due to vision reversal: Its absence in stroboscopic light. *Ann NY Acad Sci, 374*, 303–311

Mizukoshi K, Kobayashi H, Ohashi N, Shojaku H, Watanabe Y, (1985). Quantitative assessment of visual–vestibular interaction using sinusoidal rotation in patients with well–defined central nervous system lesions. *Abstracts of Barany Society (p 100)*. Ann Arbor, MI.

Möller C, Ödkvist L, White V, David C, (1990a). The plasticity of compensatory eye movements in rotatory tests: I. The effect of alertness and eye closure. *Acta Otolaryngol (Stockh), 109,* 15–24.

Möller C, White V, Ödkvist L, (1990b). The plasticity of compensatory eye movements in rotatory tests: II. The effect of vountary, visual, imaginary, auditory and proprioceptive mechanisms. *Acta Otolaryngol (Stockh), 109,* 168–178.

Monsell EM, Brackmann DE, Linthicum FH, (1988). Why do vestibular destructive procedures sometimes fail? *Otolaryngol Head Neck Surg, 99,* 472–479.

Monsell EM, Cass SP, Rybak LP, (1993). Therapeutic use of aminoglycoside in Meniere's disease. *Oto Clin North Am, 26,* 737–746.

Moore DM, Hoffman LF, Beykirch K, Honrubia V, Baloh RW, (1991). The electrically evoked vestibulo–ocular reflex. I. Normal subjects. *Otolayngol Head Neck Surg, 104,* 219–224.

Mori S, Takakusaki K, (1988). Integration of posture and locomotion. In Amblard B, Berthoz A, Clarac F, (eds.), *Posture and Gait: Development, Adaptation and Modulation (pp 341–354).* Amsterdam–NewYork–Oxford: Excerpta Medica.

Mulch G, Petermann W, (1979). Influence of age on results of vestibular function tests. *Ann Otol Rhinol Laryngol, (Suppl), 56,* 1–17.

Murphy TP, (1993). Mal de Debarquement syndrome: A forgotten entity? *Otolaryngol Head Neck Surg, 109,* 10–13.

Nashner LM, (1976). Adapting reflexes controlling the human posture. *Exp Brain Res, 26,* 59–72.

Nashner LM, (1977). Fixed patterns of rapid postural responses among leg muscles during stance. *Brain Res, 150,* 403–407.

Nashner LM, (1979). Organization and programming of motor activity curing posutral control. In Granit Right, Pompeiano O, (eds), *Progress in Brain Research. Reflex Control of Posture and Movement, 50, (pp 177–184).* Amsterdam: Elsevier Science Publishers B.V.

Nashner LM, (1983). Analysis of movement control in man using the movable platform. In Desmedt JE, (ed), *Motor Control Mechanisms in Health and Disease, (pp 607–619).* New York: Raven Press.

Nashner LM, (1993a). Practical biomechanics and physiology of balance. In Jacobson GP, Newman CW, Kartush JM, (eds), *Handbook of Balance Function Testing (pp 261–279).* St. Louis: Mosby–Year Book, Inc.

Nashner LM, (1993b). Computerized Dynamic Posturography. In Jacobson GP, Newman CW, Kartush JM, (eds), *Handbook of Balance Function Testing (pp 280–307).* St. Louis: Mosby–Year Book, Inc.

Nashner LM, (1993c). Computerized dynamic posturography: Clinical applications. In Jacobson GP, Newman CW, Kartush JM, (eds), *Handbook of Balance Function Testing (pp 308–334).* St. Louis: Mosby–Year Book, Inc.

Nashner LM, Berthoz A, (1978). Visual contribution to rapid motor responses during postural control. *Brain Res, 150,* 403–407.

Nashner LM, Cordo PJ, (1981). Relation of automatic postural responses and reaction time voluntary movements of human leg muscles. *Exp Brain Res, 43,* 395–405.

Nashner LM, Grimm RJ, (1978). Clincial applications of the long loop motor control analysis in intact man: Analysis of multiloop dyscontrols in standing cerebellar patients. *Neurophysiol, 4,* 300–319.

Nashner LM, McCoullum G, (1985). The organization of human postural movements: A formal basis and experimental synthesis. *The Behavioral and Brain Sciences, 8,* 135–172.

Nashner LM, Shumway–Cook A, Marin O, (1983). Stance posture control in select groups of children with cerebral palsy: Deficits in sensory organization and muscular coordination. *Exp Brain Res, 49,* 393–409.

Nashner LM, Woollacott M, Tuma G, (1979). Organization of rapid responses to postural and locomotor–like perturbations of standing man. *Exp Brain Res, 36,* 463–476.

Nedzelski JM, Schessel DA, Bryce GE, Pfleiderer AG, (1992). Chemical labyrinthectomy: Local application of gentamicin for the treatment of unilateral Meniere's disease. *Am J Otol , 13,* 18–22.

Norré ME, (1987). Rationale of rehabilitation treatment for vertigo. *Am J Otolaryngol, 8,* 31–35.

Norré ME, (1994). Sensory interaction posturography in patients with peripheral vestibular disorders. *Otolaryngol Head Neck Surg, 110,* 281–287.

Norré ME, (1995). Head extension effect in static posturography. *Ann Otol Rhinol Laryngol, 104,* 570–573.

Paige G, (1992). Senescence of human visual–vestibular interactions. 1. VOR and adaptive plasticity with aging. *J Vest Res, 2,* 133–155.

Paige GD, (1989). Nonlinearity and asymmetry in the human vestibulo–ocular reflex. *Acta Otolaryngol, 108,* 1–8.

Panosian MS, Paige GD, (1995). Nystagmus and postural instability after headshake in patients with vestibular dysfunction. *Otolaryngol Head Neck Surg, 112,* 399–404.

Parnes LS, McCLure JA, (1991). Posterior semicircular canal occlusion in the normal hearing ear. *Otolaryngol Head Neck Surg, 104,* 52–57.

Parnes LS, Price–Jones RG, (1993). Particle repositioning maneuver for treatment of benign paroxysmal positional vertigo. *Ann Otol Rhinol Laryngol, 102,* 325–331.

Patla AE, Koyama K, Mackintosh D, (1994). A new apparatus for studying the role of vestibular system in the control of posture and locomotion. In Taguchi K, Igarashi M, Mori S, (eds), *Vestibular and Neural Front: Proceedings of the 12th International Symposium on Posture and Gait (pp 35–42).* Amsterdam: Elsevier.

Peppard SB, (1986). Effect of drug therapy on compensation from vestibular injury. *Laryngoscope, 96,* 878–898.

Peterka RJ, Black FO, Schoenhoff MB, (1990a). Age–related changes in human vestibulo–ocular and optokinetic reflexes: Pseudorandom rotation tests. *J Vest Res, 1,* 61–71.

Peterka RJ, Black FO, Schoenhoff MB, (1990b). Age–related changes in human vestibulo–ocular reflexes: Sinusoidal rotation and caloric tests. *J Vest Res, 1,* 49–59.

Pfaltz CR, (1983). Vestibular compensation: Physiological and clinical aspects. *Acta Otolaryngol, 95,* 402–406.

Pierrot–Deseilligny C, Rivaud S, Gaymard B, Muri Right, Vermersch A–I, (1995). Cortical control of saccades. *Ann Neurol, 37,* 557–567.

Pitt MC, Rawles JM, (1988). The effect of age on saccadic latency and velocity. *Neuro–ophthalmology, 8,* 123–129.

Pompeiano O, (1994). Neural mechanisms of postural control. In Taguchi K, Igarashi M, Mori S, (eds). *Vestibular and Neural Front: Proceedings of the 12th International Symposium on Posture and Gait (pp 423–436).* Amsterdam: Elsevier.

Pompeiano O, Allum JHJ, (1988). *Vestibulospinal Control of Posture and Locomotion.* Amsterdam: Elsevier.

Pozzo T, Berthoz A, Popov C, (1994). The effect of gravity on the coordination between posture and movement. In Taguchi K, Igarashi M, Mori S, (eds). *Vestibular and Neural Front: Proceedings of the 12th International Symposium on Posture and Gait (pp 423–436).* Amsterdam: Elsevier.

Proctor Left, Glackin Right, Shimizu H, et al, (1986). Reference values for serial vestibular testing. *Ann Otol Rhinol Laryngol, 95,* 83–89.

Prudham D, Evans J, (1981). Factors associated with falls in the elderly: A community study. *Age and Aging, 10,* 141–146.

Rahko T, (1984). Optokinetic nystagmus. *Acta Ophthalmologica, Suppl, 161,* 153–158.

Raphan T, Matsuo V, Cohen B, (1979). Velocity storage in the vestibulo–ocular reflex arc (VOR). *Exp Brain Res, 35,* 229–248.

Ring C, Matthews Right, Nayak USL, Isaacs B, (1988). Visual push: A sensitive measure of dynamic balance in man. *Arch Phys Med Rehabil, 69,* 256– 260.

Roberts TSM, (1968). *Neruophysiology of Postural Mechanisms.* New York: Plenum Press.

Robinson DA, Zee DS, Hain TC, Holmes A, Rosenberg LF, (1986). Alexander's law: Its behavior and origin in the human vestibulo–ocular reflex. *Ann Neurol, 16,* 714–722.

Roydhouse N, (1974). Vertigo and its treatment. *Drugs, 7,* 297–309.

Ryu JH, (1986). Anatomy of the vestibular end organ and neural pathways. In Cummings C, Fredrickson L, Harker L, Krause C, Schuller D, (eds), Otolaryngology—*Head and Neck Surgery, vol 3, (pp. 2609–2629)* St. Louis, MO: C. V. Mosby.

Schaefer KP, Meyer DL, (1981). Aspects of vestibular compensation in guinea pigs. In: Flohr H, Precht W, (eds.). *Lesion-induced Neuronal Plasticity in Sensorimotor Systems (pp 197–207).* Berlin: Springer.

Schessel DA, Nedzelski JM, (1993). Meniere's disease and other peripheral vestibular disorders. In Cummings CW (ed.), *Otolaryngology—Head and Neck Surgery, Second edition, (pp 52–3176).* St. Louis: Mosby-Year Book.

Schuknecht HF, (1956). Ablation therapy for the relief of Meniere's disease. *Laryngoscope, 66,* 859–870.

Schuknecht HF, (1974). *Pathology of the Ear.* Cambridge, MA: Harvard University Press.

Schuknecht HF, (1991). Transcanal Labyrinthectomy. *Operative Techniques in Otolaryngology Head Neck Surgery, 2,* 17–19.

Schuknecht HF, Bartley M, (1985). Cochlear endolymphatic shunt for Meniere's disease. *Am J Otol, 6, Suppl,* 20–22.

Schwarz DWF, (1986). Physiology of the vestibular system. In Cummings C, Fredrickson L, Harker L, Krause C, Schuller D (eds), *Otolaryngology—Head and Neck Surgery, vol 3, (pp 2679–2718).* St. Louis, MO: C. V. Mosby.

Sekitani T, Ryu JH, McCabe BF, (1971). Drug effects on the medial vestibular nucleus. Perrotatory responses. *Arch Otolaryngol, 94,* 401–405.

Semont A, Freyss G, Vitte E, (1988). Curing the BPPV with a liberatory maneuver. A*dv Otorhinolaryngol, 42,* 290–293.

Sharpe JA, Zackon DH, (1987). Senescent saccades. Effects of aging on their accuracy, latency and velocity. *Acta Otolaryngol (Stockh), 104,* 422–428.

Shea JJ, (1992). The myth of spontaneous perilymph fistula [editorial]. *Otolaryngol Head Neck Surg, 107,* 613–616.

Shepard NT, Boismier TE, (1992). Variability of dynamic posturography in randomly sampled balance disorder patients. *Abstracts for Association for Research in Otolaryngology, Fifteenth Midwinter Meeting, (p 82).* St. Petersburg Beach, FL.

Shepard NT, Lawson GD, Boismier T, Oviatt DL, Wang Y, (1994a). Surface EMG response from lower leg muscles in the assessment of balance disorder patients. *Abstracts from the XIIth International Symposium on Posture and Gait, Vestibular and Neural Front.* Matsumoto, Japan.

Shepard NT, Schultz A, Alexander NB, Gu MJ, Boismier T, (1993a). Postural control in young and elderly adults when stance is challenged: Clinical versus laboratory measurements. *Ann Otol Rhinol Laryngol, 102,* 508–517.

Shepard NT, Shepard NP, Boismier T, (1994b). Fukuda stepping test: Test performance and criteria for abnormal. *Abstracts for the 18th Barany Society Meeting.* Uppsala, Sweden.

Shepard NT, Telian SA, (1995). Programmatic vestibular rehabilitation. *Otolaryngol Head Neck Surg, 112,* 173–182.

Shepard NT, Telian SA, Niparko JK, Kemink JL, Fujita S, (1992). Platform pressure test in identification of perilymphatic fistula. *The Am J Otology, 13,* 49–54.

Shepard NT, Telian SA, Smith–Wheelock M, Raj A, (1993b). Vestibular and balance rehabilitation therapy. *Ann Otol Rhinol Laryngol, 102,* 198–205.

Shepard NT, Telian SA, Smith–Wheelock M, Kemink J, Boismier T, (1993c). Vestibular rehabilitation therapy: Outpatient and postoperative programs. In Sharpe JA, Barber HO, (eds), *The Vestibulo–Ocular Reflex and Vertigo, (pp 341–346).* New York: Raven Press, Ltd.

Shimazu J, Yoshikazu S, (1992). *Vestibular and Brain Stem Control of Eye, Head and Body Movements.* Tokyo: Japan Scientific Societies Press and Basel: Karger.

Shone G, Kemink JL, Telian SA, (1991). Prognostic significance of hearing loss as a lateralising

indicator in the surgical treatment of vertigo. *J Layngol Otol, 105,* 18–20.

Shumway–Cook A, (1994). Vestibular rehabilition in traumatic brain injury. In Herdman SJ, (ed), *Vestibular Rehabilitation, (pp 347–359).* Philadelphia: F.A. Davis Co.

Shumway–Cook A, Horak FB, (1986). Assessing the influence of sensory interaction on balance. Suggestion from the field. *The Journal of American Physical Therapy Association, 66(10),* 1548–1550.

Shumway–Cook A, Horak FB, (1990). Rehabilitation strategies for patients with vestibular deficits. *Neurology Clinics, 8,* 441–457.

Silverstein H, Norrell H, Smouha EE, (1987). Retrosigmoid–internal auditory canal approach vs retrolabyrinthine approach for vestibular neurectomy. *Otolaryngol Head Neck Surg, 97,* 300–307.

Silverstein H, Smouha E, Jones Right, (1989). Natural history vs. surgery for Meniere's disease. *Otolaryngol Head Neck Surg, 100,* 6–16.

Smith PF, Curthoys IS, (1989). Mechanisms of recovery following unilateral labyrinthectomy. *Res Brain Res Rev, 14,* 155–180.

Smith PF, Curthoys IS, (1989). Mechanisms of recovery following unilateral labyrinthectomy. *Brain Res Rev, 14,* 155–180.

Smith PF, Darlington CL, (1991). Neurochemical mechanisms of recovery from peripheral vestibular lesions. *Res Brain Res Rev, 16,* 117–133.

Smith–Wheelock M, Shepard NT, Lawson G, (1996). Quantitative analysis of saccadic and smooth pursuit eye movements in normal subjects. Manuscript submitted for publication.

Smith–Wheelock M, Shepard NT, Telian SA, (1991a). Physical therapy program for vestibular rehabilitation. *Am J Otol, 12,* 218–225.

Smith–Wheelock M, Shepard NT, Telian SA, (1991b). Long–term effects for treatment of balance dysfunction: Utilizing a home exercise approach. *Seminars in Hearing, 12,* 297–301.

Smith–Wheelock M, Shepard NT, Telian SA, Boismier T, (1992). Balance retraining therapy in the elderly. In Kashima H, Goldstein J, and Lucente F, (eds), *Clinical Geriatric Otolaryngology (pp 71–80).* Philadelphia, BC Decker.

Snow JB, Kimmelman CP, (1979). Assessment of surgical procedures for Meniere's disease. *Laryngoscope, 89,* 737–747.

Sonderegger EN, Meienberg O, Ehrengruber H, (1986). Normative data of saccadic eye movements for routine diagnosis of ophthalmoneurological disorders. *Neuro–ophthalmology, 6,* 257–269.

Stelmach GE, Worringham C, (1985). Sensorimotor deficits related to postural stability. Implications for falling in the elderly. *Clinics in Geriatric Medicine, 1(3),* 679–691.

Stockwell CW, (1983). *ENG Workbook.* Baltimore: University Park Press.

Stockwell CW, Bojrab DI, (1993a). Background and technique of rotational testing. In Jacobson GP, Newman CW, Kartush JM, (eds), *Handbook of Balance Function Testing* (pp 237–248). St. Louis: Mosby–Year Book, Inc.

Stockwell CW, Bojrab DI, (1993b). Interpretation and usefulness of rotational testing. In Jacobson GP, Newman CW, Kartush JM, (eds), *Handbook of Balance Function Testing (pp 249–258).* St. Louis: Mosby–Year Book, Inc.

Suarez H, Caffa C, Macadar O, (1992). Correlation between vestibular habituation and postural recovery in cerebellar patients. *Restorative Neurology and Neuroscience, 4,* 255–259.

Taguchi K, Igarashi M, Mori S, (1994). *Vestibular and Neural Front: Proceedings of the 12th International Symposium on Posture and Gait.* Amsterdam: Elsevier.

Telian SA, Kileny PR, (1989). Usefulness of 1000 Hz tone–burst evoked responses in the diagnosis of acoustic neuroma. *Otolaryngol Head Neck Surg, 101,* 466–471.

Telian SA, Kileny PR, Kemink JL, Niparko JK, Graham MD, (1989). Normal auditory brainstem response in acoustic neuroma. *Laryngoscope, 99,* 10–14.

Telian SA, Shepard NT, Smith–Wheelock M, Hoberg M, (1991). Bilateral vestibular paresis: Diagnosis and treatment. *Otolaryngol Head Neck Surg, 104,* 67–71.

Telischi FF, Luxford WM, (1993). Long–term effecacy of endolymphatic sac surgery for vertigo in Meniere's disease. *Otolaryngol Head Neck Surg, 109,* 83–87.

Telischi FF, Rodgers GK, Balkany TJ, (1994). Dizziness in childhood. In Jackler RK, Brackmann DE, (eds), *Neurotology (pp 555–566).* St. Louis: Mosby–Year Book, Inc.

Tijssen MAJ, Straathof CSM, Hain TC, Zee DS, (1989). Optokinetic afternystagmus in humans: Normal values of amplitude, time constant, and asymmetry. *Ann Otol Rhinol Laryngol, 98,* 741–746.

Tinetti ME, Speechley M, Ginter SF, (1988). Risk factors for falls among elderly persons living in the community. *N Eng J Med, 319,* 1701–1707.

Tomlinson RD, (1988). Gaze shifts and the vestibulo-ocular reflex. In Barber HO, Sharpe JA, (eds), *Vestibular Disorders (pp 48–58).* Chicago/London/Boca Raton: Year Book Medical Publishers, Inc.

Torok N, (1970). The effects of arousal upon vestibular nystagmus. *Adv Oto Rhinolaryngol, 17,* 76–89.

Torok N, (1973). Differential diagnosis of the caloric nystagmus. *Equilibrium Res, 3,* 70–79.

Triolo RJ, Reilley WB, Freedman W, Betz RR, (1993). Development and standardization of a clinical evaluation of standing function: The functional standing test. *IEEE Trans Rehab Engineer, 1,* 18–25.

Truex RC, Carpenter MB, (1969). *Human Neuroanatomy.* Baltimore: The Williams & Wilkins Co.

Unterberger S, (1938). Neue objectiv registriebare vestibularis—K`rperdrehreaktion, erhalten durch treten auf der stelle: Der Atretversucht. *Arch Ohr–Nas–u–Kehlk–Heilk, 145,* 478.

Van de Calseyde P, Ampe W, Depondt M, (1974). The damped torsion swing test. Quantitative and qualitative aspects of the ENG pattern in normal subjects. *Arch Otolaryngol, 100,* 449–452.

Van Egmond AAJ, Groen JJ, Jongkees LBW, (1948). The turning test with small regulable stimuli. I. Method of examination: Cupulometria. *J Laryngol Otol, 2,* 63–69.

Ventre J, (1985). Cortical control of oculomotor functions. I. Optokinetic nystagmus. *Behavioural Brain Research, 15,* 211–226.

Vernick DM, (1990). Infralabyrinthine approach to the internal auditory canal. *Otolaryngol Head Neck Surg, 102,* 307–313.

Voorhees RL, (1989). The role of dynamic posturography in neurotologic diagnosis. *Laryngoscope, 99,* 940–957.

Voorhees RL, (1990). Dynamic posturography findings in central nervous system disorders. *Laryngoscope, 99,* 995–1001.

Waespe W, Cohen B, Raphan T, (1983). Role of the flocculuc and paraflocculus in optokinetic nystagmus and visual–vestibular interactions: Effects of lesions. *Exp Brain Res, 50,* 9–33.

Waespe W, Cohen B, Raphan T, (1985). Dynamic modification of the vestibulo–ocular reflex by the nodulus and uvula. *Science, 228,* 199–202.

Waespe W, Wichmann W, (1990). Oculomotor disturbances during visual–vestibular interaction in Wallenberg's lateral medullary syndrome. *Brain, 113,* 821–846.

Wall C, (1990). The sinusoidal harmonic acceleration rotary chair test—theoretical and clinical basis. *Neurologic Clinics, 8(2),* 269–285.

Wall C, Black FO, O'Leary DP, (1978). Clinical use of pseudorandom binary sequence white noise in assessment of the human vestibulo–ocular system. *Ann Otol, 87,* 845–852.

Weber PC, Cass SP, (1993). Clinical assessment of postural stability. *The Am J of Otology, 14(6),* 566–569.

Wolfson LI, Whipple Right, Amerman P, Kleinberg A, (1986). Stressing the postural response—a quantitative method for testing balance. *J Am Geriatrics Soc, 34,* 845–850.

Woollacott MH, Shumway–Cook A, (1989). *Development of Posture and Gait Across the Life Span.* Columbia, SC: University of South Carolina Press.

Woollacott MH, von Hosten C, Rosblad B, (1988). Relation between muscle response onset and body segmental movements during postural perturbations in humans. *Exp Brain Res, 72,* 593–604.

Yoneda S, Tokusasu K, (1986). Frequency analysis of body sway in the upright posture. Statistical study in cases of peripheral vestibular disease. *Acta Otolaryngol (Stockh), 102,* 87–92.

Zackon DH, Sharpe JA, (1987). Smooth pursuit in senescence: Effects of target acceleration and velocity. *Acta Otolaryngol, 104,* 290–297.

Zasorin NL, Baloh RW, Yee RD, Honrubia V, (1983). Influence of vestibulo–ocular reflex gain on human optokinetic responses. *Exp Brain Res, 51,* 271–274.

Zee DS, (1985). Perspectives on the disorder of vertigo. *Arch Otolaryngol, 111,* 609–612.

Zee DS, (1985). Perspectives on the pharmacotherapy of vertigo. *Arch Otolaryngol, 111, 609–612.*

Zee DS, (1994). Vestibular adaptation. In Herdman SJ, (ed), *Vestibular Rehabilitation (pp 68–79).* Philadelphia: F.A. Davis Co.

Zee DS, Robinson DA, (1978). A hypothetical explanation of saccadic oscillations. *Ann Neurol, 5,* 405–414.

Zee DS, Yamazaki A, Butler P, Gucer G, (1981). Effects of ablation of flocculus and paraflocculus on eye movements in primate. *Journal of Neurophysiology, 46 (4),* 878–899.

Zee DS, Yee RD, Robinson DA, (1976). Optokinetic responses in labyrinthine–defective human beings. *Brain Res, 113,* 423–428.

Zimberg S, Shepard NT, Boismier T, Telian SA, (1991). Comparison of clinical protocols for OVAR: Normative data. *Abstracts for Association for Research in Otolaryngology, Fourteenth Midwinter meeting (p 40).* St. Petersburg Beach, FL.

■ INDEX